EFFECTIVE MANAGEMENT
OF BLADDER AND BOWEL PROBLEMS
IN CHILDREN

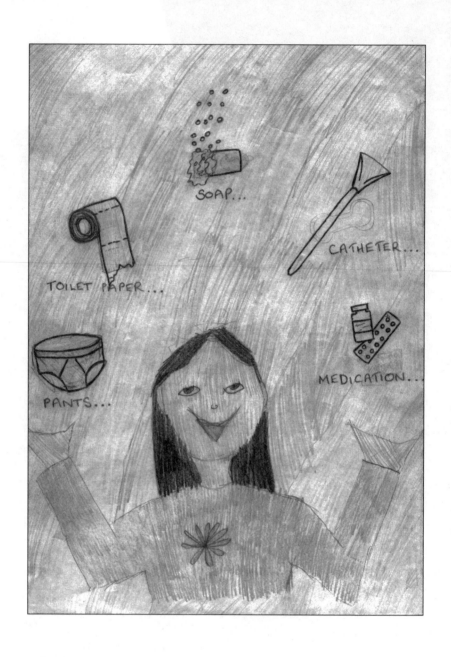

'Juggling'

EFFECTIVE MANAGEMENT OF BLADDER AND BOWEL PROBLEMS IN CHILDREN

Edited by

Liz Bonner, MSc, BSc (Hons) Health Visiting, DN Cert, RN
*Nurse Consultant, Bladder and Bowel Dysfunction,
Bedfordshire Primary Care Trust*

and

Mandy Wells, MSc, RN, RM, Dip N (London), PGCMS
Nurse Consultant, Devon Primary Care Trust

CLASS PUBLISHING · LONDON

Printing history
First published 2008

The information presented in this book is accurate and current to the best of the authors' knowledge. The authors and publisher, however, make no guarantee as to, and assume no responsibility for, the correctness, sufficiency or completeness of such information or recommendation. The reader is advised to consult a doctor regarding all aspects of individual healthcare.

The author and publishers welcome feedback from the users of this book. Please contact the publishers.

Class Publishing, Barb House, Barb Mews, London W6 7PA, UK
Telephone: 020 7371 2119
Fax: 020 7371 2878
email: post@class.co.uk
Visit our website – www.class.co.uk

A CIP catalogue record for this book is available from the British Library.

ISBN 13: 9781859591659

ISBN 10: 1859591655

10 9 8 7 6 5 4 3 2 1

Edited by Richenda Milton-Thompson

Designed and typeset by Martin Bristow

Diagrams by David Woodroffe

Index by Vicki Robinson

Printed and bound in Finland by WS Bookwell, Juva

Contents

Foreword

Professor Christine Norton

We are all born incontinent. At birth the central nervous system is too immature and the social being is too undeveloped for bladder or bowel control. A combination of maturation and socialisation enable children to acquire the complex motor and social skills required for continence. Although 'training' may facilitate and speed up acquisition of continence, most of us would become continent eventually, even in the absence of any but the most minimal prompting from adults. Yet a few do not become reliably continent. This has a variety of possible causes, from congenital and anatomical to psychosocial and situational. The consequences of incontinence vary, from minor inconvenience, through pervasive emotional and social effects on the child and family, to even more tragic events of abuse and neglect.

Childhood incontinence has often been ignored as a topic for health care professionals. There is an assumption that it is relatively trivial and most children will 'grow out of it'. And indeed most do. But for those bothered by symptoms or embarrassed by consequences, professional help is needed. This volume will guide the multidisciplinary team towards practical, evidence-based care for those who need it. It sets the topic firmly within the context of modern healthcare and society, giving equal weight to bladder and bowel care. It is the first comprehensive text covering both clinical and legislative issues, exploring the child, parent, school and health service perspectives.

The editors are to be congratulated on assembling an excellent panel of contributors, and for recognising that a text on this issue of great importance to children and their families is long overdue.

Christine Norton

Acknowledgements

This book could not have been published without the efforts of Class Publishing especially our editor Richenda Milton-Thompson, admirable administrative assistance from Christine Sinfield, and the time and effort of our wonderful team of contributors.

We are grateful our friends and family members for their support while we were working on the book, and Liz would like a particular thank you for her long-suffering husband Terry.

David Woodruffe produced the illustrations from a wide variety of briefs and sketches. And a special mention should be made of our young artists, Lindsey Kirwan and Abigail Horrod, who kindly produced the pictures you will see opposite the title page and in Chapter 12. Many thanks indeed to them.

The General Teaching Council for England, the General Social Care Council and the Nursing and Midwifery Council have kindly allowed us to reproduce their 2007 Consultation Document on inter-professional values underpinning work with young people. This appears as Appendix 3.

The excerpt from 'The Eloquent Young Elephant' in Chapter 19 has been used with permission of the author Sheree Fitch. The original poem is from her book *If You Could Wear My Sneakers*, illustrated by Darcia Labrosse and published in 1992 Doubleday, Canada.

We would also like to thank Ray Addison and Dr Ursula Butler for their insightful reviews of the 'work in progress', Dr Adrian Wagg for advice on the Glossary entries, and Professor Christine Norton for her support of this project and for kindly writing a Foreword.

Liz Bonner and Mandy Wells

About the contributors

Sue Affleck, RGN, RSCN
Clinical Nurse Specialist:
Paediatric Continence,
St Georges Hospital NHS Trust,
London

Jim Beattie, MBCHB, FRCP (Glas),
FRCPCH
Consultant Paediatrician
and Nephrologist,
Royal Hospital for Sick Children,
Glasgow

Maddie Blackburn, MSc,
GRAD Dip Law, GRAD Legal Practice,
RN, RM, Higher Dip HV, Cert.HEd
Head of Children's Strategy:
Healthcare Commission

Su-Anna Boddy, MS, FRCS
Consultant Paediatric Urologist
(with special interest in
neuropathic bladder and bowel),
St Georges Hospital NHS Trust,
London

Liz Bonner, MSc, BSc (Hons) Health
Visiting, DN Cert, RN
Nurse Consultant,
Bladder and Bowel Dysfunction,
Bedfordshire Primary Care Trust

Lynne Conboy, BEd, BA
Assistant Headteacher,
Uffculme School,
Birmingham

Christina Chi Ding, MB, BS,
BSc (Hons), MRCOG
Senior Specialist Registrar
(Obstetrics & Gynaecology)
and Clinical Research Fellow,
Royal Infirmary of Edinburgh

Penny Dobson, MSc, RGN, CQSW
Director, ERIC (Education and
Resources for Improving Childhood
Continence)

Melinda Edwards, BSc, Dip Clin Psych
Consultant Paediatric
Clinical Psychologist,
The Evelina Children's Hospital,
Guy's and St Thomas'
NHS Foundation Trust

Ruth Emery, RGN, RSCN, BSc(Hons):
Health and Social Care Practice
Children's Continence Nurse
Specialist, Bradford and Airedale
Teaching Primary Care Trust

Anton Emmanuel, MD, FRCP
Senior Lecturer in
Neurogastroenterology,
Consultant Gastroenterologist,
Director of Physiology Unit,
University College Hospital, London

Debra Evans
Information and Knowledge Manager/Product Specialist, PromoCon, Disabled Living, Manchester

Jonathan Evans, FRCP, FRCPCH
Consultant Paediatric Nephrologist, Nottingham University Hospital NHS Trust

Rosie Kelly, MSc Nursing, RSCN
Lead Nurse: Childrens' Services, Ulster Hospital, Belfast

Charlotte Kerslake, RGN
Paediatric Continence Adviser, Bedfordshire Continence Service

Edward Kiely, FRCSI, FRCS
Honorary Senior Lecturer, Institute of Child Health, and Consultant Surgeon, Great Ormond Street Hospital for Children NHS Trust

June Rogers, MBE, RN, RSCN, BA (Hons), BSc
Paediatric Continence Adviser, Director PromoCon, Disabled Living, North West

Caroline Sanders, BSc (Hons), PGD, RCN, RN
Paediatric Urology Nurse Specialist, Royal Liverpool Children's Hospital NHS Trust

Mark Slack, MB CH, M.Med, FCOG (SA), FRCOG
Consultant Urogynaecologist, Addenbrookes Hospital, Cambridge, Cambridge University Teaching Hospitals Trust

Stella Snell, RGN, RSCN
Clinical Nurse Specialist – Paediatric Continence, St George's Hospital, London

Lizi Snushall, BEd (Hons)
Head of Lower School, Uffculme School, Birmingham

Julie Vickerman, Dip. COT
Clinical Specialist/Research Occupational Therapist, Central Lancashire Primary Care Trust and PromoCon, Disabled Living, Manchester

Mandy Wells, MSc, RN, RM, Dip N (London), PGCMS
Nurse Consultant, Devon Primary Care Trust

Mary White, MA, RGN, Dip Counselling Studies, SN (Cert), Dip Special Needs in Education
Specialist Continence Adviser, Disabled Living, Manchester

Kenneth Wilkinson, BSc, DCH, FRCPCH
Consultant General Paediatrician, with a Special Interest in Childhood Continence Problems, Airedale General Hospital NHS Trust

Introduction

Mandy Wells and Liz Bonner

Principle 2 of the United Nations Declaration of the Rights of the Child states that:

> The child shall enjoy special protection, and shall be given opportunities and facilities, by law and by other means, to enable him to develop physically, mentally, morally, spiritually and socially in a healthy and normal manner and in conditions of freedom and dignity. In the enactment of laws for this purpose, the best interests of the child shall be the paramount consideration. (UNHCHR, 1997)

What does this have to do with continence, or perhaps a better way of putting it might be: 'what impact might continence problems have on this principle?'

Under normal circumstances, a healthy child will gain control of his or her bladder and bowels by the age of four. If, for whatever reason, this is doesn't happen, there will be impacts on the child's self-image, dignity, freedom to socialise, schooling and wider relationships. Prolonged exposure to urine or faeces can cause irritation of the skin and, in time, damage to its integrity. Problems maintaining cleanliness can lead to urinary tract infections, and reflux problems can cause permanent damage to the kidneys. So, incontinence can be seen to have serious effects on the child's social, mental and physical health. Clearly, health professionals have a duty of care to enable any continence problems to be overcome as far as possible.

Difficulties with bladder and bowel function in children can affect their normal growth and development. Their effects can go beyond the merely physical (which is not to diminish the importance of physical problems) and lead to considerable social and psychological impairment. In addition, there is the effect on the wider family, which must never be underestimated.

A study of around 3000 primary schoolchildren was carried out by school nurses in London. They found that there was more chance of children having health problems if they were being bullied. Symptoms reported included poor sleep, bed-wetting, feeling sad, headaches and stomach pains (Williams *et al.* 1996). The researchers didn't look at whether any of these symptoms predated the bullying (in which case they may well have been a causative factor, even if indirect), but they

1

did find that, as the frequency of bullying increased, so did the risk of having these health problems. Where difficulties with wetting or soiling are concerned, it is often hard to tell which comes first, the continence problem or the problems with the way the child is treated.

An extreme example of the horrifying impact continence problems can have on a child's well-being can be found in Lord Laming's report on the Victoria Climbié Inquiry (Laming 2003). A summary of the references to continence can be found at the end of the book, as Appendix 2. Reading this summary makes it clear that there was a circular relationship here between incontinence and abuse. Wetting the bed is a normal reaction for a young child to being far from home and unhappy. The report suggests that Victoria's 'problem' was well within normal limits at the start, but as the abuse escalated, her control over her bladder and bowels deteriorated proportionately. It should be pointed out, however, that the report contains no reference to a professional assessment that included a continence assessment or identified incontinence as a problem.

The Government responded to the Laming Report with the 'Every Child Matters' initiative (DfES 2003a, 2003b). A need for radical change to the whole system of children's services was identified, including the improvement and integration of universal services in early years settings, schools and the health service. Identifying and benchmarking of good practice has been identified (NHSME 2003) so that we as health professionals know what it is we are aiming for. The Children's Act (2004) gives a clear focus and the new status to children's services. The NSF for Children, Young People and Maternity Services (DH 2004) is integral to implementation, setting out a ten year plan to stimulate long term and sustained improvement in children's health and well being. Although these aims are not yet fully realised (Shribman 2007), they are at least now firmly on the agenda.

This book has been written for all health, education and social services professionals with an interest in promoting continence in children. It looks at the problems of continence in children and what can be done about them. Overarching issues such as protecting children and ensuring good practice are tackled, but so too are the ways of actually making children's lives better. In many cases, this will begin with a thorough assessment and identification of the cause of the child's incontinence. For some children, this may be something as simple as a urinary tract infection that can be treated with appropriate antibiotics. Sometimes a behaviour training programme will be what is required, but in other cases surgery may be necessary. Children who do not have the anatomical ability for controlling the flow of their urine or faeces may need to learn to manage a catheter or stoma – preferably in such a way that their ability to lead a normal life like their peers is not compromised. But even children with loving and supportive families and other networks will find living with continence problems difficult. The frontispiece to this book shows one young girl's experience of continually juggling – tablets, products, timing, etc. There is not a lot of time for relaxing.

This book has been written by a wide range of professionals from a range of disciplines – nursing, medicine, surgery, psychology, occupational therapy and education. Something they all have in common is that they believe passionately in the right of the child to live a life of freedom and dignity undamaged by continence problems. They are also concerned to raise awareness of the associated issues and improve standards of care provision. While there may be some overlap in subject area between chapters, our aim as Editors has been to provide an insight into the complexity of this subject area, without ever losing sight of the plight of the child at the centre.

Each chapter opens with a 'Key Point' box and where appropriate with a 'Health Promotion Point' box also. Readers will find references at the end of each chapter and a glossary and Resources list at the end of the book.

We hope that will find this volume helpful, practical and thought-provoking. If you would like to send us any comments or feedback please feel free to contact us c/o Class Publishing, Barb House, Barb Mews, London W6 7PA.

References

Department for Education and Skills (2003a) *Every Child Matters.* Norwich: The Stationery Office. Website: www.everychildmatters.gov.uk

Department for Education and Skills, Department of Health, Home Office (2003b) *Keeping Children Safe: The Government's response to the Victoria Climbié Inquiry Report and Joint Chief Inspectors' Report on Safeguarding Children.* Norwich. The Stationery Office

Department of Health (2004) *The National Service Framework (NSF) for Children and Young People.* London: DH

Laming WH (Chair) (2003) *The Victoria Climbié Inquiry.* Norwich: Crown Copyright. Website: www.victoria-climbié-inquiry.org.uk

NHS Modernisation Agency (2003) *Good Practice in Paediatric Continence Services – Benchmarking in Action.* London: Department of Health. Website: www.modern.nhs.uk

Shribman S (2007) *Making it Better for Children and Young People: Clinical case for change.* London: Department of Health

United Nations High Commissioner for Human Rights (1997) *Declaration of the Rights of the Child.* Geneva: UNHCHR

Williams K, Chambers M, Logan S, Robinson D (1996) Association of common health symptoms with bullying in primary school children. *British Medical Journal,* 313 (7048): 17–19

Safeguarding children and young people with continence difficulties

Maddie Blackburn

Key points

- Abuse of children is frighteningly common, and may be emotional, physical, sexual or a combination of these in nature.

- Health professionals have a duty to do everything they can to safeguard children.

- Continence problems can have a damaging association with abuse as demonstrated in the landmark case following the death of Victoria Climbié.

In the 1990s, I was awarded a research fellowship by the Association for Spina Bifida and/or Hydrocephalus (ASBAH). This was for undertaking research into, among other matters, the sexual knowledge and experiences of young people with those conditions. Sixty per cent of the 100 people interviewed in that study had continence difficulties. Key findings were the young person's lack of understanding of the differences between urinary and bowel incontinence, lack of understanding of the difference between sperm and urinary incontinence, as well as managing continence in personal relationships. Of particular concern, 10% of young people reported that they had been abused at some point during their childhood (Blackburn 2002). This convinced me that safeguarding children and young people with continence difficulties is an important consideration in this highly challenging area of work. Safeguarding young people with continence difficulties still remains an important consideration for me in my current work in relation to local and national policy surrounding the safeguarding agenda.

The Victoria Climbié Inquiry Report, which was published by Lord Laming in January 2003, made reference to Victoria 'lying in her own urine and faeces' (1.4, page 1), and being 'tied up' in 'a plastic bag full of excrement'. Children who are abused or neglected are often incontinent of urine or faeces. The significance of continence to the safeguarding agenda therefore cannot be ignored. The horrific death of this little girl in February 2000 makes us aware not only of how a young, innocent child suffered a catalogue of abuse, but also of how *all* professionals must respond to a child's needs. This report was described as a 'beacon pointing the way to securing the safety and well-being of all children in our society' (Laming 2003: 13). How much have we applied to our learning since the publication of this report?

Definitions

For the benefit of this chapter, **continence** is defined as: 'the process by which you control the disposal of urine and faeces. If you can control this process, you are continent, if you have difficulties, you are incontinent' (Simage Communications 1993).

Safeguarding and promoting the welfare of children is defined for the purposes of this chapter as:

- Protecting children from maltreatment;

- Preventing impairment of children's health or development;

- Ensuring that children are growing up in circumstances consistent with the provision of safe and effective care;

- Undertaking this role so as to enable those children to have optimum life chances and to enter adulthood successfully.

Child protection is an essential part of the wider definition of safeguarding and refers to the responsibilities to protect children who are at risk of suffering or who are suffering significant harm (HM Government 2006).

Promoting welfare means ensuring that children and young people have the opportunities to achieve physical and mental health. For most children and young people, once they have survived the hurdles of potty training, their bodies will signal when they need to go to the toilet. However for some children and young people, particularly those with complex disabilities such as spina bifida, or children with emotional difficulties, and particularly those who have been abused, they may lose control of their bladder and bowels, albeit temporarily.

Accurate data about the prevalence of abuse is difficult to ascertain but a reliable indication is that by the time children and young people reach 18 years of age, 750,000 children in the UK will have been abused. According to a study carried out for the NSPCC, about

400,000 of these will have been sexually abused (Cawson *et al.* 2000). Statistics collected for the Departments for Education and Skills suggest that the percentage of abused children falling into the different categories of abuse is as indicated in Table 1.1. The same research also suggests that the number of children being sexually abused was 2 per 10,000 for both boys and girls in the population as a whole (DfES 2006).

Table 1.1 Statistics showing the percentage of abused children suffering different types of abuse

Types of abuse	Percentage
Neglect	43
Emotional abuse	21
Physical abuse	16
Sexual abuse	8
Mixed abuse	11

Source: DfES (2006) *Referrals, assessments and children and young people on child protection registers, England. Year ending 31 March 2006.* These statistics are updated annually, the figures given in this table were the most recent available at the time of going to press.
NB: In the future, the Child Protection Register will be replaced by the Integrated Children's System (ICS).

Legislation underpinning the safeguarding of children and young people

Changes in the organisation and delivery of services for children and young people and the safeguarding agenda follow the legal and policy guidance largely enshrined in the following:

■ Children Act 1989;

■ Education Act 2002;

■ Every Child Matters 2003;

■ The National Service Framework (NSF) for Children and Young People 2004;

■ Children Act 2004;

- The Education and Inspections Act 2006;
- Safeguarding Vulnerable Groups Act 2006.

'Children' generally refers to children and young people who have not yet reached their eighteenth birthday. However, the Children Act 2004 underpins the wider children's strategy for improving the outcomes in children's lives. The Act defines children and young people as those aged 0–19 years but also includes those receiving services, such as those leaving 'care' (Children Act 1989: S23c–24d), those over 19 years of age but under 25 with learning difficulties within the meaning of the Learning and Skills Act 2000 (i.e. those who are receiving services under that Act).

Children Act 2004

Fundamental to this legislation is the encouragement of integrated planning, commissioning and delivery of services as well as positive interdisciplinary working, reducing the burden of work and inspection in all councils and their partnerships in England. These partnerships include health providers. This Act is pivotal to the safeguarding agenda and has fundamentally changed the organisational context for safeguarding children in England.

Section 10 of the Children Act 2004 came into force in April 2005 and **placed a duty on local authorities and relevant partners in order to improve the well-being of children in their area.**

Well-being covers physical, emotional and mental well-being (as well as protection from harm and neglect), education, training and recreation, etc. The notion of **co-operation** means understanding the needs of the local childhood population – yet surprisingly general practitioners to date are not included in the list of *relevant partners.*

Section 11 of Children Act 2004 places a duty on Strategic Health Authorities, designated Special Hospitals, Primary Care Trusts, NHS Trusts and NHS Foundation Trusts to make arrangements to ensure that in discharging their functions, that they have regard of the need to safeguard and promote the welfare of Children (and ensure particularly those with chronic and complex conditions such as urinary and bowel continence are not ignored.

Section 11 and **Section 28** place a **general duty of care on services to safeguard and promote the welfare of children.** This includes Strategic

Health Authorities (reformed in 2006), PCTS, NHS or Foundation Trusts.

Children Act 1989

This is still current law and places a duty on Councils with Social Services responsibilities (CSSRS) to ensure children and young people 'in need', are safeguarded in their area.

Section 17 promotes the upbringing of such children by their families, by providing a level of services appropriate to those children's needs. In addition, it places a specific duty on other local authority services and health bodies to co-operate in the interests of children 'in need'. Children with continence difficulties may be considered to be 'in need' of appropriate management of their continence from education, health, and social care services.

Section 27 places a specific duty on other local authority services and health bodies to co-operate in the interests of children in need. Children with continence difficulties may be considered to be 'in need' of appropriate management of their continence from education, health, and social care services.

Section 47 covers the investigation of child abuse allegations.

The NSF and safeguarding children

The NSF, published in 2004, set out a ten-year programme to improve the quality of services for children, young people and pregnant women, putting them at the heart of service development and delivery. The expectation is that the standards would be met in full within ten years. The way in which local agencies are moving towards the fulfilment of these standards is an important aspect of any inspection of healthcare services for children.

The NSF contains 11 Standards and many markers of good practice designed to bring about that shift.

Progress in delivering the NSF has begun through performance assessment frameworks (PAF) developed by Strategic Health Authorities, through the Healthcare Commission's Children's Hospital Improvement Review (published at the end of February 2007), Joint Area Reviews (JARs) and the Commission's ongoing work in maternity services and through the Healthcare Commission's Annual Health Check. Some PCTS have developed their own NSF implementation plans. The Department of Health is currently working on a common set of measurement criteria that can reflect progress at local, regional or national levels in order to assist organisations in planning, commissioning and delivering services as well as those involved in assessing their progress.

After much debate, paediatric continence was also incorporated into the NSF. Delivering the NSF is a major part of the *Every Child Matters: Change for Children Programme*. It also complements other key government publications (DH 2003; 2004a; 2006). Safeguarding children is a theme running throughout all the 11 standards of the NSF, but Standard 5 specifically addresses 'safeguarding as well as promoting the welfare of children and young people'. Standard 5 states that:

> all agencies work to prevent children suffering harm and to promote their welfare; provide them with the services they require to address their identified needs and safeguard children who are being or who are likely to be harmed.

The vision and outcomes of this standard aim to ensure that children and young people are safeguarded from harm and are able to achieve their optimal outcomes throughout childhood, adolescence and into adulthood. In addition children and young people should be able to grow up in circumstances and environments where they feel safe and supported by those caring for them and that all children requiring specialist support can receive those services, such as children with continence difficulties.

Clearly, agencies and professionals should work in partnership with each other, service users and members of their local community, in accordance with their agreed Local Safeguarding Children Board annual business plans. Other markers of good practice include:

- The development, implementation and evaluation of effective policies, procedures and practices for safeguarding children, including the recruitment and vetting of staff (see above).

- Where there are concerns about a child or young person, then an assessment is carried out in accordance with the Framework for the Assessment of Children in Need. The Common Assessment Framework (CAF) is a key component in the *Every Child Matters: Change for Children* programme. The aim is to identify, at the earliest opportunity, children's additional needs that are not being met by the universal services they are receiving, and provide timely and co-ordinated support to meet those needs. The CAF is:

☐ a simple **pre-assessment checklist** to help practitioners identify children who would benefit from a common assessment;

☐ a **process for undertaking a common assessment**, to help practitioners gather and understand information about the needs and strengths of the child, based on discussions with the child, their family and other practitioners as appropriate;

☐ a **standard form** to help practitioners record, and, where appropriate, share with others, the findings from the assessment in terms that are helpful in working with the family to find a response to unmet needs (Every Child Matters: Fact Sheet) ideally with full co-operation with the child and his or her carers.

■ All staff are aware of the increased likelihood of harm being suffered by disabled children, those with complex needs, or children living in special circumstances.

Possible indicators in relation to this Standard are the numbers of children showing symptoms of failure to thrive; emotional abuse, which might be demonstrated through enuresis; or soiling problems.

Markers of good practice should ensure that the needs of children with complex needs, and this should include young people with continence difficulties, are met through a multi-agency approach. So for example, the school age child with a disability, or who uses a wheelchair and has both urinary and bowel incontinence, should be able to access appropriate toileting facilities and support in the school environment.

Several organisations (such as ERIC – Education and Resources for Improving Childhood Continence) have campaigned widely for better child-centred NHS continence services. The importance of acknowledging continence difficulties in children should not be underestimated. There should be a focus on early intervention and prevention – as well as the provision of accessible and integrated services. The successful 'Water is Cool in School Campaign' aimed to improve the quality of provision and access to fresh drinking water for children in UK primary and secondary schools. Doctors had been telling us for many years that children did not drink enough during the school day, and that the resulting dehydration contributed to a number of short and long-term health problems. In order to find out more about the water situation in schools, ERIC, in conjunction with the Royal College of Paediatrics and Child Health, carried out a survey of drinking facilities in primary and secondary schools in two education districts. The results, published in the *Nursing Times* (Haines *et al.* 2000), revealed that drinking facilities and access to water in many British schools were highly unsatisfactory. In response to these findings, the Water is Cool in School Campaign was launched in October 2000, with a press launch at the House of Commons in March 2001.

This was followed by an audit of school toilets. The Bog Standard campaign aimed to promote better toilets for pupils (Vernon 2002). There were three key aims: to increase awareness of the health benefits of better toilets for pupils, encourage schools to improve the condition of pupils' toilets and to allow pupils to use them, and to bring about reforms. School toilets can affect children's physical and psychological health. Toilets which are unpleasant, or out of bounds, may cause serious, long-term health problems. In order to raise awareness, and to implement the NSF, ERIC, in collaboration with the RCN Paediatric Nurses Forum, have designed a 'toolkit' to assist PCTs in establishing integrated paediatric continence services. (See the ERIC website, also Bonner and Dobson 2005.)

'Every Child Matters'

Health professionals and organisations have a key role to play in active promotion of the health and well-being of children. As part of the *Every Child Matters* agenda (DfES 2003), Joint Area Reviews (JARs) are currently being conducted under arrangements made by Her Majesty's Chief Inspector of Schools and agreed with other participating inspectorates and commissions (including the Healthcare Commission) under the requirements of Section 20 of the Children Act 2004. Section 112 of the Education and Inspection Act 2006 lists the key functions of the 'Office for Standards in Education, Children's Services and Skills'. This is now known as New Ofsted, and will continue to lead these inspections from April 2007. These reviews began in September 2005. A JAR is and will be carried out in each Children's Services Authority in England until 2008.

The JAR focuses on the experiences of children and young people in a Children's Services Authority. It sets out to describe the extent to which they are *healthy, safe, enjoy and achieve, make a positive contribu-*

tion and are well prepared to secure economic well-being, the five outcomes in *Every Child Matters* (2003). In doing so, the JAR examines a range of agencies to assess the outcomes for children. In particular, judgements are made on how services work together to improve outcomes for children and young people.

To date, nearly half of the planned inspections have been undertaken. The *Staying Safe* outcome addresses the health, social and education implications of safeguarding children and young people in their local community.

In relation to health, the arrangements for ensuring that looked-after children can access health services and assessments are monitored. In addition, these inspections are designed to ensure that there are robust policies and key personnel, such as arrangements for key named and designated health personnel, are in place in the NHS economies are assessed.

The first Joint Chief Inspectors' Report on JARs was published in March 2007 and features some of the key findings and learning from the safeguarding agenda. Although continence is not specifically reviewed in the current JARs methodology, a recent review of the JARs methodology has indicated the need to focus the JAR, not only on safeguarding and looked-after children, but including more targeted work on groups with poor outcomes, in particular those with learning difficulties or disabilities.

The Healthcare Commission annual health check

Standards for Better Health was published by the Department of Health in 2004, and sets out the standards that currently apply to all NHS organisations. The Healthcare Commission's annual health check (AHC) aims to promote continuous improvement. In 2006/2007: trusts will be asked to make a declaration on three developmental standards as well as the 24 Core Standards. Core Standard 2 specifically addresses children's safeguards. Trusts must declare their overall progress for each domain in which they are being assessed. In 2006/7, some data related to continence will also be included in the annual health check.

Safeguarding vulnerable people following the Bichard Inquiry: the Vetting and Barring Scheme

The new Vetting and Barring Scheme, under the Safeguarding Vulnerable Groups Act 2006 will be introduced from Autumn 2008. Recommendation 19 of the Bichard Report stated:

> New arrangements should be introduced requiring those who wish to work with children, or vulnerable adults, to be registered. The register would confirm that there is no known reason why an individual should not work with these client groups. (Bichard 2004)

This scheme will be a comprehensive, integrated, continuously updated system of pre-employment vetting and referral-based barring for all those seeking to work in, or who are already working in, the child or vulnerable adult related workforce. Barring decisions made prior to employment will also be able to be made. (The term 'employers' refers to both employers and managers of volunteers; the term 'employees' refers to both paid and unpaid volunteer work and/or activities.)

An expert board, independent of Ministers, is being established and will be given statutory responsibility for all discretionary barring decisions. Information from a wider range of agencies will be assessed centrally by the new vetting and barring board. A new independent body will take barring decisions: The Independent Barring Board (IBB). The new scheme's operation will build on the current Criminal Records Bureau (CRB) infrastructure. Online checks will be able to be undertaken and will be cheaper and easier to update. Employers, inspectorates and professional regulators will be able to use the system; but most of all parents and carers will also be able to check the status of, for example, a childminder or nanny if they so wish.

The Safeguarding Vulnerable Groups Act 2006, which received Royal Assent at the end of 2006, provides the legal framework for the new Vetting and Barring Scheme. The new Scheme will replace the current List 99, Protection of Children Act (PoCA) and the Prevention of Vulnerable Adults (PoVA) and Disqualification Orders through a single approach to barring individuals.

It is essential that there is a joint approach placed on all agencies working with children and that these expectations are applied consistently with the Government's response to the recommendations of the Bichard Inquiry (2004), *Safeguarding Children* (Joint Chief Inspectors 2005), and the Safeguarding Vulnerable Groups Act 2006.

In summary:

- Local Safeguarding Children Boards must fulfil their duties to work to ensure that the recruitment and Human Resource practices of organisations take account of the need to safeguard and promote the welfare of children.

- All agencies should be able to explain their recruitment processes and ensure that they undertake the appropriate vetting procedures to safeguard children and young people.

- For inspection purposes, the agency/organisation should be able to provide a list recording the checks undertaken, including the name of the person, the date of the check, the nature of the check (standard or enhanced) and the reference number.

At present, the Criminal Records Bureau (CRB) is an Executive Agency of the Home Office. Since March 2002, the CRB has had the responsibility for carrying out criminal records checks in England and Wales. These checks are currently called 'Disclosures' and have replaced 'police checks'. The CRB provides access to criminal record information in order to help organisations make safer recruitment decisions by identifying candidates who may be unsuitable for certain work.

In future, the CRB will administer automatic inclusions on the list and cases where there is no information, provide the facility for online checks and continuous updates, as well as gather and monitor information on behalf of the IBB.

The CRB currently offers two types of Disclosure. The **Standard Disclosure** details the current and spent convictions, cautions, reprimands and warnings that are held on the Police National Computer. In the case of a post that involves working with children, The Protection of Children Act List, and information that is held under section 142 of the Education Act 2002 – commonly known as List 99 – is searched but, as previously stated, will be replaced once the Safeguarding Vulnerable Groups Act is fully implemented.

The **Enhanced Disclosure** contains the same information as the Standard Disclosure, but with the addition of any relevant information held by local police forces, such as details of acquittals, pending prosecutions or other non-conviction information. All agencies and inspectorates recommend that an Enhanced Disclosure should be applied for by any person who is appointed to a post in which normal duties involve regularly caring for, training, supervising or being in sole charge of children and young people aged under 18, when they:

- Take up a new appointment with a different employer;

- Are appointed as a governor of a school;

- Have had a break in service of three months or more;

- Have moved to a post of significantly greater responsibility for children and young people;

- Have moved within the agency or organisation;

- Are employed as a locum or agency staff before being able to work (for example supply teachers, locum doctors, bank nurses or social workers who work in schools, hospitals or social services departments).

Human Resource Departments should ask supply teachers, and/or bank health or social care staff to produce an Enhanced Disclosure and to check the recruitment processes that are in place in the particular locum or recruitment agency.

There are no straightforward answers to some of these questions, which may be compounded by the requirements of registration and service-specific regulations that suggest that all staff in establishments such as children's homes (including domestic and administrative staff) should have a CRB check. The provisions of the CRB scheme itself may also be problematic as they only allow for checks to be run on a limited number of job descriptions. These do not currently include jobs involving access to information about children, which could involve many layers of administrative and support staff who may not ever have direct access to children, except in the specific case of those with responsibility for monitoring Internet contact between children in chat rooms.

The current scheme offers little protection where staff were appointed some time ago, at a time when the police/CRB check may have been satisfactory. In theory, they might have committed subsequent offences or engaged in activities that might lead to a renewed CRB check being unsatisfactory. This will under the new legislation be replaced through a policy of regularly repeated CRB checks.

Recommendation 13 of *Safeguarding Children* (Joint Chief Inspectors 2005), stated that all agencies directly involved with children should audit their recruitment and staff-checking procedures so that the following practices are carried out consistently:

- References are always verified and properly recorded in staff files;

- A full employment history is available on file for every member of staff;

- Any gaps in employment history are checked and accounted for and qualifications are checked; and

- Enhanced CRB checks are consistently undertaken on new staff and those working with children who have not previously been subject to checks, including temporary, agency or contract staff, prior to the establishment of the centralised vetting and barring scheme, which will come into place, in response to the Bichard Inquiry (2004) report recommendations.

The DfES is continuing to work with the Home Office and the CRB to ensure that enhanced checks are still available for, and consistently undertaken on, new staff and those working with children who have not previously been subject to checks. These include temporary, seasonal, agency, voluntary or contract staff. This will be taken forward in response to Recommendation 21 of the Bichard Inquiry and, in the interim, as part of the List 99 review. In terms of overseas workers, the CRB is seeking to improve links with overseas authorities and build on its Overseas Information Service so that employers have access to the necessary information before employing applicants from abroad (Bichard 2004). There will be duties on police, employers, professional and regulatory bodies, and local authorities to provide relevant information. The aim is to ensure that individuals who are known to pose a risk of harm to children and vulnerable adults are barred from the workforce at the earliest possible opportunity. Barring decisions will be updated as soon as any new information becomes available. It will be a criminal offence for a newly barred individual to continue working with children/vulnerable adults.

Checks through the new scheme will be mandatory for certain positions and in certain settings that offer close contact with children and vulnerable adults. Where the contact is occasional or irregular and the setting is not directly targeted at children or vulnerable adults, the need for a check will be left to the discretion of the employer.

The Government is looking at the options for checking those already in post as part of a phased implementation strategy. In the interim, the Government is not recommending retrospective checking. However, if an employer is concerned about the suitability of an employee to work with children, they can request that the individual apply for a CRB disclosure.

Practical responses

The Healthcare Commission has a duty to uphold the rights and Welfare of Children under the Health and Social Care Act (Community Health and Standards) 2003. The Healthcare Commission receives a number of enquiries related to children's safeguards and through its regional offices will respond promptly to these, in collaboration with other agencies, when indicated. Sometimes NHS, Independent Healthcare Organisations, members of the public, children and parents themselves contact the Healthcare Commission for advice about safeguarding measures. Although the query will usually be handled by someone with particular expertise in safeguarding children, it is important that all staff have a basic awareness of the principles of children's safeguards, adhering to the guidance of *Working Together to Safeguard Children* (HM Government 2006). Figure 1.1 shows a card, issued by the Healthcare Commission for its own staff, providing them with advice if they receive a concern about a child who may be being

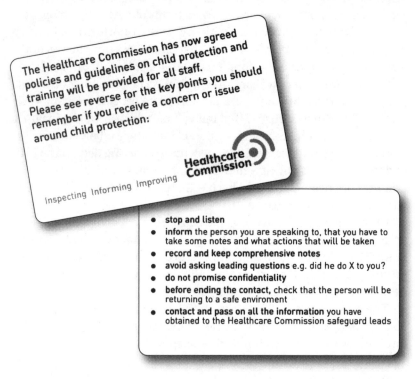

The Healthcare Commission has now agreed policies and guidelines on child protection and training will be provided for all staff. Please see reverse for the key points you should remember if you receive a concern or issue around child protection:

Healthcare Commission

Inspecting Informing Improving

- **stop and listen**
- **inform** the person you are speaking to, that you have to take some notes and what actions that will be taken
- **record and keep comprehensive notes**
- **avoid asking leading questions** e.g. did he do X to you?
- **do not promise confidentiality**
- **before ending the contact,** check that the person will be returning to a safe enviroment
- **contact and pass on all the information** you have obtained to the Healthcare Commission safeguard leads

Figure 1.1 Smart card issued by the Healthcare Commission to all health professionals working with children abused. Please note that this card *is not* issued to Health professionals outside the Healthcare Commission. The card is available for Healthcare Commission staff only. Referrals will be made to Social Services by the Healthcare Commission when necessary.

Case history examples

In order to understand some of the safeguarding concerns for children with continence difficulties, it is helpful to look at cases from clinical experience. Some examples are given below.

CASE STUDY

Nisha

Nisha is a 13-year-old girl who lives with her Asian family, in a two-bedroomed flat in South London. She has two brothers who share one of the bedrooms. Nisha shares the other bedroom with her parents. Nisha has spina bifida and uses a wheelchair. She has poor bladder and bowel control. She uses clean intermittent catheterisation (CIC) to empty her bladder. The bathroom is cramped and Nisha regularly has to carry out the CIC procedure in the main living room. This is difficult as it is also the centre of family activity; being used as the dining room, TV room and for other social and work activities. Nisha's Mother previously assisted Nisha with her bladder and bowel management but her Continence Adviser has now taught Nisha to carry this out herself. On one occasion, Nisha's older brothers arrived home from school and found Nisha carrying out her CIC management in the living room and complained at her for doing this. Nisha said she did not have enough space to do this in either the bathroom or the bedroom.

Comments: This case highlights a number of issues for professionals: the lack of space, and limited privacy, as well as dignity issues in the family home for both the 13-year-old girl and her siblings and parents. It potentially raises safeguarding concerns. Nisha has to share a bedroom with her parents and risks being viewed by her older brothers while emptying her bladder when carrying out CIC. Her brothers also witness her carrying out this procedure in their main living room.

Clearly the family would benefit from an extra bedroom as well as additional privacy for Nisha to perform her CIC.

CASE STUDY

Johnny

Johnny is 12 years of age. He has been 'looked after' on a voluntary basis by a series of foster carers since he was eight. His mother has regular bouts of depression and hallucinations and has previously been sectioned under the Mental Health Act. Johnny's father has 'not really been around' since Johnny was a year old. Johnny was excluded from school recently and has just received a police caution. He has had regular nocturnal enuresis since he was five years old. He previously attended an enuresis clinic but, given that he has had a range of foster parents, it has been difficult to link him to a regular enuresis clinic. Furthermore, the area where he is currently living has recently withdrawn its enuresis service in the local clinic.

Comments: Johnny has a mother who is not always well enough to look after him. He has had a number of different carers and a lack of continuity in managing his bed-wetting because of his frequent moves. He has recently received a Police Caution and has been excluded from school. There are a number of safeguarding concerns that need to be addressed here which may or may not have contributed to his bed-wetting.

CASE STUDY

Jasmine

Jasmine is 13 years old, and of mixed parentage. She has two older brothers and one sister. All the children have been on the child protection register at sometime or other during their lives. Jasmine's parents have not lived together for three years. Her father has a Residence Order for all the children (under Section 8 of the Children Act 1989). Jasmine started running away from her father's home some months ago. Each time she has been returned to the care of her

> father by the Police and Social Services but Social Services believe that she is 'getting out of control'. Jasmine 'bed wet' as a young child and has recently started wetting the bed again. There is a question as to whether she and her friends may be being 'abused through prostitution', as she is often seen out in the streets late at night. A strategy meeting is to be convened at the request of health professionals.

Comments: There are a lot of unknown answers in this case history, although it highlights the fact that Jasmine previously wet the bed and has started bed-wetting again. We need to ask what is causing the bed-wetting. Are there social, emotional or physical factors? Are there concerns within the family? Where is Jasmine's mother and does she ever see her daughter? Is Jasmine being abused through prostitution or are other family members abusing her? If she is being abused through prostitution, who or what brought her into contact with this form of abuse? If the children have previously been on the child protection register, for what reasons were they registered? How has Jasmine been monitored and supported since her name was removed from the child protection register?

Summary: what next?

This short chapter has touched on some of the key legislation and policies which impact on safeguarding children, while acknowledging that those with continence difficulties have specific needs that must be addressed.

Safeguarding children and young people requires that staff in all agencies make every effort to overcome barriers to communication with those engaged in assessing or supporting vulnerable children and families in need. This should include children and young people with continence difficulties who have very significant needs.

Let us not forget that Victoria Climbié was severely emotionally abused and neglected and died at 8 years of age from that abuse. During the latter part of her life (see Appendix 2), Victoria was also incontinent of both urine and faeces. While this memorable, landmark case exposed a catalogue of abuse on one individual, vulnerable child, the association between severe emotional abuse and neglect with incontinence cannot be ignored. While there are other less extreme examples which may trigger temporary or long-term enuresis or soiling (for example, changes in family circumstances, bullying, changes to the child's environment, such as moving schools or following a bereavement), assessing the safeguarding needs of the child in need, as well as the child in need of protection, cannot and should never be ignored.

Note

Please note that while this chapter is written with the knowledge of the Healthcare Commission, the contents may not necessarily reflect the views of the Healthcare Commission. It is also written with the knowledge that Maddie Blackburn will not receive any royalties for this chapter. We are concerned though that it should be helpful for professionals and, through them, for young people with continence difficulties themselves.

References

Bichard M (Chair) (2004) *The Bichard Inquiry Report*. Norwich: HMSO.
    Website: www.bichardinquiry.org.uk/report
Blackburn MC (2002) *Sexuality and Disability*. Oxford: Butterworth Heinemann
    (now Elsevier)
Bonner L, Dobson P (2005) *Promoting Continence in Children with Disabilities:
    Minimum standards of practice for treatment and service delivery*. Bristol: ERIC
Cawson P, Wattam C, Brooker S, Kelly G (2000) *Child Maltreatment in the United
    Kingdom. A Study of the Prevalence of Child Abuse and Neglect*. London: NSPCC
Department for Education and Skills (2003) *Every Child Matters*. Norwich: The
    Stationery Office. Website: www.everychildmatters.gov.uk
Department for Education and Skills, Department of Health, Home Office (2003)
    *Keeping Children Safe: The Government's response to the Victoria Climbié Inquiry
    Report and Joint Chief Inspectors' Report on Safeguarding Children*. London: The
    Stationery Office. Website: www.everychildmatters.gov.uk
Department for Education and Skills (2004) *Safeguarding Children in Education*.
    London:DfES.
    Website: www.teachernet.gov.uk/wholeschool/familyandcommunity/childprotection/guidance
Department for Education and Skills (2004) *The Local Safeguarding Children Boards
    Regulations 2006: Statutory Instrument No 90*. Norwich: Crown Copyright
Department for Education and Skills (2006) *Referrals, assessments and children and
    young people on child protection registers, England. Year ending 31 March 2006*.
    London: DfES. Website: www.dfes.gov.uk/rsgateway/DB/SFR/s000692/CPRCommentary.doc

Department of Health (2003) *Tackling Health Inequalities: A Programme of Action.* London: DH

Department of Health (2004a) *Choosing Health: Making healthier choices easier.* London: DH

Department of Health (2004b) *The National Service Framework (NSF) for Children and Young People.* London: DH

Department of Health (2006) *Our Health, Our Care, Our Say: A new direction for community services.* London: DH

Department of Health and Department for Education and Skills (2004) National Service Framework for Children, Young People and Maternity Services. London, Department of Health. Website: ww.dh.gov.uk/PolicyAndGuidance/HealthAndSocialCareTopics/ChildrenServices/ChildrenServicesInformation/fs/en

Department of Health, Department for Education and Skills, Home Office, Department for Culture, Media and Sports, Office of the Deputy Prime Minister and the Lord Chancellor's Department (2003) *What To Do If You're Worried a Child Is Being Abused.* London: DH

Haines L, Rogers J, Dobson P (2000) A study of drinking facilities in schools. *Nursing Times Supplement,* 5th October, 96(40): 2–4

HM Government (2006) *Working Together to Safeguard Children: A guide to inter-agency working to safeguard and promote the welfare of children.* Norwich: The Stationery Office

Joint Chief Inspectors (2005) *Safeguarding Children: The second Joint Chief Inspectors' report on arrangements to safeguard children.* Norwich: The Stationery Office. Website: www.safeguardingchildren.org.uk

Laming WH (Chair) (2003) *The Victoria Climbié Inquiry.* Norwich: Crown Copyright. Website: www.victoria-climbie-inquiry.org.uk

Simage Communications (1993) *You, your partner and continence; an introduction to sexuality, disability and continence for adults with spina bifida and/or hydrocephalus, other adults with continence difficulties, carers and trainers.* Training video, booklet and cassette (Principle Adviser: Maddie Blackburn). Wembley Park: Simage Communications

Vernon S (2002) *School Toilets: ERIC Says.* Bristol: ERIC

Legislation
Children Act 1989
Education Act 2002
Children Act 2004
Education and Inspections Act 2006
Safeguarding Vulnerable Groups Act 2006

2 Involving and communicating with patients

Ruth Emery

Key points

■ We need to begin by understanding what makes communication 'effective'.

■ There are a number of recognised barriers to communication which need to be addressed.

■ Good communication strategies can be learned.

■ Communication takes place within a social context.

Health promotion points

■ It is very important to encourage parents to use objective, non-judgemental language with their children, so that children will realise it is their difficulties with continence and not they themselves that are the problem.

■ Demonstrate and encourage use of positive language with both parents and children.

This chapter focuses on communicating with children and families, and on the interactions between children and their parents. The role of the health professional as communicator, facilitator, interpreter and teacher is explored.

The chapter draws on current, limited research, but it also makes use of anecdotal evidence and practical experience.

What is communication?

Communication can be defined as 'information sharing' and 'exchanging ideas in an interactive manner'. Mullally (2002) defines the term as:

> . . . the exchange of information between at least two people, usually accomplished by using verbal language, which can be spoken, written, word processed, typed, printed or displayed on a screen, or non-verbal, which transmits attitudes, values and beliefs relevant to the information exchanged.

Poor communication, on the other hand, can be summed up by the following widely available slogan:

> I know you believe you understand what you think I said, but I am not sure you realise that what you heard is not what I meant.

Effective health promotion employs a range of strategies to persuade people to change their behaviour. 'Persuasion' being the key word here, it should be evident that sensitivity and tact are particularly important if you are working with children and young people who have a bladder or bowel problem. A sensitive and individualised programme of assessment and treatment is needed if the young person is to be motivated to become a partner in their own care. The approach should be patient-centred and should focus on the particular sensitivities and needs involved. It is vital that anyone involved in paediatric healthcare understands how to share information in an age-appropriate and respectful manner, starting at a point alongside the young people themselves. A positive, no-blame approach is necessary if children are to be able to overcome their feelings of helplessness (see also Chapter 12 by Melinda Edwards).

Getting to know your patient

Initial contact

Beginnings are important, and a first contact acknowledgement letter to the child's family, accepting the referral, helps the child and family to become aware that their concerns and difficulties have been acknowledged and taken seriously. They can now take comfort from realising that help and support are about to become available to them. It is simply good practice for all families to be offered the opportunity both to rearrange the appointment and to book a language interpreter in advance if English is not their first language.

Communication during the assessment process

As assessment of the child's problem will take place early in the course of the therapeutic relationship, it is particularly important that good communication underlies this. The importance of information sharing in an age-appropriate and respectful manner cannot be over-emphasised. Nor can the necessity of ensuring that the information given is sensitive to the individual needs of the child.

The assessment needs to be patient-focused, reflecting the young person's experience of life, to have achievable outcomes, and set attainable goals. It needs to be carried out in a way that acknowledges cultural diversity and ethnicity, recognising that approaches to toilet training or dealing with continence problems differ greatly from one country or culture to another. Children need structure, demystification of the problem, appropriate advice and consistent positive reinforcement if they are to be empowered to overcome their incontinence. Celebrating success is important to keep the sense of achievement alive. A non-judgemental manner is crucial, making the child and parents feel accepted whatever they look like, whoever they are. Trust and acceptance are the basis for establishing a helping relationship.

We need to understand that children and young people who suffer continence problems are likely to experience enormous embarrassment and shame, coupled with a sense of overwhelming failure. If they are not given support, they can suffer permanent, life-long consequences such as poor self-esteem, lack of confidence and other damaging consequences. A more detailed examination of the psychological consequences of incontinence is given in Chapter 12 by Melinda Edwards.

To help children and their parents feel at ease, it is a good idea to ensure they have information about what to expect *before* their first clinic visit. Children, and their parents too, are likely to be anxious and embarrassed, so it is important to ask questions in a way which can be clearly understood and won't prejudice the answers. Listening carefully to the child's answers will show him or her that you are genuinely interested in them as well as in their problem.

Non-verbal communication

Reading a child's non-verbal signals will help you make a thorough and holistic assessment. Body language can convey powerful messages. For example, excessive fidgeting or poor eye contact may demonstrate a high level of anxiety that is not revealed in what the child actually says. More extreme behavioural examples may include apparent lack of ability to hear, pulling clothes over the face, or walking away to play with toys, for example.

Communication during the treatment process

Treatment should reflect assessment, and needs to be easily incorporated into the young person's family context. Providing good information before the first clinic appointment can help to allay fears and cultivate expectations. Charting of fluid intake and recording episodes of wetting or soiling helps the family engage with the idea of tackling the problem. It can be very useful to let children themselves lead the way, by showing the professional their records and charts. This can give them a sense of ownership and taking control, while helping them to understand what information can be revealed about the cause of their problem. Written care plans can be integrated into the child's care pathway. Individual care pathways for the assessment and management of childhood enuresis can be shared documents which function as 'route maps' of the child's journey to completion of treatment. If agreements or contracts of agreed action plans are written up in the presence of the child and parents, and given to them to take away, this can help to motivate them between appointments. Motivation to engage in treatment is more important than the child's chronological age.

Practical barriers

Language problems

Useful strategies to employ if the child or parents do not have English as their first language include the use of interpreters (if available), audiovisual aids, diagrams, pictures and drawings, play therapy and anatomical dolls or teddy bears. Alternatively, symbols such as those in Widgett (see Figure 2.1) may be useful.

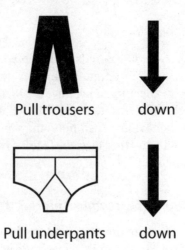

Pull trousers   down

Pull underpants   down

Figure 2.1 Step Chart using Widgett symbols

Learning difficulties

The term 'learning difficulty' is an umbrella term for a wide variety of genetic, social or specific medical conditions which result in a restricted capacity to learn. These may include the autistic spectrum, attention deficit disorder, and global developmental delay. Many children with problems such as these have other difficulties – such as hearing loss or visual impairment – which present a particular challenge to the process of communication (Cokerill 2002).

Both faecal and urinary incontinence have been found to be common in children with additional special needs (Butler and Price 2001). Every child is a complex individual, whose continence cannot be considered in isolation from their other problems. Developmental delay and other difficulties (such as dyspraxia or attention deficit disorder) will interfere with a child's ability to recognise the need to pass a bowel movement or urine.

The prevalence of continence problems in children with physical disabilities in the UK is not known (Brookes 1997). Figures for children with Down's syndrome, however, show attainment of continence to be delayed, but not drastically (Rogers 1998).

It should not be presumed, however, that children with learning difficulties are unable to achieve continence or a higher degree of control, nor that they are unable to become involved in decision-making. The social and family support available will have a major impact on a child's ability to cope with continence problems.

Negative feelings

During the normal development process, very young children create their own identity and self-realisation by those positive and negative reflections given to them by their parents, families and peers. This process continues for many years, until adulthood.

During this process, young children will 'externalise' their feelings onto an inanimate object (such as a teddy, doll or other toy) for example by saying 'Teddy is hungry, Teddy is tired' if they are. So, understandably, if they are given the message that faeces are dirty, smelly and bad, they may associate not yet being toilet trained, wet or soiled with being 'dirty, smelly and bad'. If not treated with great care, this can cause feelings of inadequacy, unworthiness and shame to develop with consequent damage to self-confidence and self-esteem.

Visualise this image: an infant has had a bowel action in his nappy. He is handed from one grimacing parent to the other with the words, 'Ohhh . . . he's done a pooh . . . what a stink! You can change him this time . . . eeeurgh, yuck!' If the child develops control and the ability to inhibit the urge to void until a more acceptable time and place occurs (i.e. is toilet trained in a positive manner) this negative reinforcement will have been short lived, and not detrimental to his emotional well-being.

Some children are not so fortunate, however, and if control takes longer to develop, the negative messages being communicated by the parents will start to take their toll on the child's consciousness. So one of our roles as health professionals is to tackle communication patterns that damage a child's self-esteem and teach parents more positive ways of expressing themselves (see also Chapter 12 by Melinda Edwards).

Rewarding success and ignoring accidents is a positive and usually successful method adopted by parents in toilet training. It is also a method which often encourages healthy children to develop the skill of inhibiting the urge to void when they first recognise the message sent from the bladder or bowel to the brain signalling the need for emptying. Children who become enuretic or constipated or soilers may not have had this training. Alternatively, they may have been told 'dirty' is 'bad' and 'clean' is 'good', and have overdeveloped 'holding on' or deferment techniques which fail ultimately, leaving them incontinent.

It is important to stress here, however, that it should *never* be assumed by professionals that this lack of training is the sole cause of a child's incontinence. A sensitive assessment of the parents' attitudes and abilities regarding the way in which toilet training was or is managed can be very revealing. An open approach and a non-judgemental attitude may uncover much more information about previous attempts to train the child and teach independent toileting skills. For example, many parents display exasperation at failure, or despair when their child wets or soils. It may seem to be a natural response (especially with a child who is old enough to be expected to have control) to demand the child explains 'why' the accident has occurred. Parents are unlikely to find coping with an incontinent child easy, and every effort should be made to help them deal with this problem in a constructive and supportive way (Butler *et al.* 2005).

This is the point at which parents can develop parental intolerance and reinforce the child's sense of bewilderment, shame and isolation, as they do not usually know of anyone else with the same problem (Butler *et al.* 2005). This does not mean they do not know anyone else who shares their problem, simply that they are likely to be unaware that others may be affected too, because incontinence is generally kept deeply private and socially taboo.

Anecdotal evidence suggests that a high percentage of parents believe their children are 'not bothered' by their continence problems, but children rarely feel able to share how they truly feel until they are asked in a safe, caring and positive environment. This is the environment to try to create in a children's continence clinic or during a planned home visit.

When children *are* asked how they feel, the replies would indicate they certainly are bothered! Yamamoto and colleagues (1987) researched perceived stressfulness of events to 1814 school-aged children from six countries. The research involved a questionnaire which described 20 life events and the participants were asked to rate how stressful they thought this experience would be on a scale of one to seven. There was considerable similarity across nationalities in terms of the types of life events identified as stressful, and in the actual experiences of the young people in the study. Without exception, the experience of losing a parent was rated as the most stressful experience imaginable. Listed among the other potential stressors were: 'hearing my parents quarrel and fight'; 'wetting myself in class'; 'being caught stealing something'; 'telling the truth and having no one believe me'. This indicates that children are stressed by incontinence, and that those for whom this is not actually a problem do fear it happening to them. Children who do suffer in this way need to be given a definite message that we, as healthcare professionals, believe in their problem and value their need to attain continence.

What makes a good communicator?

At the centre of good communication and engaging patients is the motivation to establish a connection with young patients, in a way that empowers them to become active partners in regaining control of their bladder and bowel function. It is important that you are able to win the confidence of the child and family. They must be able to trust you not to judge them or betray their confidences. So beginning by greeting them with warmth and a smile, and establishing their right to confidentiality early in the first interview, will get you off to a good start.

Body language and facial expression

Non-verbal presentation and appropriate body language at the initial meeting can convey respect, empathy and sincerity. Engaging the child and parents in direct eye contact and smiling, as appropriate, help to inspire confidence. So too does sitting in an 'open' posture – non-threatening, facing the other person, and with the arms and legs unfolded. There should not be any large objects (such as a desk) dividing the space between the professional and the child and family. It is important to respect the others' personal body space boundaries too.

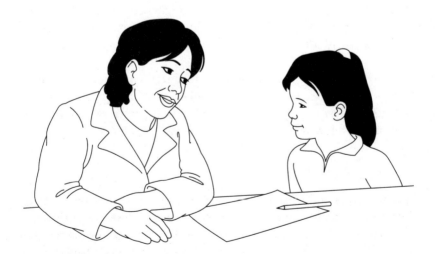

Figure 2.2 Appropriate posture and positioning will help to make communication effective

The art of listening

The most important aspect of your two-way communication with the child and family is the way you listen. It is not only important that you do listen, you need to let your conversation partners know that you do. There are various techniques you can employ to reinforce this. For example, by reflecting back what has just been said (repeating a couple of words from the end) you let your patient know you have heard them. Or you can ask them to elaborate, for example by asking 'So you enjoyed that, did you?'

A similar, but slightly different technique, is that of *paraphrasing*. This involves repeating back to the child or parent what they have just said but in slightly different words. This gives you as a professional the chance to check that the speaker means what you think they do, and can also help them to be a little more objective.

What we hear when we listen is our primary source of information. It also provides clues as to the emotional impact that continence problems are having both on the child him or herself, and on the parents. Active listening and appropriate response conveys empathy, which can be a powerful means of inspiring confidence in children and their parents.

Appropriate questioning

It can be helpful to begin by asking the child, 'What do *you* want to change?' Following this up by asking the parents the same question will rapidly bring parental attitudes to light; intolerance, lack of understanding of the problem and misconceptions will then be out in the open where they can be addressed.

In exploring further, it is important to use 'open questions', ones that do not encourage a yes or no response (see Table 2.1).

This is a technique that can be immensely useful in helping children to expand their own thinking about their situation.

Exploring available options

We can use various responses to open up and develop what is important for the child – for example, 'Could you say more about this?' As health professionals, we need to curb our desire to ask or respond from our own curiosity. Once assessment, diagnosis and possible treatments have been discussed, it is time to put together a contract of mutually agreed actions.

Table 2.1 Open and closed questions

Closed questions	Open questions
'Are you doing well in school?'	'How are things going at school?'
'Did you fill in your record chart?'	'Can you tell me about your record chart?'
'Do you feel OK?'	'I am wondering how you feel?'
'Did you cry when you wet yourself?'	'It would really help me to understand how you felt when you wet yourself. Do you think you could try to tell me?'

When the issue being addressed is complex or audiences are easily distracted, messages that contain a conclusion or recommendations are more effective (Linder and Worchel 1970). Each choice of available options and the consequences of each treatment option need to be explored considering all the family dynamics, expectations and abilities. Children will need reassuring that the planned change will not increase their likelihood of failure, as 'moderate or high fear may actually interfere with change' rather than motivating it (Leventhal *et al.* 1983). This is the point at which arrangements should be made to meet again, and clear information given about how to contact a named adviser between agreed meetings or appointments.

At the end of any clinic appointment, it is important to give simple conclusions by summing up the most important topics discussed. Recommendations can become the basis for a plan of action. It may also be appropriate to use a checklist here, provided that the checklist is regarded as a tool to be adapted for individuals and their circumstances, not as something to be followed slavishly.

Communicating in a social context

A gulf between perspectives

Will parents and children meet professional prejudice? Healthcare professionals may inadvertently minimise and diminish parents' concerns or even worse dismiss them outright. After all, they are not the ones who have to live with the problem, day in and day out. Professional potential for disillusionment and 'burn out' is higher than in some other fields of nursing, perhaps due to lack of support in the recognition of the extent of the problem and financial constraints affecting service delivery. Barriers that reduce or prevent effective communication between families and health professionals are legion, but the following are deserving of a special mention.

- **Apathy** on the part of professionals, parents, other family members or the young people themselves, is a significant factor, along with lack of awareness about the services available.

- **Containment** of incontinence versus promotion of continence.

- **Problems with communication skills and levels of understanding** – it may well be health professionals themselves whose communication skills are at fault, especially if they have not judged the child's ability to understand correctly.

- **Mobility problems** on the part of the child.

- **Fear of incontinence, leading to a high level of anxiety** which simply makes the situation worse.

- **Poor access to health promotion** for people with learning disabilities – as has been recognised at government level (DH 1995). Guidance for health professionals on the provision of primary care services, including health promotion, to people who have learning disabilities can be found in the document *Once a Day* (NHSE 1999) and on the BBC website (Spink 2006).

Multi-agency involvement

While collaborative working across a number of professional groups has much to recommend it, this situation can present real challenges to consistent patient involvement and effective communication. A large number of different health, education and social care professionals can be involved, all with their own professional culture and each one with a separate, defined, role with regard to the child (see Table 2.2).

It is important that people who are part of the child's life in any sort of long-term or consistent manner should be involved in the communication process. Children often have significant people in their lives who they nominate as their 'family' whether or not they are actually blood relatives. Failures of communication between a child and any of

Table 2.2 The main individuals concerned with caring for children

Birth and infancy	Antenatal/midwifery team Special care nursing and medical staff	Acute care sector
Early years	Health visitors Nursery nurses Childminders	'Sure Start' early learning projects Pre-school nurseries
Primary years	School nurses Classroom teachers Learning support staff Rainbows, Cubs, Brownies and similar organisations	Primary school sector (especially if child is 'statemented')
Secondary years	School/college staff Adolescent groups such as 'Connexions' Local youth groups Scouts, guides etc. Youth education centres Family planning clinics Child and adolescent mental health services	Education services Social groups Health services
Young adulthood	Probation and young offenders' teams Police officers Legal services Community centres Pharmacists, Paediatricians, senior and junior house officers Extended schooling and home tuition provision Many allied health professionals	Community and hospital
Throughout the age span	Hospital-based centres for child development or learning disabilities Children's wards and outpatient departments Paediatric accident and emergency departments Speech and language therapists Dietitians Psychologists	

Table 2.2 The main individuals concerned with caring for children
(*continued*)

Throughout the age span	Social services, as residential guardians of some children in care (now known as 'looked after children') Churches, mosques and other places of worship Voluntary and non-statutory organisations

these significant figures can cause unnecessary additional stress, with a knock-on adverse effect upon treatment outcomes.

It is not just the children themselves who suffer when communication breaks down. Parents can feel disempowered and inadequate, unable to cope. They can feel they personally have failed to improve their child's quality of life and experience. Social isolation, exhaustion and depression can set in, as the parent's sense of self-worth and value as a caregiver evaporates. Some of this can be pre-empted by 'recognising the worth and value of other agencies including child and adolescent mental health teams, voluntary organisations and support groups' (The Children Act 1989).

Service provision

Changes within the nursing profession pose a challenge to the future care of children and adolescents with continence problems. For example, although there were 7,520,000 nurses working in the NHS in 2003 (Hutton 2004), there were only 622 continence advisers, and and some of these were not registered nurses.

Demographic changes mean fluctuations in both the workforce and in demand for services. Such changes may also change the way in which care is delivered, and affect opportunities for one to one communication.

Communicating information about the service

Often the most effective way that good news spreads is by word of mouth. So patients and families may themselves be your best ambassadors – but often in a way that is invisible and impossible to measure.

Bear in mind too that they may be too embarrassed to tell others that this socially taboo and deeply humiliating health problem has affected them so closely.

Practical experience suggests that most parents of children with any bladder or bowel dysfunction start by simply wanting to know who can they talk to about their concerns. They are then likely to ask *what* to do about the problem, *what* help is available to them and *why* this is happening to their child. Parents will search newspapers, websites, magazines and radio media to find out how they can resolve their child's problem. The national Health Needs Assessment programme, a new method of asking school-age children at specified points in time about their health needs and related worries, may help to address some of these concerns. A Health Needs Assessment programme, which is delivered by school nurses, includes age-appropriate questions about continence within the general context of many other health-related questions (Hall 1996). This allows children and young people to identify their own concerns in a confidential manner.

Conclusion

Children learn what they are taught by adults. Being incontinent can have a drastic effect on a child's quality of life, especially if they find themselves on the receiving end of a great deal of negative emotion. Both the child and the family may become dependent on health professionals. Interventions to help resolve issues of incontinence should not target the problem in isolation, but take an holistic approach with the aim of improving general, physical and emotional and spiritual well-being. Children who regain control of their previously lost continence can develop other problem-solving skills and grow into well-balanced individual adults.

At the centre of good patient involvement is the motivation to engage and communicate with the young patient, thereby enabling him or her to become the driving force behind the ability to regain control of bladder and bowel function. Communication, and the feelings of empowerment it can engender, are central to this. It is up to us as specialists, both in continence promotion and relating to children and adolescents, to take a lead role in communicating positively with our patients. What a privilege and rewarding experience it can be for us to be able to walk alongside them in this process. They have the right to our help in regaining or controlling the function of their bladder and bowel, something that is essential to allowing them to realise their full potential.

References

Brookes E (1997) Independent Means. *Nursing Times,* 93 (July 23): 30
Butler RJ, Golding J, Heron J, ALSPAC Study Team (2005) Nocturnal enuresis: a survey of parental coping strategies at 7½ years. *Child: Health Care and Development,* 31: 659–67
Butler U, Price K (2001) Bowel and bladder management in children with disabilities. *Current Paediatrics,* 11:143–8
Cokerill H (2002) Supporting communication in the child with a learning disability. *Current Paediatrics,* 12(1):1–8
Department of Health (1991) *The Children Act 1989: an introductory guide for the NHS.* London: HMSO
Department of Health (1995) *The Health of the Nation: strategy for people with learning disabilities.* London: HMSO
Department of Health (2003) *Not Complacent, Still a Long Way to Go.* (Press Release No 2003/0242). London: Department of Health
Department of Health (2004) *National Service Framework for Children, Young People and Maternity Services. Part 1: the NSF Emerging Findings consultation document 10/04/03.* London: HMSO
ERIC (Regularly updated) *Education and Research for the Improvement of Childhood Continence Catalogue.* Available as hard copy from ERIC or downloadable from the website
Hall R (1996) Health for all children. *Nursing Standard,* 11 (Oct 2): 33
Hutton J, MP (2004) Speech to Allied Health Professionals by the Minister of State for Health, 31 March, House of Commons
Linder D, Worchel S (1970) Opinion change as a result of effortfully drawing a counter-attitudinal conclusion. *Journal of Experimental Social Psychology,* 6: 42–8
Leventhal H, Safer M, Paganis D (1983) The impact of communications on health beliefs, decisions and behaviours. *The Health Education Quarterly,* 1 0: 1–29
Mullally S (2002) *Dictionary of Nursing.* Edinburgh: Churchill Livingstone
Morgan R (1996) *Guidelines for the minimum standard of practice in the treatment of childhood enuresis.* Bristol: ERIC
National Health Service Executive (1999) *Once a Day.* London: Department of Health
Pollock D (2002) *Director of the Continence Foundation: Memo of Evidence to The House of Commons Health Committee.* London: HMSO
Rogers J (1998) Promoting continence: the child with special needs. *Nursing Standard,* 12 (13) May 13: 47–55
Rustin M (2004) Learning from the Victoria Climbié Inquiry. *Journal of Social Work Practice,* 18 (1): 9–18
Scott L (2002) Child Protection: the role of communication. *Nursing Times,* 98 (18 April): 34–6

Simons J, Macdonald L (2004) Pain assessment tools: children's nurses' views. *Journal of Child Health Care*, 4 (December): 264–78

Spink GA (2006) Disabled suffer healthcare gap. Age and Disability Correspondent, www.bbc.co.uk

Yamamoto K, Suliman A, Parsons J, Davies OL Jr (1987) Voices in unison: stressful events in the lives of children in six countries. *Journal of Child Psychology*, 28 (6): 855–64

3 Embryology of the urogenital tract and pelvic floor

Christina Chi Ding and Mark Slack

Key points

- The human embryo arises from three basic germ layers: ectoderm, mesoderm and endoderm. The urogenital system arises from the mesoderm.

- The majority of organ systems are formed between the third and the eighth week.

- Developmental anomalies of urinary and genital system often coexist.

- There are three different phases of development of the kidneys and ureters – namely pronephros, mesonephros and metanephros. Most parts of the adult kidney are formed from metanephros and mesonephros.

- The bladder and the urethra arise from the urogenital sinus.

- The Y chromosome is crucial for gonadal development, and the SRY gene on the Y chromosome influences sexual differentiation.

- The external genitalia in males and females develops from two genital folds, two genital swellings and one midline genital tubercle.

- The presence of fetal androgen is the key factor in the development of male external genitalia. Female external genitalia develops in the absence of fetal androgen.

A wide spectrum of congenital abnormalities of the urinary and genital tract can occur in females. These abnormalities commonly co-exist. Treatments of such problems depend upon the understanding of both normal and abnormal embryological development of the urogenital tract.

From a functional point of view, the urogenital system can be divided into two sub-systems: the urinary system and the genital system.

By the third week after conception, the embryo consists of three germ layers known as ectoderm, mesoderm and endoderm. The ectoderm gives rise to skin, central and peripheral nervous systems. The endoderm forms the epithelial lining of the respiratory tract, gastrointestinal tract, urinary bladder, liver and pancreas. The mesoderm forms smooth and striated muscle, connective tissue, cardiovascular systems (heart, arteries, veins, blood cells, bone marrow) and the urinary and genital systems (kidney, gonads).

The period between the third week and the eighth week is known as the embryonic period, during which specific tissues and organs are developed. The main organ systems are established by the end of this period. This also represents the time period when the fetus is at greatest risk from external factors such as drugs or medications.

During the fourth week of gestation, both urinary and genital systems originate from a common mesodermal ridge (i.e. intermediate mesoderm) which is made up of two parts on each side of the aorta: the urogenital ridge and the nephrogenic ridge. The urogenital ridge will give rise to the genital system (gonads, genital ducts and external genitalia) while the nephrogenic ridge forms the urinary system (kidney, ureter, bladder and urethra). Excretory units of both systems enter a common cavity called the cloaca. These two systems are closely associated and interwoven both embryologically and anatomically (Moore and Persaud 2003; Sadler 2004). As a result, developmental abnormalities of one system will often be associated with abnormalities in the other.

Development of the urinary system

The urinary system consists of the following components:

- Kidneys;
- Ureters;
- Urinary bladder;
- Urethra.

In addition to the development of these four components, in this section we will also briefly describe the development of the pelvic floor.

Development of the kidneys and ureters

During the development of the embryo, three different but slightly overlapping kidney systems are formed within the nephrogenic ridge:

- The **pronephros:** a rudimentary and transitory kidney develops early in the fourth week but is not functional.

- The **mesonephros:** a structurally well-developed kidney, functions briefly between the fourth and the eighth week and lays the foundation of the urinary collecting system.

- The **metanephros:** permanent kidney appears in the fifth week and starts to function from the ninth week.

In the first phase of kidney development, the pronephros appears as a series of tubules and ducts formed in the uppermost portion of the nephrogenic ridge. It soon undergoes regression.

In the second phase, the mesonephric tubules and ducts develop at the centre of the nephrogenic ridge. By the end of the first trimester, the majority of the mesonephros has degenerated. However, the mesonephric duct (also known as the *Wolffian duct*) that drains the mesonephric tubules continues in the male in the form of the *efferent ductules* of the testes, but disappears in the female.

In the third phase, the metanephros forms at the most distal part of the nephrogenic ridge and eventually becomes the kidney and collecting system in adults. The metanephros develops its own excretory tubules and nephrons. However, its collecting system originates from the ureteric bud, which is an outgrowth of the mesonephric duct developed at the second phase. This ureteric bud evolves to become the entire collecting system (including the major and minor calyces, the renal pelvis, the ureter and approximately one to three million collecting tubules).

Development of the bladder and urethra

Both the bladder and urethra are developed from the cloaca, a transient embryological structure evolving from the primordial gut system. It is a common cavity into which the digestive, urinary and reproductive tracts open.

For descriptive purposes, the primordial gut system is divided into three parts: the foregut, the midgut and the hindgut. The hindgut not only forms most part of the colon, the rectum and the superior part of the anal canal, but also forms the epithelium of the urinary bladder and most of the urethra.

Figure 3.1 Congenital anomalies (1)

Connection between the collecting and excretory tubule systems is essential for normal fetal development. Failure to connect may cause congenital cystic diseases and renal agenesis. Forty per cent of renal failure cases in childhood result from developmental anomalies of the ureteric bud and the metanephros. Timing of the ureteric bud division is also important. If it occurs too early, it may result in bifid or supernumerary kidneys with ectopic ureters.

Congenital anomalies of the kidneys and ureters occur in 3–4% of newborn infants. The most common anomalies are abnormal shape and position, e.g. malrotated kidney, horseshoe kidney. Others such as Renal Agenesis (unilateral and bilateral), cystic kidney disease (autosomal recessive polycystic kidney disease or ARPKD, multicystic dysplastic kidney or MDK) have been extensively studied and reported (Sadler 2004).

Renal agenesis (RA)

There are two types of RA:

- Unilateral RA occurs in 1/1000 births, and usually affects the male infant. The missing kidney is often the left one and is commonly associated with compensatory hypertrophy of the other kidney.

- Bilateral RA is much more rare, occurring in only 1/10,000 births. This condition is incompatible with postnatal life. The lack of amniotic fluid secondary to anuria is usually detected by routine ultrasound scan during the antenatal period. Over three quarters of these cases are associated with other major structural abnormalities such as cardiac, neurological or genital abnormalities, tracheal or duodenal atresia, cleft lip and/or palate.

Congenital polycystic kidney disease (PKD)

This is characterised by multiple non-functional cysts. It often has autosomal recessive inheritance. Autosomal recessive polycystic kidney disease occurs in 1 in 5000 births. It is a progressive disease in which the kidney becomes very large, often leading to renal failure early in childhood. Autosomal dominant PKD occurs in 1 in 500–1000 births and usually does not cause renal failure until adulthood.

Figure 3.2 Development of the cloaca into the anterior primitive urogenital sinus and the posterior rectum. Further development of the primitive urogenital sinus into three parts: the bladder, the pelvic urethra and the definitive urogenital sinus

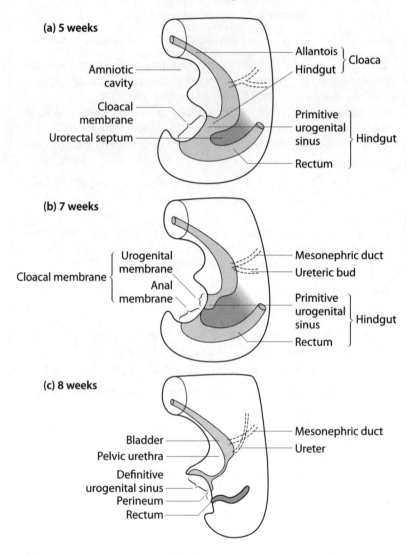

At the beginning of the fourth week, the primordial gut system is closed at both the top and bottom ends. The bottom end is closed by the cloacal membrane, which separates the cloaca from the amniotic cavity. The cloacal membrane is further divided into the urogenital membrane in the front and the anal membrane at the back. The cloaca is

Figure 3.3 Congenital anomalies (2)

Bladder defects may take the form of urachal cysts or urachal fistulae, where urine will escape from the umbilical orifice as a result of persistence of the lumen of the allantois.

More severe abnormalities include:

- **Extrophy of the bladder** (a condition where the trigone of the bladder and the ureteric orifices are exposed and urine leaks intermittently from the everted bladder);

- **Epispadias** (where the urethra opens on to the posterior aspect of penis).

---

composed of two portions, a closed hindgut at the back and a sausage-shaped allantois in the front.

The perineum is formed when the urorectal septum (i.e. perineal body in the adult) reaches the cloacal membrane.

Between the fourth and the seventh week, the distal end of the cloaca is further divided into a primitive urogenital sinus in the front and rectum at the back. The primitive urogenital sinus can be divided into three parts:

- The urinary bladder which is the upper part;

- The narrow pelvic urethra, which develops into the prostatic and membranous parts of the urethra in the male, and forms the membranous (entire) urethra in the female;

- The definitive urogenital sinus, which forms the penile urethra in the male and vestibule of the vagina in the female.

The further development of the definitive urogenital sinus differs greatly between the two sexes.

The allantois is a sausage-shaped out-pouching from the bottom end of the yolk sac extending into the connecting stalk. It plays a key role in early embryological vascular development and its blood vessels become the umbilical arteries and veins.

The bladder is initially continuous with the allantois. Later, as the bladder enlarges, the allantois constricts, looses its lumen and becomes a thick fibrous cord called the urachus. The urachus extends from the

Figure 3.4 Urachal anomalies: **(a)** Urachal cyst; **(b)** Urachal sinus, which may open into the bladder or at umbilicus; **(c)** Urachal fistula, connecting the bladder and the umbilicus

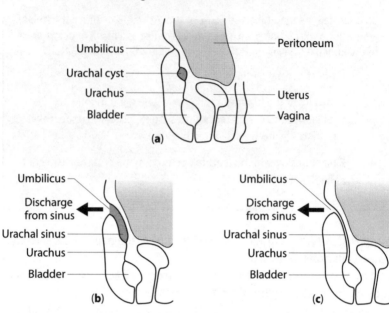

dome of the bladder to the umbilicus and later becomes the median umbilical ligament in the adult.

Development of the pelvic floor

Each urogenital structure is surrounded by mesenchymal tissues, which will further differentiate into smooth and striated muscle cells to form sphincter structures. This forms the basis for later development of the deep and superficial pelvic floor.

The differentiation of the striated muscle cells occurs during the fetal period, while that of the smooth muscle cells occurs later during the neonatal and infant period. The formation of the deep perineal structures and the important sphincter structures surrounding the anal canal and the urethra take place by the end of the second month of gestation (Gearhart and Jeffs 1998).

Figure 3.5 Congenital anomalies (3)

Anomalies of the urinary, genital and anorectal structures are often results of defective partition of the cloaca.

Congenital anomalies may cause incontinence via a number of mechanisms:

- Anomalies that affect the function of the sphincter mechanism, such as female epispadias or urogenital sinus anomalies;

- Duplicated ectopic ureters (which open into the vagina) giving rise to urinary stress incontinence or continuous leakage;

- Bladder extrophy, which causes abnormal bladder storage. This is caused by the failure of the cloacal membrane to be reinforced by invagination of mesoderm during the fourth week, resulting in the incomplete closure of the inferior abdominal wall. It is a rare but serious anomaly occurring in 1 in 10,000 to 50,000 births, and more commonly affects male infants;

- Other abnormalities which cause abnormal bladder storage, such as cloacal extrophy and myelomeningocele (spina bifida), and which include incontinence among their more obvious symptoms.

Incontinence may also be caused by sphincter-bypass anomalies such as bilateral single ectopic ureters.

Patients often have multiple anatomical defects involving the anterior abdominal wall and the anterior wall of the urinary bladder. As a consequence, the posterior wall of the bladder is often exposed. They may have other abnormalities involving abdominal and pelvic muscles, the bony pelvis, umbilical fascia defects, anorectal defects and hernias. Genital or uterine ligament defects may result in uterine prolapse in later life.

Muscular defects include the absence of the rectus muscle and the deficiency of external or internal oblique and the transverse abdominal muscles. The levator muscle may also be affected. The anterior segment of the levator ani is often shorter, and the posterior segment usually longer. Thus 70% of the levator muscle is posterior to the rectus, which results in the lack of anterior pelvic muscular floor. The puborectal sling may also be markedly flatter (Bourdelat 1987).

Development of the genital system

The three components of the genital system are:

- **Gonads** further differentiation controlled by SRY gene on the Y chromosome;

- **Genital ducts** further differentiation under the influence of sex hormones;

- **External genitalia** further differentiation under the influence of sex hormones.

The fetus at the seventh week only has genetic difference and could potentially develop either as male or female. All three components (gonads, genital ducts and external genitalia) go through a stage in which they are identical (indifferent stage) and can develop into either male or female.

The primordial germ cells are found in the yolk sac. These cells migrate from the yolk sac to the primitive gonads. The migration is completed by day 42. This process is regulated by the SRY gene on the Y chromosome, which is an auotosomal gene crucial for gonadal development. The factors that determine whether the fetus develops into a male or a female include presence of the SRY gene on the Y chromosome, presence or absence of the anti-Müllerian hormone and fetal androgen production.

If the primordial germ cells fail to reach the indifferent gonad, the gonad remains indifferent or is absent.

Development of gonads

There are three sources from which the gonads are derived:

- The mesothelium (mesodermal epithelium) which lines the posterior abdominal wall;

- The underlying mesenchyme (embryonic connective tissue);

- The primordial germ cell.

Indifferent gonad

Primordial germ cells reach the primitive gonads by the fifth week and invade the genital ridges.

Sex determination
The chromosomal (genetic) sex is established at fertilisation. The Y-induced histocompatibility antigen (H-Y) is found to be essential for subsequent male development. The sex-determining region on the Y chromosome (**SRY**) is the DNA basis of sex-determination. Their presence enables the development of indifferent gonads into testes.

Development of testes
Under the influence of the SRY gene on the Y chromosome, the primitive sex cords develop to form the testis. The tunica albuginea develops from further medullary growth. Solid testis cords consist of primitive germ cells and sertoli calls, surrounded by interstitial cells of Leydig which produce testosterone by the eighth week. At puberty, the testis cords canalise and become the seminiferous tubules and are joined to the ductus deferens by rete testis cords.

Development of ovaries
Gonadal development occurs two weeks later in female embryos. In the absence of the SRY gene, the gonadal cortical layer containing the germ cells further develops, while regression occurs in the medullary layer resulting in the formation of ovaries.

By week 20, the division of the germ cells allows the primordial follicles to reach a peak of 5–7 million. These germ cells arrest in the first meiotic division, with only one million remaining by birth.

Genital ducts

At the indifferent stage of genital duct development, two different duct systems exist in both male and female embryos:

- The mesonephric duct – Wolffian system (male);

- The paramesonephric duct – Müllerian system (female).

According to the sex, one system will develop further while the other will regress. The development of the Wolffian system requires the positive presence of adequate androgen. The development of the Müllerian system is passive.

Differentiation of the indifferent genital ducts is controlled by the sex hormones produced by the functioning fetal gonad. In the male, secretion of testosterone by the Leydig cells in the fetal testis stimulates the development of the Wolffian system. At the same time, secretion of

Figure 3.6 Congenital anomalies (4)

Various forms of uterine and vaginal anomalies are the result of developmental arrests during the eighth week of embryonic life.

This includes different degrees of *incomplete fusion of the paramesonephric ducts* (Müllerian system). In its extreme form it may present as double uterus (*uterus didelphys*). If duplication only involves the top part of the uterus, bicornuate uterus results. In its mildest form with only slight indentation in the middle of the uterine body it is called an *arcuate uterus*.

Developmental failure of one or both paramesonephric ducts (Müllerian system)
If one paramesonephric duct fails to develop, a unicornuate uterus (a uterus with one uterine tube) is formed. Failure of development in both paramesonephric ducts (i.e. Rokitansky-Kuster-Hauser Syndrome) may lead to Müllerian agenesis (absence of uterus, tubes and the upper two-third of the vagina).

Incomplete canalisation of the vaginal plate
This results in vaginal septum at different levels (e.g. imperforate hymen).

Müllerian inhibitory factor will result in regression of the Müllerian system. The mesonephric duct persists (Wolffian system) and forms the epididymis, seminal vesicle, ductus deferens and ejaculatory duct.

In the female, the paramesonephric ducts (Müllerian system) fuse and develop into uterine tubes, uterus, cervix, and upper two thirds of the vagina. Degeneration of the Wolffian system occurs at the same time. The distal end of the fused paramesonephric ducts meets the urogenital sinus, forming the paired sinovaginal bulbs, which further fuses to form the vaginal plate. Later the cells central to this plate break down in the process of canalisation. By the fifth month of fetal life, the canalisation of the vagina is complete, forming the lumen of the lower third of vagina. The membrane separating the lumen of vagina from the urogenital sinus is called the *hymen.*

This embryological development is reflected in the anatomical supports described by De Lancey (1992). It is divided into levels I, II and III. At level III the vagina is tightly adherent to the surrounding structures and differs from the supports at levels II and III.

Figure 3.7 Illustrations of various types of uterine anomaly:
(**a**) Normal; (**b**) Uterine didelphys (double uterus and vagina);
(**c**)Bicornuate uterus; (**d**) Septate uterus; (**e**) Unicornuate uterus

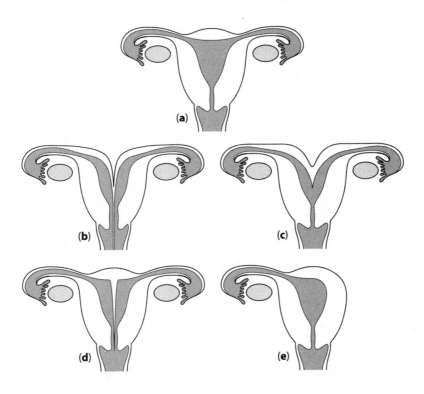

- The upper quarter (i.e. level I) is suspended by the cardinal and uterosacral ligaments.

- The middle two quarters (i.e. level II) is maintained by lateral attachment, anteriorly to the arcus tendinous fascia pelvis and posteriorly to the pubococcygeus and iliococcygeus fascia.

- The lower quarter of the vagina (i.e. level III) is maintained by fusion of the lower vagina to the urogenital diaphragm anteriorly and the perineal body posteriorly.

External genitalia

By the sixth week, the external genitalia at the indifferent stage consist of:

- Two genital folds;
- Two genital swellings;
- One midline genital tubercle.

Fetal dihydrotestosterone is the influencing factor in the male development of external genitalia. By the second trimester, the genital tubercle forms the glans, genital folds elongate and fuse forming the penis and urethra and the genital swellings form the scrotum.

In female, in the absence of androgen the above changes do not occur, so oestrogen will influence the development of the clitoris from the genital tubercle, labia minora from the genital folds and the labia majora from the genital swellings.

Abnormalities of development in the male genitalia

Hypospadias
Hypospadias is the most common anomaly of the penis (1 in 300 male infants). It is due to incomplete fusion of the urethral folds in the male,

Figure 3.8 Hypospadias: an anomaly of the penis resulting from incomplete development

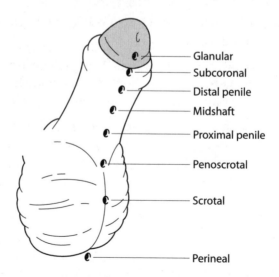

- Glanular
- Subcoronal
- Distal penile
- Midshaft
- Proximal penile
- Penoscrotal
- Scrotal
- Perineal

resulting in an abnormal urethral opening on the posterior surface of the penis. It is the result of inadequate production of androgens by the fetal testes while differences in the timing and degree of hormonal failure account for various forms of hypospadias.

Epispadias
This rare condition occurs in 1/30,000 male infants. The urethra opens onto the anterior aspect of the penis. It is often associated with extrophy of the bladder.

Micropenis
Micropenis results when androgen stimulation of the external genitalia during its development is insufficient, often the result of primary hypogonadism (hypothalamic and/or pituitary level dysfunction).

Abnormalities of sexual differentiation

Abnormalities in sexual differentiation can present in the early neonatal period or may only become apparent with delayed onset of puberty or with the inability to establish normal sexual relationships. Sex differentiation defects include Klinefelter syndrome, gonadal dysgenesis, true hermaphroditism, pseudo-hermaphroditism and androgen insensitivity syndrome.

Klinefelter syndrome
As the most common major sexual differentiation abnormality, Klinefelter syndrome (47, XXY or other variants such as XXXY) occurs in 1/500 males. The main characteristics of this syndrome include infertility, gynecomastia, impaired sexual maturation of various degrees and (in some cases) under androgenisation.

With normal sexual differentiation, the external and internal genitalia should be consistent with the sex chromosome complement.

Hermaphroditism
Hermaphroditism is the result of inconsistency between the appearance of the external genitalia and the morphology of the gonads. Hermaphroditism can be classified into true hermaphroditism and pseudo-hermaphroditism according to the appearance of the gonads.

The condition is poorly understood. Genetic constitution of this group of patients is varied with 70% of them being 46, XX, 20% being 46, XX/46, XY mosaic, and the remaining 10% being 46, XY.

True hermaphrodites have both ovarian and testicular tissue, thus resulting in an individual with characteristics of both sexes. They have ambiguous external genitalia and are often raised as female.

Pseudo-hermaphroditism can be further divided into female pseudo-hermaphroditism with ovaries and male pseudo-hermaphroditism with testes.

Female pseudo-hermaphroditism (46, XX) is usually caused by congenital adrenal hyperplasia (CAH). The gonads (ovaries) are normal, however, the external genitalia undergo virilisation as the result of excessive androgen exposure during the development of the female fetus. The principal fault lies in the defective enzyme (21-hydroylase) involved in adrenal steroidogenesis. This results in decreased steroid hormone production and increased androgen hormone production. Masculinisation of the external genitalia results in clitoral hypertrophy and partial fusion of the labia. Other rather rare causes of female pseudo-hermaphroditism (non-CAH) include ingestion of androgenic agents during pregnancy.

Male pseudo-hermaphroditism (46, XY) is caused by genetic defects in the enzymatic synthesis of testosterone by the fetal testes resulting in inadequate virilisation of the male fetus.

Androgen insensitivity syndrome

Androgen insensitivity syndrome (46, XY) is an X-linked recessive disorder that occurs in 1/20,000 live births. The defect lies at the level of the androgen receptor. As a result of this defect, androgens produced by the testes are unable to induce the differentiation of male genital ducts and external genitalia. The testes can consequently fail to descend, remaining in the abdomen or inguinal canals. Malignancies may develop in these undescended testes which should therefore be removed after puberty.

The Müllerian system is suppressed due to the presence of testes, thus although the external genitalia is female, the vagina is usually a blind pouch with no uterus or fallopian tubes. At puberty, the secondary sexual characteristics develop in response to oestrogen but, as there is no uterus, menstruation does not occur. The upper two-thirds of the vagina do not develop, only the lower third. Clinically these patients appear to have normal female external genitalia, but with a short blind vagina.

Acknowledgement

We would like to thank Dr Meera Sunder and Dr S. Zhou for their help and support during the completion of this chapter.

References

Bourdelat D (1987) The cloaca, reelect and metaphors: cloacal thinking. *Sexologies*, VI (25): 16–23 (French language)

De Lancey JO (1992) Anatomical aspects of vaginal eversion after hysterectomy. *American Journal Obstetrics and Gynecology*, 166:1717–28

Gearhart JP, Jeffs RD (1998) Extrophy of the bladder, epispadias and other bladder anomalies. In: Walsh PC, Retik AB, Stamey TA, Darracott Vaughan E Jr (eds) *Campbell's Urology*, Vol. 2, 6e. Baltimore: WB Saunders

Moore KL, Persaud TVN (2003) *The Developing Human: Clinically Oriented Embryology*, 7e. Baltimore: WB Saunders

Sadler TW (2004) *Langman's Medical Embryology*, 9e. Lippincott, Williams and Wilkins

4 Anatomy and physiology of the urinary system, and some common problems

Caroline Sanders

Key points

- Bladder management and attainment of continence is a skill that the majority of children will be able to develop during toddler years.

- Failure to achieve continence during this time may indicate physiological problems in the lower urinary tract. It is important therefore that health professionals understand normal physiology.

- Psychological issues can also affect bladder control.

Health promotion point

- Children should be taught good voiding habits. Routine, ease of access and attention to hygiene are all important aspects of toilet training.

The urinary system comprises of two kidneys, which filter and excrete the waste products that accumulate as a consequence of cellular metabolism. The urine is subsequently drained from the kidneys via the ureters into the bladder where it is stored until it is periodically eliminated via the urethra.

Ureters

Two ureters lie behind the peritoneum and extend from the renal pelvis (pelvic ureteric junction – PUJ) to the posterior wall of the bladder. An incomplete collar of detrusor smooth muscle, separated from the

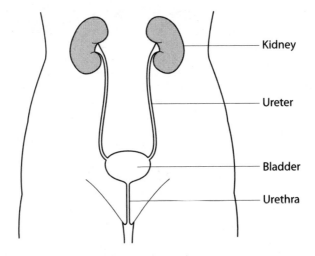

Figure 4.1 The bladder and urinary system in females

ureteric muscle coat by connective tissue, surrounds the distal end of each ureter. The ureters penetrate the posterior aspect of the bladder and run obliquely through its wall for a distance of 1.5–2.0 cm before ending at the ureteric orifices (Dixon and Gosling 1994). The length and diameter of the ureter(s) will change over time as the child grows,

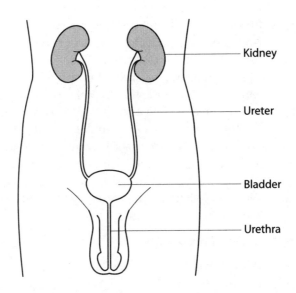

Figure 4.2 The bladder and urinary system in males

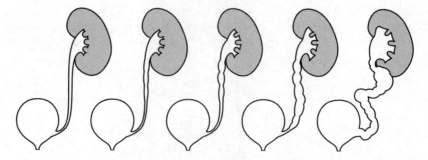

Figure 4.3 What happens in reflux

to an average of 30 cm (length) and 0.5 cm (width) in adulthood. The ureter is comprised of three layers:

- Mucosa (inside) – transitional epithelium;

- Muscularis - mostly inner longitudinal and outer circular layers of smooth muscle;

- Serosa – fibrous connective tissue.

Peristaltic contractions push the urine from the kidney through the ureters (vesico-ureteric junction – VUJ) into the bladder. The inner ureteric smooth muscle of the VUJ has a dual innervation by cholinergic (parasympathetic) and noradrenergic (sympathetic) nerves (Dixon and Gosling 1994). The ureters enter the bladder on the trigone, the length of the intramural and submucosal ureter results in a 'flap valve' mechanism, which prevents the urine from going back up the ureter. Insufficiency in ureter length entering the bladder results in a failure of the 'flap mechanism' and predisposes to vesico-ureteric reflux, or VUR (Thomas 2002). As the submucosal tunnel length increases with age and growth there is often a resolution of VUR. VUR is clinically significant in that it plays a role in urinary tract infection, which in turn can lead to ill health, failure to thrive, renal scarring (reflux neuropathy) and possibly dysfunctional voiding coupled with continence problems in childhood. In the longer term, renal scarring can lead to hypertension, complications in pregnancy and end-stage renal failure.

Abnormalities of the ureters

Hydronephrosis is a descriptive term for the dilatation noted in the renal pelvis and calyces. If the ureter is also dilated this is termed *hydroureteronephrosis*. Dilatation could be secondary to obstruction at the pelvic-ureteric junction, where the kidney joins the ureter (PUJ) or the vesico-ureteric junction, where the ureter enters the bladder (VUJ) or due to stones somewhere in the collecting system. Dilatation could also be secondary to dysplastic kidney or to another developmental abnormality in the kidney such as duplex kidney or horseshoe kidney. Ureteric dilatation (*megaureter*) can be obstructed, non-obstructed, non-refluxing or refluxing.

Complete duplication of a ureter can occur in embryonic life. There are varying degrees of duplication such that only the renal pelvis and upper ureter are involved or a complete duplication may exist with both ureters opening into the bladder (duplex) or other area either inside or outside of the bladder (ectopic).

An ureterocele is a cystic dilatation of the distal ureter at its insertion (normal or ectopic) into the bladder (Cullinane 1997). It appears as a thin-walled, often translucent structure, in either a single collecting system or the ureter to the upper pole of a duplex system. The ureterocele that is entirely contained within the bladder is often small and associated with a single collecting system. However, an ectopic ureterocele can be bigger and extend into the bladder neck or urethra. It can be distressing for a parent to see the ureterocele when changing a nappy. It may also be difficult for them to convince others due to the possible intermittent nature of urethral presentation. Ureteroceles are not inevitably obstructive.

The bladder

The bladder is a hollow, oval-shaped, muscular organ that sits in the abdominal cavity in infants and young children. This can make palpation of a full bladder easier than in adults and furthermore facilitates the suprapubic aspiration of urine (Yeung 2001). Both alpha-receptors (receptors associated with the stimulation and contraction of smooth muscle) and beta-receptors (receptors associated with the inhibition and relaxation of smooth muscle) are located in the bladder. The bladder has been described as a unique organ in that it has a double function, in the storage and co-ordinated emptying of urine (Yeung 2001). When the bladder is fully distended it is spherical in shape but when partly full it approximates to a more cuboid outline (Patel and Rickards 2005). Also, with full distension, the normal bladder neck may be seen as a slightly open funnel at the base of the bladder.

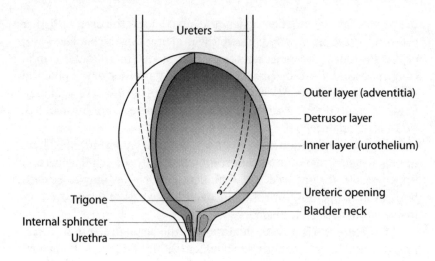

Figure 4.4 The bladder

The bladder has been described as being made up of three different layers; firstly, an inner layer, the bladder mucosa, which is transitional epithelium (urothelium). This urothelium lines the inner part of the muscle layer and is continuous with the urothelium of the ureters and urethra. The bladder mucosa is made up of folds called *rugae*, which allows it to stretch as it fills with urine. The inner surface is smooth on full distension, but corrugated when not distended except around the trigone. Mucus protects the bladder from the urine with the submucosal layer having both a nerve and blood supply.

The middle layer is the detrusor, which is characterised as a meshwork of smooth muscle bundles arranged to make it possible to act as a singular functioning unit (Yeung 2001). This meshwork of the detrusor consists of smooth muscle fibres layered in many directions (outer longitudinal, middle circular, inner longitudinal), which serve to aid its contractility. It is the ability of this muscle to repeatedly stretch, fill with urine from the kidneys and subsequently store urine at low pressure, which maintains the safety of the urinary system. When the bladder behaves in this way it can be described as *bladder stability*.

The trigone is an area in the floor of the bladder; the two posterior corners contain the ureteric openings and the anterior corner the internal urethral orifice. The superficial trigone muscle is a sensitive area of the bladder with relatively few cholinergic (parasympathetic) nerves yet many noradrenergic (sympathetic) nerves. The interior surface of the trigone is smooth as it is a fixed structure.

Fibres of the detrusor muscle fuse and surround the opening to the urethra, forming an internal urethral sphincter (alpha-receptors are located in this bladder neck area). In males the internal urethral sphincter encircles the upper prostatic urethra. Also in males the prostate gland lies between the bladder neck and the external urethral sphincter, with the seminal vesicles and rectum as the posterior structures, the rectovesical pouch lies between (Patel and Rickards 2005). In females the external urethral sphincter of striated muscle is described as thickest in the middle third of the urethra and it lies just below the bladder neck with the uterus posteriorly (the space between being the pouch of Douglas or the rectovesical pouch) (Dixon and Gosling 1994).

The outer lining (adventitia) of the bladder is serosa, fibrous connective tissue, with the superior surface of the bladder covered by the peritoneum.

The smooth muscle fibres from the bladder base and trigone travel through the bladder neck area and extend towards the proximal urethra. At micturition, the bladder base, neck and proximal urethra all contract at the same time, resulting in a widening of the bladder neck. At the same time this happens the levator ani muscles of the pelvic floor relax and there is a funnelling effect, which opens the bladder outlet and initiates voiding (Yeung 2001; McLaren 1996).

Abnormalities of the bladder

These can be congenital, such as bladder exstrophy in which there is an embryonic failure of closure of the lower anterior abdominal wall resulting in the bladder being exposed at birth (see also Chapter 4 by Mark Slack and Christina Ding). An unstable bladder or hyper-reflexic bladder can be secondary to neuropathic problems, damage to the nerves that supply the bladder. A neuropathic bladder can also be due to a birth defect such as spina bifida or spinal cord injury or acquired post-viral infection, i.e. transverse myelitis.

Over-activity of the bladder can be idiopathic in nature or secondary to urinary tract infection or dysfunctional voiding (Rigby 2003). Symptoms can include frequency, nocturia, urgency and incontinence. Incontinence can have detrimental effects on the child and family (DH 2004).

Stones can also be present in the bladder, either from travelling down the system or formation in the bladder.

The urethra in boys

The urethra extends from the neck of the bladder to the external urethral opening and is the passage for eliminating urine and ejaculation
of semen. It consists of two layers, inner mucous membrane (stratified
squamous epithelium) and outer sub-mucous tissue surrounded by the
external sphincter, which comprises of striated muscle. The length of
the urethra will change with age; it passes through the prostate, prostatic glands and ejaculatory duct area. The urethra can be differenti-
ated into areas, the prostatic, membranous, bulbar and spongy or
penile area. The external sphincter is in the membranous region.

Abnormalities of the urethra (boys)

Posterior urethral valves (PUV) cause outflow obstruction and can
cause long-term damage to upper renal tracts. A PUV consists of 'an
obliquely orientated membrane with a small eccentric aperture,
which arises from the verumontanum, extends through the zone of
the external sphincter and attaches anteriorly to the urethral wall'
(Duffy 2002: 87).

   Hypospadias is a failure of the urethral folds to close resulting in the
external urethral orifice opening somewhere along the underside (ventral) of the penis (Sanders and Baird 2003). Epispadias is when the
urethra open on the top (dorsal) aspect of the penis (see Chapter 3 by
Mark Slack and Christina Chi Ding, page 53).

The urethra in girls

A girl's urethra consists of three layers, inner (mucosa), middle (a thin
layer of smooth muscle) and outer (a layer of serosa, which is a continuation of the bladder serosa). The smooth muscle of the female urethra is associated with few noradrenergic nerves but it is believed to
have a cholinergic parasympathetic nerve supply identical to the
detrusor. It is suggested that competence of the female bladder neck
and proximal urethra is not solely due to smooth muscle activity in the
absence of a separate anatomical sphincter. The innervation and longitudinal orientation of most of the muscle fibres suggest that urethral
smooth muscle in the female is active during micturition, serving to
shorten and widen the urethral lumen.

   The external urethral orifice is located between the clitoris and vaginal opening. The female urethra runs down and along the anterior wall of the vagina. The space between the bladder and the uterus or anterior wall of the vagina, that is not enclosed in the peritoneum, is referred to as the pouch of Douglas.

Abnormalities of the urethra (girls)

Urogenital conditions exist which are secondary to embryonic failure, such as a persistent cloaca resulting in a common openings for urine, stool and vagina (see Chapter 3 by Mark Slack and Christina Chi Ding, page 47). A urogenital sinus may exist where the urethra opens in to the vagina, this can be of a low or high confluence. Some girls can experience vaginal pooling of urine, which can lead to episodes of incontinence as the urine dribbles out once voiding is finished (Mattsson and Gladh 2003).

The pelvic floor

The pelvic floor in females is described as consisting of two specific components, the levator ani and the coccygeus (Dixon and Gosling 1994). The coccygeus forms a triangular structure the top of which attaches to the spine of the ischium and is the musclotendinous internal surface of the sacrospinous ligament and does not contribute to active movement in the pelvic floor (Dixon and Gosling 1994). The levator ani forms the effective contractile structure in the pelvic floor and assists in maintaining continence and producing a forceful occlusion of the urethra such as during coughing).

Storage of urine

In the urethra

A tension is exerted along the urethra by the smooth muscle and within the striated muscle around the urethral wall. This compresses the inner urethral connective and vascular tissues making a water-tight seal, which aids continence. The resting intra-urethral pressure has been suggested as 50–100 cm H_2O (Mundy and Thomas 1994). The sphincter-active urethra is supported by the muscles and ligaments of the pelvic floor. The musculature of the anterior pelvic floor when contracted can elevate, lengthen and compress the urethra, which contributes to continence. The bladder neck mechanism that has no demonstrable sphincter relies on the integrity of normal detrusor function. If the detrusor muscle does not contract, the bladder neck remains closed irrespective of any rise in bladder pressure (such as coughing). Only when the detrusor contracts does the bladder neck open (Mundy and Thomas 1994).

In the bladder

The bladder is able to hold increasing volumes of urine without a corresponding rise in intravesical pressure due to the elasticity of its musculature. The ratio of change in intravesical volume to the change in intravesical pressure is called compliance. Any process that alters the elasticity can alter the compliance of the bladder. The bladder normally fills at a rate of about 1 ml per minute from each ureter, but this can be increased with kidney disease or increased fluids or pharmacology. Initially there is no sensation of the bladder filling; as the filling progresses this sensation becomes more apparent and voiding normally takes place. If the bladder is allowed to continue to fill and desires to void ignored then a sensation of lower abdominal distention occurs.

Box 4.1 Abnormal bladder symptoms

Abnormal bladder symptoms associated with storage difficulties can present as:

- Increased daytime frequency;
- Nocturia;
- Urgency;
- Incontinence;
- Abnormal bladder sensation.

Post-voiding symptoms include:

- Incomplete emptying;
- Post-micturition dribbling;
- Vaginal pooling.

If filling continues the child suddenly feels that voiding is imminent. This sensation is thought to originate in the urethra or peri-urethral striated muscles (Mundy and Thomas 1994).

Innervation and neuro-transmitters and voiding

The activation and co-ordination of the bladder and sphincter region are controlled through three sets of peripheral nerves. These are:

- The sacral parasympathetic nerves;

- The sympathetic nerves;

- The somatic motor and sensory nerves.

The sacral parasympathetic nerves

These nerves supply via the pelvic nerve, which comprises of sensory (*afferent* – nerves that carry impulses towards the central nervous system) and motor (*efferent* – nerves that carry impulses away from the central nervous system) fibres. The sensory fibres supply the detrusor and the bladder neck area and as the bladder stretches signals are sent to the sacral segment of the spinal cord (S_2–S_4). From here they are transmitted in the ascending ventral columns of the cord to the higher centres of the brain. Therefore when these nerves are stimulated during micturition, they bring about the contraction of the detrusor muscle and the funnelling effect of the bladder that initiates voiding. Acetylcholine is the chemical transmitter that relays the signal from the parasympathetic nerve fibres to the smooth muscle of the detrusor (facilitating contraction during the voiding phase). During the filling phase the cholinergic receptors should be blocked allowing the detrusor to relax and allow it to fill with urine. Other drugs can interfere with the reception of acetylcholine (for example, atropine used in anaesthesia). This can cause a temporary failure in the message system and the detrusor does not contract, leading to retention of urine.

The sympathetic nerves

Sympathetic nerves also consist of motor and sensory fibres, originating in a different region of the spinal column (T_1–L_2). It is thought that these nerves influence the inhibition cycle in the bladder. It is thought sensory nerve fibres relay impulses in response to painful stimuli (over-distension, spasm, inflammation, stones). The chemical transmitter is noradrenaline.

The somatic motor and sensory nerves

Somatic motor and sensory nerves supply the wall of the urethra and the pelvic floor (levator ani), primarily from S_3 (but also to some degree S_4 and S_2) becoming the pudendal nerve. The pudendal nerve is mixed carrying both motor and sensory fibres and is derived from the sacral plexus.

Micturition and bladder control

Bladder control is dependent on physical and cognitive maturation and is actively learnt. Often rewarding incentive behaviour helps the child develop the ability to voluntarily inhibit and delay voiding.

At a physiological level, control of micturition requires three key areas to develop:

- The bladder has to have grown, such that there is an ongoing increase in the functional storage capacity of the bladder. Formulae have been developed to estimate the average bladder capacity of a child at different ages (see below, Yeung 2001).

- Maturation in control over urethral sphincter muscle. This is dependent upon the development and co-ordinated activity of parasympathetic, sympathetic and somatic nerves.

- Development and mastery of control over the bladder and sphincter in unison, therefore allowing the child to voluntarily initiate or inhibit micturition. Furthermore the ability to control this reflex will be dependent upon intact receptors and chemicals (neurotransmitters) and a complete neuro/sensory pathway between the bladder, spinal cord and brain. Higher brain centres in the cerebral, basal ganglia, and reticular formation control micturition. Reflex control of micturition is to be found S_2–S_4. The reflex control in the spinal cord connects the nerves, which descend from and ascend to the higher centres, and also the parasympathetic and somatic nerves, which supply the bladder (McLaren 1996).

Voiding

Voiding pattern changes during the neonatal period from an infrequency immediately after birth for the first few days to a rapid increase after the first week of life. This peaks at about once an hour somewhere between 2–4 weeks after delivery. At about 6 months the frequency has levelled at approximately 10–15 times per day (Yeung 2001). Over the next 2–3 years there is a continual decrease in voiding frequency coupled with an increase in volume voided and development of a non-interrupted flow. In both male and female infants there is a formula suggested by Holmdahl and colleagues (1996), which is commonly used [bladder capacity (ml) = 38 + (2.5 × age in months)] or weight (kg) × 7 (Fairhurst *et al.* 1991). Other formulae exist for older children: [bladder capacity (ml) = age × 30] + 30 (Hjalmas 1976; Koff 1983), or for children up to 12 years [age (years) × 30] + 50 (Rickwood 1994).

Initially, voiding causes a momentary fall in the urethral pressure. Then, at a sustained rise above a certain level in intravesical pressure, the bladder neck opens and voiding begins (Mundy and Thomas 1994). When voiding is complete the distal sphincteric mechanism closes up towards the bladder neck and the cycle starts again.

Problems with voiding present as:

- Slow stream;

- Hesitancy;

- Insufficiency frequency.

Furthermore, voiding difficulties can be witnessed as holding manoeuvres and reluctance to use the toilet. Factors that contribute towards voiding difficulties include poor fluid intake, constipation and dysuria (Shaikh 2004).

Good voiding habits

Training
Development of bladder control is often described as a process that occurs in stages, usually when the child is between the ages of 2–3 years. Toilet training should not be undertaken too early, with guidelines suggesting training from 27 months of age (Blum *et al.* 2004). Daytime control is usually mastered first, followed by night control.

Parents will often seek a range of healthcare advice if successful toilet training is delayed. Being incontinent or late to attain continence can be stressful both for children themselves and for their parents (DH 2004). It can also lead to issues of social exclusion, for example if children are unable to participate in pre-school groups. A fully toilet-trained child has the ability to inhibit and restart urine flow, to relax the external sphincter and void on demand (Berry 2005; Jansson *et al.* 2005). Regularly asking children to void when they do not need to empty their bladder can encourage the development of dysfunctional voiding, so should be avoided. Pain associated with toileting (urine or stool) can cause a regression in toilet training, and this too can lead to the development of dysfunctional voiding habits (Berry 2005).

Access

Good toileting routine should be fostered in children by their parents' or carers and access to clean, safe, well-lit toilets is made available (Lundblad and Hellstrom 2005). Toilet paper and good hand washing facilities should be available and children should be encouraged to develop good levels of hand hygiene after using the toilet. Some public toilets are of a poor hygienic standard and no toilet paper is available, therefore parents can be encouraged to take wipes to clean the facilities and ensure their child has toilet paper. Children should be given time to void in a relaxed manner on average between 5–8 times per day, depending on fluid intake (Bloom *et al.* 1993). Good positioning on the toilet can be important; when small children are progressing from a potty to a toilet they should have adequate support for seating and also to support their feet if they are sitting to void. Crouching to void has been suggested in women's studies as a voiding technique that encourages a reduction in functional bladder capacity (Moore *et al.* 1991).

Good routine and hygiene

Children should be discouraged from holding on to urine when they have a desire to void as this may increase their chance of developing urinary tract infections or episodes of incontinence (Bakker *et al.* 2002). Also children should not be forced to void when they are not ready, by pushing out their urine or running taps to encourage them to void as this behaviour has the potential to cause lasting voiding problems for the child (Bakker *et al.* 2002). Girls should be taught how to wipe from front to back in order to reduce the likelihood of ascending urinary tract infection. Boys should be taught how to clean their foreskin properly. Good hygiene of the perineum will help minimise ascending infections, therefore management of soiling is important (Berry 2005). Children should be encouraged to change wet underwear promptly, in a supportive and uncritical environment. Sitting in wet or damp underwear can lead to excoriated skin, as well as urinary tract infection which. in turn, can cause dysfunctional voiding.

Good fluid intake is important to maximise the efficiency of the lower urinary system, minimise bacturia and maximise bladder capacity. Some fluids can irritate the bladder; these include caffeine-based drinks, as they can act as both and irritant and stimulant to increase the filling phase of the bladder.

References

Bakker E, Van Gool JD, Van Sprundel M, Van der Anwera C, Wyndaele JJ (2002) Results of a questionnaire evaluating the effects of different methods of toilet training on achieving bladder control. *British Journal of Urology International* 90(4): 456–61

Berry A (2005) Helping children with dysfunctional voiding. *Urologic Nursing,* 25(3): 193–200

Bloom DA (1993) Toilet habits and continence in children: an opportunity sampling in search of normal parameters. *Journal of Urology,* 149(5): 1087–90

Blum NJ, Taubman B, Nemth N (2004) Why is toilet training occurring at older ages? A study of factors associated with later training. *Journal of Pediatrics,* 145(1): 107–11

Cullinane C (1997) Pathology of the kidney and urinary tract in infancy. In Thomas DFM (ed.) *Urological Disease in the Fetus and Infant Diagnosis and Management.* Oxford: Butterworth-Heinemann

Department of Health (2004) National Service Framework for Children and Young People. London: The Stationery Office

Dixon JS, Gosling JA (1994) The anatomy of the bladder, urethra and pelvic floor. In Mundy AR, Stephenson TP, Wein AJ (eds) *Urodynamics: Principles, practice and application.* London, Edinburgh: Churchill Livingstone

Duffy PG (2002) Posterior urethral valves and other urethral abnormalities: In Thomas DFM, Rickwood AMK, Duffy PG (eds) *Essentials of Paediatric Urology.* London: Martin Dunitz

Fairhurst JJ, Rubin CME, Hyde I, Freeman N, Williams JD (1991) Bladder capacity in infants. *Journal of Pediatric Surgery,* 26 55–7

Hjalmas K (1976) Micturition in infants and children with normal lower urinary tract: A urodynamic study. *Scandinavian Journal of Urology and Nephrology,* 37: 9–17

Holmdahl G, Hanson E, Hanson M, Hellstrom A-L, Hjälmas K, Sillen U (1996) Four-hour voiding observation in healthy infants. *Journal of Urology,* 156: 1809–12

Jansson UB, Hanson M, Sillen U, Hellstrom AL (2005) Voiding pattern and aquistion of bladder control from birth to age 6 years – a longitudinal study. *Journal of Urology*, 174(1): 289–93

Koff SA (1983) Estimating bladder capacity in children. *Urology*, 21: 248

Lundblad B, Hellstrom AL (2005) Perceptions of school toilets as a cause for irregular toilet habits among schoolchildren aged 6 to 16 years. *Journal of School Health*, 75(4): 25–8

Mattsson S, Gladh G (2003) Urethrovaginal reflux – a common cause of daytime incontinence in girls. *Pediatrics*, 111(1): 136–9

McLaren SM (1996) Renal function. In: Hinchliff SM, Montague SE, Watson R (eds) *Physiology for Nursing Practice*, 2e. London: Baillière Tindall

Moore KH, Richmond DH, Sutherst JR, Imrie AH, Hutton JL (1991) Crouching over the toilet seat: prevalence among British gynaecological outpatients and its effect upon micturition. *British Journal of Obstetrics and Gynaecology*, 98(6): 569–72

Mundy AR, Thomas PJ (1994) Clinical physiology of the bladder, urethra and pelvic floor. In: Mundy AR, Stephenson TP, Wein AJ (eds) *Urodynamics: principles, practice and application*. London, Edinburgh: Churchill Livingstone

Patel U, Rickards D (2005) *Imaging and Urodynamics of the Lower Urinary Tract*. Oxford: Taylor & Francis

Rickwood AMK (1994) Neuropathic bladder in childhood. In: Mundy AR, Stephenson TP, Wein AJ (eds) *Urodynamics: principles, practice and application*. London, Edinburgh: Churchill Livingstone

Rigby D (2003) The overactive bladder. *Nursing Standard*, 11(39): 45–52

Sanders CD, Baird AD (2003) Current practice in hypospadias repair. *Current Opinions in Urology*, 9(3): 61–7

Shaikh N (2004) Time to get on the potty: are constipation and stool toileting refusal causing delayed toilet training? *Journal of Pediatrics*, 145(1): 12–13

Thomas DFM (2002) Vesicoureteric reflux. In Thomas DFM, Rickwood AMK, Duffy PG (eds) *Essentials of Paediatric Urology*. London: Martin Dunitz

Yeung CK (2001) Pathophysiology of bladder dysfunction. In: Gearhart JP, Rink RC, Mouriquand PDE (eds) *Pediatric Urology*. London: WB Saunders

Anorectal anatomy and physiology

Anton Emmanuel

Key points

- An understanding of the physiology of the normal colon is necessary to understand normal defecation and faecal incontinence;

- Normal defecation depends on an interplay between motor and sensory function in the gut and pelvic musculature;

- Maintenance of continence depends on the balance between rectal contraction pressure and anal sphincter resisting pressure;

- Patients whose sensation is reduced due to illness, injury or other cause will find it hard to recognise the body's cues for the need to defecate, potentially leading to evacuation difficulties or faecal incontinence.

Health promotion point

- Teaching children and adults how best to position themselves on the toilet, and how to perform the Valsalva manoeuvre, will help them to defecate more easily.

The colon

The colon is a hollow muscular tube with an internal mucosal lining. The twin functions of the colon can broadly be summarised as being to propel intestinal content distally, at the same time as reabsorbing liquid from that content. The anal sphincter is a relatively simple structure that performs an extraordinarily complex function. Not only do the anal sphincters regulate faecal continence, but also they are increasingly recognised as controlling defecation. As such, the colon is involved in presenting the rectum with a faecal bolus derived from ingested food and gastrointestinal secretions, while the rectum is involved with controlling the emptying of that content from the rectum. Knowledge of the interplay between the anal sphincter, rectum and pelvic floor is required for understanding of the physiology of defecation and continence. The motor component of the mechanism involves both involuntary and voluntary muscle, and the sensory component is modulated by pelvic nerves which also have a somatic (voluntary nerve) function. This highlights a key concept of this chapter: there is an interplay between motor and sensory function, mediated through pelvic muscle and pelvic nerves.

Throughout this chapter, the pathophysiology of anorectal function in the spinally injured patient will be highlighted. This is because an understanding of the changes in the spinal patient helps shed light on 'normal' physiology, and also because such patients have a large burden of symptoms with regard to continence and bowel function.

Colonic motility

The colon comprises two layers of muscle underlying the colonic mucosa, namely the inner circular and outer longitudinal layers. Co-ordination of contraction of these muscles occurs through the local 'enteric' nervous system. Contraction of the circular muscle results primarily in mixing ('ring contractions') of faecal matter, while contraction of the longitudinal muscle ('sleeve contractions') results in propagated peristaltic movement of that faecal matter. The right side of the colon primarily serves a reservoir and mixing function, helping to make the faecal content more solid by allowing time for water re-absorption (Ambroze *et al*, 1993). In the transverse and descending colon, contractions are mostly peristaltic in the form of episodic 'mass movements'. This activity delivers the relatively solid faecal matter into the rectum and sigmoid colon which act as a further reservoir. When there is filling of the rectum and sigmoid to a critical level, the urge to defecate is initiated.

Anatomy

The rectum

The two layers of colonic muscle are smooth muscle structures and receive no external somatic (voluntary) nerve input. Hence, the muscle of the rectum is not under voluntary control. Rather the nerve supply to the rectum is from extrinsic autonomic nerves which act upon the intrinsic ('enteric') nerves at submucosal plexuses. The combined effect of these nerves is to allow the rectal muscle to relax and gradually accommodate increasing content as faecal material enters the rectal ampulla. This phenomenon is known as rectal compliance and is dependent upon the function of rectal muscle and its nerve supply. It is known to be mediated at spinal level since, in spinally injured patients, rectal compliance is normal. This is in contrast to the loss of bladder tone that is seen in patients with a chronic spinal injury.

Traditionally anorectal pressures are expressed in centimetres of water (cm H_2O); 1 cm H_2O is approximately equal to 0.75 mm mercury (Hg). Resting pressure in the rectum is low, between 5 and 20 cm H_2O. To put this in context, this pressure is similar to that seen in the venous system. Rectal pressure does not increase appreciably with increasing rectal content – this phenomenon is termed 'compliance' and is important in that it means that each increase in rectal content is *not* associated with an increase in rectal pressure and hence urge to defecate. If there is poor rectal compliance there are frequent urges to defecate, and this loss of compliance explains some of the increased bowel frequency seen in patients with radiotherapy-induced damage to the rectum and in ulcerative colitis or Crohn's disease.

The internal anal sphincter

The inner layer of rectal smooth muscle, namely the circular muscle layer, becomes about three times thicker at the distal end of the rectum. This condensation of muscle is the internal anal sphincter. It is approximately 3 cm long and 3 mm wide, being slightly longer in men and getting thicker with age. It does not extend downwards as far as the skin of the anal verge, ending some 10 mm above it. Like all smooth muscle sphincters, the internal anal sphincter is able to maintain tonic contraction for long periods of time.

The internal sphincter has an intrinsic, sinusoidal 'slow wave' activity with a frequency of 20–40 cycles per minute. The continuous activity of the sphincter is primarily responsible for the resting tone of the anus. The internal sphincter contributes about 85% of the resting anal sphincter pressure, which is measured at between 60–110 cm H_2O in health. Weakness or disruption of the internal anal sphincter results in the passive leakage of faecal contents and incontinence of flatus. The resting tone is greatest in the lower internal sphincter, and the importance of this in anorectal 'sampling' is discussed below.

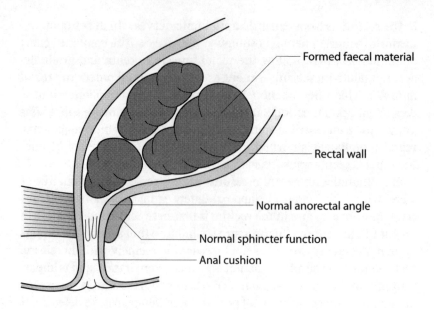

- Formed faecal material
- Rectal wall
- Normal anorectal angle
- Normal sphincter function
- Anal cushion

Figure 5.1 A diagrammatic representation of the structures involved in the mechanisms of defecation and continence

Distension of the rectum results in a reflex relaxation of the internal anal sphincter (the recto-anal inhibitory reflex). This reflex is mediated at spinal level. The extent of the relaxation depends on the degree of distension – with large volume rectal distension the internal sphincter relaxation can be prolonged, and with slight distension only partial sphincter relaxation occurs (see the section on anorectal sampling below).

The external anal sphincter

The external anal sphincter is a striated muscle and as such is under voluntary control, its nerve supply being provided by the pudendal nerve. It surrounds the internal anal sphincter and extends down to the skin at the anal verge. Also, unlike the internal sphincter, it is a fatigable muscle. The external anal sphincter is composed of both tonically contracting 'slow twitch' fibres and phasically contracting 'fast twitch' fibres.

The external sphincter contributes a small part (about 15%) towards resting anal tone. Rather, it is primarily responsible for the voluntary contraction of the sphincter. Pressures of between 60 and

250 cm H_2O (well above systolic blood pressure!) are generated during a voluntary anal squeeze in normal subjects.

Rectal distension results initially in a progressive increase in external anal sphincter activity, which temporally precedes the relaxation of the internal sphincter. However when distension is increased (usually above 200 ml) the external sphincter activity then disappears, resulting in loss of pressure in both anal internal and external sphincters. This too is a reflex mediated at spinal level, being present in spinally injured patients.

There is one further important aspect of external sphincter contraction to consider. When traction is applied to the external sphincter (by pulling gently but firmly away from the anus with a gloved finger at the anal verge) there is an initial increase in contraction which is then exaggerated when the traction is released. This is termed the 'closing reflex' and is the basis on which the anal sphincter snaps shut at the end of rectal evacuation. In patients with spinal injury, traction results in external sphincter relaxation, and this is the basis of some spinal patients employing digital anal stimulation to achieve evacuation. The difference in this reflex in spinal patients illustrates that there is a descending cortical influence upon it.

Reflex anal dilatation was at one time thought to be caused by child abuse, and in the 1980s was put forward as a method of identifying abused children. Although this theory has been discredited, it did lead to the Cleveland scandal in 1987, in which 121 children were diagnosed as abused and removed from their families. Ninety-six of these charges were found to have no basis at appeal (Pragnall 2002).

The pelvic diaphragm (pelvic floor)

This is a striated muscular layer, with a central ligamentous structure, that surrounds the rectum, vagina and urethra. The pelvic diaphragm is composed of a number of muscles, all of which can be considered as acting in concert. The puborectalis muscle component of the diaphragm, in particular, contributes to maintenance of the anorectal angle which is held to be important in preserving continence. Although there are known to be certain changes in the pelvic diaphragm during straining in the laboratory setting, the correlation with events during normal defecation is uncertain. However, it seems clear that the whole pelvic diaphragm mechanism works in tandem with the external anal sphincter during defecation.

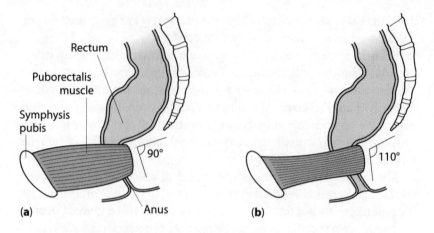

Figure 5.2 The pelvic floor (**a**) at rest and (**b**) during defecation. In the resting state, the puborectalis muscle, and the remainder of the pelvic diaphragm, are at an angle to the rectum which maintains continence. During defecation, the puborectalis muscle relaxes and this angle straightens out, opening up the rectum to allow passage of faeces

Physiology

Nerve supply of the rectum and anus

The rectum and internal anal sphincter receive an extrinsic autonomic innervation from lumbar (sympathetic) and sacral (parasympathetic) nerve roots. This innervation conveys information in each direction between the hindgut (lower bowel) and the brain. There is also a dense network of 'local' enteric neurones in the gut wall which mediate the fine processing of information from brain to rectum and anus. This enteric nervous system (ENS) comprises a dense network of neurones connected to each other by a series of plexuses within the gut wall. The ENS is second only to the central nervous system in complexity and quantity of nerve tissue. The ENS is the only region of the peripheral nervous system that is capable of mediating reflex activity without input from the central nervous system (CNS). Peristalsis is the result of descending influences from the CNS integrated with local reflexes elicited within the gut wall by luminal content.

The motor supply to the striated (voluntary) muscle of the external anal sphincter is from the second to fourth sacral spinal cord segments via the pudendal nerves. The spinal nuclei for this nerve output are directly influenced by descending input from the higher centres in the brain.

Sensory information from the ano-rectum travels in afferent fibres of the pudendal nerve and is handled in two ways – firstly it is relayed to the central nervous system by these extrinsic autonomic nerves and secondly it initiates local reflex arcs. The combination of these two systems results in the potential for both conscious and subconscious processing of gut feelings. This can be demonstrated by balloon distension of the rectum. Initially balloon distension in the rectum activates mucosal receptors resulting in patients' first perception of rectal sensation ('threshold sensation'). Further distension then stimulates the mechano-receptors (stretch receptors) in the muscular layer of the mucosa resulting in the sensation of need to defecate ('urge sensation'), and distension beyond that point results in activation of serosal mechano-receptors and nociceptors (pain receptors) ('maximum tolerable volume').

Rectal compliance

The normal rectum is capable of accommodating increases in volume with only minor alterations of pressure. This phenomenon of compliance is most pronounced at lower volumes of rectal filling. As the maximum tolerable volume is approached, even small increments in volume are accompanied by changes in rectal pressure. Thus sensory perception of anorectal activity depends on both luminal content and also the state of contractility, or compliance, of the rectum. In conditions where the rectum is inflamed (inflammatory bowel disease, infection, radiation proctitis) there is reduced compliance (namely a stiffer, more contractile rectum) and an associated increase in sensitivity.

For more information about rectal problems and constipation, see Chapter 8 by Kenneth Wilkinson.

Anorectal sampling

It is known that a local anaesthetic, lidocaine, when applied to the anal canal results in a reduced ability to maintain external anal sphincter contraction. This is evidence of the close link between anorectal sensation and motor function in the maintenance of continence. This association between sensation and motor function is characterised by the phenomenon of anorectal sampling. With progressive rectal filling

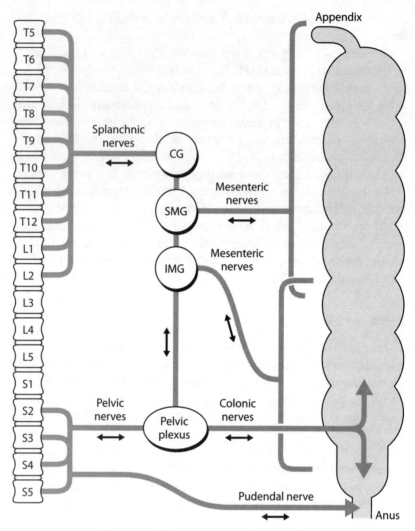

Figure 5.3 Nerve pathways to the colon

reflex relaxation of the upper internal anal sphincter occurs. This happens every eight to ten minutes as rectal contents are presented to the anal sensory mucosa. Since the lower internal sphincter exhibits higher resting pressure, incontinence does not occur. In fact the slow wave activity in the lower part of the sphincter complex, coupled with contraction of the external anal sphincter and puborectalis results in the contents being returned back to the rectum. Each of these episodes lasts less than 10 seconds. The importance of this anal 'sampling' is that it allows the sensory epithelium of the anal canal the opportunity to distinguish solids from liquids from gas, important in the maintenance of perfect continence.

The physiology and pathophysiology of defecation and continence

The dynamics of continence

Normal stool output per day is of the order of 200 gm. The proximal (upper) colon defines the consistency and volume of delivery of contents to the rectum. The rectum has a reservoir function to accommodate this content until such time as defecation is socially and practically appropriate. As rectal filling gradually proceeds, anorectal sampling occurs allowing subconscious perception of the consistency of the content. An intact anal sphincter, especially in the lower part, ensures continence; in situations where this has been damaged (typically iatrogenically after anal dilatation or lateral sphincterotomy) passive loss of anal contents may occur.

Anorectal sensation of the build up of rectal contents is relayed centrally by autonomic nerves. These afferents result in both conscious perception and activation of local reflexes such as the recto-anal inhibitory reflex to begin relaxation of the internal anal sphincter. In health, reflex voluntary external sphincter contraction then maintains continence until voluntary defecation is possible. By contrast, spinally injured patients who are unable to contract their external anal sphincter experience incontinence when the internal sphincter relaxes. A similar but reflex activation of the external sphincter to maintain continence occurs when there is a rise in abdominal pressure, for example with coughing. Partial external sphincter contraction is also observed during passage of flatus, and coupled with intact anorectal sensation this is the mechanism by which faecal continence during passage of gas is maintained. The voluntary passage of flatus depends on reflex relaxation of the internal anal sphincter and partial voluntary relaxation of the external anal sphincter.

Patients who have either loss of sensation or impaired perception (for example in diabetes, following stroke, or with a rectal prolapse) may become incontinent due to the loss of recognition of 'normal' anorectal sensation and its relationship to continence. Thus the preservation of continence depends on the normal functioning of anorectal sensation, the appropriate perception of that sensory information, the integrity of local and higher reflex arcs, and the action of the internal and external anal sphincters.

The dynamics of defecation

Defecation commences with rectal sensory awareness of a critical level of filling which is relayed to the cerebral cortex as the perception of the need to evacuate the rectum. The actual volume depends on the nature of the contents (volume, consistency) and the rectum (mucosal inflammation, rectal wall compliance). When the subject is in a socially appropriate context for defecation, the person adopts a sitting, or squatting, position. The latter position results in straightening of the rectal angle and allows more effective propulsion of contents. The external sphincter and puborectalis relax. The rectal contents provoke reflex relaxation of the internal anal sphincter and the subject then performs a Valsalva manoeuvre (holding the breath and forcibly trying to exhale against a closed glottis, creating a pushing down effect). Abdominal pressure is raised, and the muscles of the anterior abdominal wall tense up to funnel the pressure down to the pelvis. The relaxation of the pelvic floor then allows some stool to enter the lower rectum. This in turn tends to initiate a spontaneous giant recto-sigmoid contraction, which pushes stool through the relaxed anal canal. Further large propulsive contractions of the rectum occur until the rectum is empty. A sensory input from the anus maintains this propulsive activity until the rectum is fully voided. This seems to be a reflex mediated at spinal cord level since even spinally injured patients can void a complete stool from the rectum, once the process has been initiated. Such patients tend to use digital rectal stimulation to initiate the propulsive contractions of the recto-sigmoid. As the stool passes through the anal canal, it stretches the external anal sphincter creating a traction force upon it. After the last bolus of stool is passed, the 'closing reflex' of the external sphincter is stimulated by the release of traction. In this way anal continence is maintained after the act of defecation.

It can be seen that the mechanisms controlling continence and defecation are complex. This chapter has presented a basic overview of the subject, the emphasis being to highlight the synergy of structure to function in these complex processes.

References

Ambroze WL, Pemberton JH, Bell AM, Brown ML, Zinsmeister AR (1993) The
    effect of stool consistency on rectal and neorectal emptying. *Diseases of the
    Colon and Rectum*, 34:1–7
Christensen J (1987)Motility of the colon. In Johnson LR (ed.) *Physiology of the
    Gastrointestinal Tract*, 2e. New York: Raven Press
Dickinson VA (1978) Maintenance of anal continence: a review of pelvic floor
    physiology. *Gut*, 19: 1163–9
Duthie HL (1982) Defecation and the anal sphincter. *Clinical Gastroenterology*, 11:
    621–8
Longo WE, Ballantyne GH, Modlin IM (1989) The colon, anorectum and spinal
    cord patient: a review of the functional alterations of the denervated hindgut.
    Diseases of the Colon and Rectum, 32: 261–7
Miller R, Bartolo DCC, Cervero F, Mortensen NJM (1988) Anorectal sampling: a
    comparison of normal and incontinent patients. *British Journal of Surgery*, 75:
    44–7
Pragnell C (2002) The Cleveland child sexual abuse scandal: an abuse and misuse
    of medical power. Children Webmag, October 2002. Accessed on
    www.childrenuk.co.uk/choct2002
Read NW, Harford WV, Schmulen AC, Read MG, Santa Ana C, Fordtran JS (1979)
    A clinical study of patients with faecal incontinence and diarrhoea.
    Gastroenterology, 76: 747–51
Speakman CTM, Kamm MA (1991) The internal anal sphincter – new insights
    into faecal incontinence. *Gut*, 32: 345–53
Sun WM, Read NW, Miner PB (1990) Relationship between rectal sensation and
    anal function in normal subjects and patients with faecal incontinence. *Gut*,
    31: 1056–61
Swash M, Snooks SJ, Henry MM (1985) Unifying concept of pelvic floor disorders
    and incontinence. *Journal of the Royal Society of Medicine*,78: 906–13

6 Investigations for bladder problems
Rosie Kelly

Key points

- Detailed assessment is crucial as a first step in investigating bladder problems.

- More specific information can be gained from urine tests (see Chapter 10), radiological investigations and blood tests.

There are a number of different methods of investigating incontinence in children, and these are presented in this chapter. The primary aim of such investigations is to identify evidence of renal impairment requiring immediate treatment. Where there is no evidence of renal impairment, the secondary aim of such investigations is to establish the degree of incontinence and possible treatment modalities. Identification of the reasons for incontinence, and the various approaches to its treatment, are covered elsewhere in the book.

Invasive procedures should be avoided in children wherever possible. Where they are necessary, however, careful preparation is extremely important. Invasive procedures can be frightening and traumatic for children, especially if they have not been given explanatory information beforehand, pitched at a level they can understand. So patient education is important (see Chapter 3), and all procedures should then be carried out as efficiently as possible, by professionals who are experienced in working with children.

Assessment

A comprehensive assessment of the child is not only the starting point, it is also the most important step you will take in the process of identifying the cause of the child's incontinence. Many continence services have designed continence assessment forms, which are completed jointly by the health professional and patient (Ross 1994). Children should be assessed using an appropriate paediatric tool, to be completed by the health professional, child and parents.

Increasingly, the lead professional in this assessment process is a nurse who has received appropriate training, and is familiar with all the relevant issues (Kaschak Newman 1996).

The following components should be included as part of any paediatric continence assessment (Bankhead *et al.* 2000; Winder 2001; Royal College of Physicians 2003):

General

Patient details.

Composition of family.

Birth history:

- Traumatic delivery,
- Prematurity,
- Neonatal resuscitation.

Medical history:

- Congenital abnormalities.

Family medical history:

- Diabetes,
- Spina bifida,
- Childhood illnesses.

Developmental history:

- Walking – define mobility problems,
- Talking,
- Dressing – define manual dexterity problems,
- Understanding commands.

Medication.

Allergies.

Continence

- Daytime continence achieved   YES/NO
- Night-time continence achieved   YES/NO
- Fluid intake/24 hours
- Bowel habit.

Symptoms

Ask about the symptoms listed in Table 6.1. All answers should be recorded.

Table 6.1 Symptoms relating to childhood incontinence

Day	Night	Bowels
Urgency	Frequency per night/week	Frequency day/week
Frequency	Volume	Consistency – Bristol stool chart
Significant leakage	Time of last drink	Soiling – overflow encopresis
Constant dribbling	Time of last void	Diet
Giggle incontinence		Awareness of need to defecate
Infrequent voiding		
Vincent's curtsey*		

*Vincent's curtsey is a manoeuvre designed to counteract urinary leakage by crouching down and pressing the heel of one foot into the perineum (Fisher and Frank 2000:129; Rickwood 2002)

Social and psychological aspects

Enquire about the toilet facilities at home and at school. You will also need to include in your assessment psychological and quality of life issues including:

- Embarrassment;
- Fear;

- Isolation;

- Avoidance of social situations;

- Refusing to go to the toilet.

It is also important to ask about *sexual function* in older adolescents:

- Although the age at which adolescents become sexually active varies, it is not common practice in paediatric urology to ask for a sexual history in those under the age of 16, unless the physical examination warrants it.

You will also need to record details of any previous investigations and management, including the use of incontinence products.

Physical examination

The following all need to be checked:

- Height/weight;

- Blood pressure;

- Mid-stream urine specimen;

- Abdomen:

  □ inspect for normal contours and taut skin;

  □ palpate for faeces/mass/tenderness;

- Genitalia (NB: genital examination must be carried out by a trained practitioner only):

  □ penis/meatus/scrotum;

  □ labia majora/labia minora/urethral meatus/vaginal orifice;

- Neurology:

  □ asymmetrical buttocks;

  □ subcutaneous lipoma;

  □ abnormal hair growth over lower spine;

  □ reduced perineal sensation.

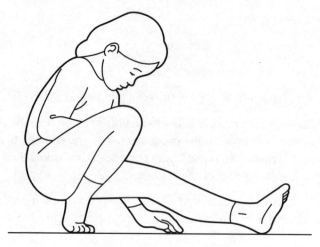

Figure 6.1 Vincent's curtsey

- Residual urine volume (which should be 10% of bladder capacity) – preferably using a portable bladder scanner (Frederickson *et al.* 2000).

The child (or parent) should be advised to complete a bladder and bowel diary for one week (ICCS 2005):

- Use a plastic jug to measure accurately all voided urine. Also record episodes of voids not measured to reflect frequency (children will not want to take a jug to school).

- Include fluid intake (1–1.5 litres per day is advised for school-aged children).

- Include bowel movements – less than three bowel movements per week, or evidence of soiling, may indicate constipation (Issenman *et al.* 1999).

The chart should be completed by the parents and child together whenever possible. In the case of a child under the age of 5 years, or a child with learning difficulties, the parents should be asked to complete the chart.

If the child is not yet toilet trained, or has severe incontinence, the *nappy test* may be used. Using the same type of nappy throughout, weigh a dry nappy first. All subsequent dry nappies will weigh the same. Weigh all subsequent wet nappies and subtract the dry weight to obtain the total amount of urine passed at each nappy change.

> *Bladder capacity can be estimated using the following formula:*
> **30 mls per year of life + 30 mls**

This formula is used for children up to the age of 10 years; after that age the bladder is expected to be of adult proportions. Maximum capacity is harder to identify in children under the age of 2 years because of the reflex action of voiding causing constant filling and emptying episodes (Silverstein 2004), but the following formula may be used as a guide:

> **Weight (kg) × 7**
> (See Rickwood and Malone 2002: 136)

Referral for further investigation

The results of the assessment should be evaluated and discussed with the family. If the results warrant further investigation, medical advice should be sought after consultation with the family.

Such results may include:

- Abnormal voiding pattern indicating obstruction;

- Incomplete bladder emptying associated with neurological signs (see physical examination);

- Persistent dribbling of urine (suggesting a possible anatomical defect such as ectopic ureter).

Any evidence of sexually transmitted disease or genital abnormality must be investigated. If the patient is a sexually active teenager, the patient's permission must be obtained before giving any information to the parents or carers. If permission is not forthcoming, advice should be sought from a senior paediatric clinician. This is an extremely difficult area of paediatric practice that requires a sensitive and tactful approach to both patient and the family.

Plan

An appropriate plan should be agreed with the child and family. This may be either an *action* plan or a *management* plan.

Action plan

This will include any further investigations required. Information can be given to the child and family at the time of assessment, with confirmation after consultation with the medical team.

Management plan

This should cover the following:

- Anticholinergic medication;
- Regular toileting programme;
- Increased fluid intake;
- Biofeedback for dysfunctional voiding;
- Prophylactic antibiotic therapy for recurrent UTIs;
- Laxative therapy for constipation;
- Clean intermittent catheterisation for incomplete bladder emptying.

A review date should be agreed with the child and family at the end of the assessment. If further investigations are planned, the review should be planned after all the results are available. If a management plan has been instigated, the review date should be approximately 4–6 weeks later.

Radiological investigations

NOTE: The investigations are described with the least invasive first.

Ultrasound

Ultrasonography of the upper and lower urinary tract is a non-invasive, low radiation method of identifying the following possible causes of urinary incontinence:

- Vesico-ureteric reflux (VUR);
- Bladder wall thickness;

- Incomplete bladder emptying;

- Hydronephrosis;

- Residual volume of urine.

Research has demonstrated that carrying out renal ultrasound following a first urinary tract infection is of little clinical benefit (Alon and Ganapathy 1999). So renal ultrasound should only be used on selected patients where there is evidence of recurrent UTIs or congenital abnormalities of the upper/lower urinary tract or spinal cord. To be most effective, ultrasound should be performed both before and after micturition.

CASE STUDY

Claire

Claire is a 5-year-old girl who was referred to clinic with incomplete bladder emptying, recurrent urinary tract infections and an inverted right foot. Claire's foot problem had been noted at birth and she had been seeing a physiotherapist for two years to try and straighten her foot through the use of strengthening exercises and serial casting. Claire's mother had noticed that recently Claire did not seem to use the toilet very often, but could be wet several times a day. On further questioning, her mother revealed that Claire had never had very wet nappies, and had always been prone to constipation, which her mother had managed with a high fibre diet.

Claire is the eldest of three children, she has a three-year-old brother and a one-year-old sister. Claire's mother is a housewife and her father works full time outside the home. There are no medical problems in the family and Claire is otherwise fit and well. She has just started primary school where she has settled in well.

On physical examination, Claire was found to have a small lump at the base of her spine and her ankle reflexes were difficult to elicit. A bladder scan showed incomplete bladder emptying. The findings were discussed with Claire's parents and a decision was made to carry out a magnetic resonance imaging (MRI) scan of Claire's spinal cord, and videourodynamic (VUD) studies. Claire was given a general anaesthetic for the MRI scan to ensure good quality images of her spinal cord. The urethral and rectal catheters required for the VUDs were inserted while Claire was anaesthetised to make it less traumatic for her. The VUD study was carried out later the same day, when the effects of the anaesthetic had worn off.

The MRI scan revealed a sacral lipoma (closed sac containing sacral nerves) and a tethered spinal cord. The VUD study demonstrated a large capacity bladder with detrusor sphincter dyssynergia (disturbance in the coordination of the internal and external urinary sphincters) and incomplete bladder emptying. These results confirmed that Claire had a neuropathic bladder secondary to her sacral lipoma.

Claire's parents were naturally upset by these results, but were seen by a neurosurgeon very promptly. He spoke to them at length about the MRI results and possible treatment options. After considering the risks and benefits of surgery, Claire's parents agreed that her spinal cord should be untethered.

Following the procedure, Claire developed urinary retention and had to have a urethral catheter reinserted. Three days later, and together with her parents, she was seen by the nurse specialist who discussed clean intermittent catheterisation as an option. Claire was very keen to do this as she did not like the indwelling catheter. Within two days, Claire had learnt to self-catheterise and was able to go home. She continues to self catheterise three times a day.

Urodynamic studies

Urodynamics should only be undertaken under the following circumstances:

- Where there is evidence of a neurological or urological abnormality;

- Where there is a discrepancy between symptoms and clinical findings;

- Where initial treatment has failed;

- Prior to surgery;

- Where there is evidence of large residual volumes of urine postmicturition;

- If nocturnal enuresis in an adolescent fails to respond to treatment.

Features of a urodynamic study

Urine flow rate is measured by (Norgaard *et al.* 1998; Hoebeke *et al.* 2001):

- Cystometry – measures the pressure/volume relationship of the bladder, and is used to assess detrusor activity; sensation; capacity and compliance.

- Slow fill cystometry (5–10 ml/min), which is used for young children, suspected small capacity or suspected detrusor overactivity.

- Medium fill cystometry (10–25 ml/min) is used for adolescents; large capacity or atonic bladders.

- An optional video film of the bladder filling or emptying. This can be used to identify vesicoureteric reflux or spincter performance.

- Urethral pressure profile (UPP) is an optional method for identifying sphincter incompetence in the presence of a normal electromyography reading.

- Electromyography (EMG) is another optional method which measures the activity of the urethral sphincter during the filling and voiding phases.

Plain or ambulatory urodynamics may be undertaken in a designated clinic setting, supervised by an experienced nurse specialist. Video-urodynamics take place in the X-ray department under the supervision of an appropriately trained radiologist.

Urodynamics involve invasive procedures requiring patients to be catheterised using either the urethral or suprapubic route. If video is used, there is also exposure to radiation and the instillation of uro-grafin for the procedure. Urografin is a radioisotope solution which appears as an opaque solution on the X-ray screen. Saline 0.9% may be instilled for plain urodynamics.

Preparing the patient

Children generally co-operate more fully with investigations if they have been given age-appropriate information beforehand. This information should be given by professionals familiar with the procedure.

It may not be possible to prepare very young children for this procedure, so parents should be given both verbal and written information. Figure 6.2 lists some crucial points.

Figure 6.2 What to consider when preparing children
for videourodynamics

Children under 5 years old

Young children need:

- To be able to see and touch the parent/carer at all times
- A familiar toy from home to provide comfort
- A story book for the parent or carer to use as distraction
- A bottle of juice or milk for very young children
- A calm environment with low voices

Children over 5 years old

Older children need:

- An explanation of the test with the use of photographs
- A visit to the X-ray department
- To be able to examine and handle the urodynamic catheters
- An explanation of the use of local anaesthetic gel
- The use of a video or DVD player on which to watch a favourite film as distraction for the duration of the procedure
- Provision of written information, to be taken away from the clinic
- Provision of a contact number for further questions/information

---

Videourodynamics takes around one hour – which is a very long time for the child who has to undergo the procedure. No aspect of the procedure should be rushed, and the child should be offered constant reassurance throughout. It should only be performed by appropriately trained professionals, experienced in working with children.

A report of the study should be compiled by the professional carrying out the procedure, in conjunction with an experienced doctor or paediatric urologist. This report should then be forwarded to the professional who requested the investigation for discussion with the family.

A treatment course of antibiotic cover should be arranged for two days, commencing on the day of the procedure before the procedure is carried out as follows:

- Children with normal upper tracts – trimethoprim 4 mg/k twice a day;

- Children with renal impairment – one dose of IV gentamicin 6 mg/kg.

(**NOTE:** The adjustment is made for weight.)

Micturating cysto-urethrogram (MCUG)

An MCUG is used most commonly to confirm the presence of vesico-ureteric reflux or VUR (Carty 2002: 25) in a child with a previously proven UTI. It can also be used to identify suspected anomalies such as posterior-urethral valves, antenatal hydronephrosis and pelvi-ureteric junction obstruction (Hunter 2002).

- **This investigation should only be carried out if videourodynamics are not available or are not being planned.**

The patient has to be catheterised, usually in the X-ray department, so that urografin can be instilled into the bladder. The catheterisation procedure is similar to that for urodynamics, and must only be carried out by an experienced practitioner. A pre-contrast image of the urinary tract is taken. Contrast is slowly instilled via the catheter from a hanging bottle or hand-held syringe, and the patient is screened regularly as the bladder fills with contrast and during micturition. Routine antibiotic cover should be arranged, especially for younger children, as for videourodynamic studies.

Intravenous urography (IVU)

IVU has been less frequently used since the improvements in ultrasonic scanning (Smellie 1994: 164). It can, however, prove useful for diagnosing pelvic–ureteric junction obstruction prior to surgical intervention, and for detailed anatomy of duplication anomalies.

A full-length control film of the entire urinary tract is taken prior to injection of a contrast medium. Films are taken subsequently at 3 minutes post injection (renal areas only), and a full length film at 15 minutes.

Dimercaptosuccinic acid (DMSA)

(The name of the radioactive tracer gives its name to the test.)
DMSA is a radiological tracer, injected intravenously, to provide static images of both kidneys. It is the most reliable method of identifying cortical renal scarring occurring after upper urinary tract infections. Reproduction of DMSA images also means that anomalies such as horseshoe kidney, duplex kidneys and multicystic dysplastic kidneys can be identified.

No special preparation is required for this investigation, but the child must be weighed in order that the amount of tracer can be calculated. Scanning takes place approximately three hours after the tracer has been administered. Renal function is considered abnormal if the differential function between the two kidneys is greater than 10% (Rossleigh 2002), or if there is a distortion of the normal renal outline.

DMSA imaging should not be carried out while the patient has a UTI, as residual scan abnormalities can persist for up to three months. Most specialist centres advocate a time lapse of two to three months after a confirmed UTI before carrying out the study.

Diethylene pantacetic acid (DTPA)

(The name of the radioactive tracer gives its name to the test.)
DTPA is a glomerular tracer used in dynamic renal imaging. It is considered the gold standard for identifying split renal function, because it reflects the glomerular filtration rate (GFR). It is particularly useful in identifying acute urinary tract obstruction or renal artery stenosis. The radiation dose is generally low.

Patients are asked to void prior to the study. Screening is commenced at the time of tracer injection, and the study is completed in approximately 20 minutes.

> For both DMSA and DTPA studies, parents should be advised that radioactive tracers are being used. Pregnant mothers should not accompany the child for the procedure, and should not come into contact with the child's body fluids for 24 hours after the procedure.

Magnetic Resonance Imaging (MRI)

MRI uses magnetic waves, which can be transferred to a multi-dimensional visual image. It can clearly define organ structures. It is also valuable in diagnosing diseases of the brain and spinal cord, cardiovascular disease, and musculoskeletal abnormalities. There is no exposure to radiation.

The patient must be placed entirely into the cylinder containing the magnet. Many children find this frightening, and most will need sedation or a general anaesthetic for the procedure. All metallic objects such as jewellery, must be removed prior to scanning, and particular care must be taken with patients who have pacemakers fitted.

Blood tests

The primary aim of carrying out blood tests in children with bladder dysfunction is to assess renal function. Blood tests are unpleasant for children, and should only be undertaken if absolutely necessary. All children, regardless of age, should be offered local anaesthetic cream or spray prior to the procedure. Venepuncture or cannulation should be carried out by an experienced practitioner, in a child-friendly environment. Figure 6.3 lists what such an environment should include.

Figure 6.3 Providing a child-friendly environment for venepuncture

Try to ensure the following are available:

- A quiet area with privacy from other patients

- Means of distraction, such as toys or story books

- A comfortable chair for the child to sit in, or where a parent can sit with the child on her knee

- Input from a play specialist

- A sticker box as a means of reward

Full blood count (FBC)

This is particularly useful in identifying infection (raised white cell count), or anaemia (low haemoglobin). Normal values are given in Table 6.2.

Table 6.2 Blood count: normal values and what any deviation might indicate

Full blood count	Normal values	Suspected pathology
White Cell Count	$4.5–13.5 \times 10^9$	**Elevated:** infection, malignancy, emotional stress **Decreased:** rickets, drugs and chemicals, anaphylactic shock
Red blood cells	$4.10–5.40 \times 10^{12}$	**Elevated:** dehydration, acute poisoning, haemorrhage **Decreased:** blood loss, iron deficiency, leukaemia
Haemoglobin	11.5–14.5 g/dl	**Elevated:** dehydration, congestive heart failure **Decreased:** anaemia, hyperthyroidism
Platelets	$150–400 \times 10^9$	**Elevated:** leukaemia, trauma, Rheumatoid arthritis **Decreased:** aplastic anaemia, HIV, allergic reaction
Packed cell volume	0.320–0.450 l/l	**Elevated:** severe dehydration, shock **Decreased:** anaemia, leukaemia

Urea and electrolytes

Children with suspected compromised renal function or who have undergone bladder reconstruction need regular evaluation of creatinine, urea and electrolytes. Normal values are given in Table 6.3.

Glomerular filtration rate (GFR)

GFR is the rate at which plasma is filtered through the glomeruli in one minute, thereby defining renal efficiency. The figure obtained after laboratory analysis is the measurement of total renal function. GFR may be evaluated by measuring 24 hour urine creatinine clearance, or by estimating creatinine clearance from plasma creatinine. Urinary clearance may be unreliable, so plasma creatinine clearance is preferred (Durand and Prigent 2002). Normal GFR levels for infants and children are shown in Table 6.4.

Table 6.3 Urea and electrolytes: normal values and what any deviation might indicate

Urea and electrolytes	Normal values	Suspected pathology
Sodium	135–145 mmol/l	**Elevated:** dehydration, diabetes insipidus, Cushing's syndrome **Decreased:** diarrhoea, vomiting, severe nephritis
Potassium	3.5–5.0 mmol/l	**Elevated:** renal failure, acidosis, diabetes **Decreased:** diarrhoea, malabsorption, renal tubular acidosis
Calcium	2.27–2.69 mmol/l	**Elevated:** hyperparathyroidism, malignancy; respiratory acidosis **Decreased:** coeliac disease, rickets, hypoparathyroidism
Phosphate	1.1–1.8 mmol/l	**Elevated:** renal insufficiency, severe nephritis, hypocalcaemia **Decreased:** rickets, hyperparathyroidism
Creatinine	40–90 umol/l	**Elevated:** impaired renal function, chronic nephritis, muscular dystrophy, urinary tract obstruction
Urea	2.5–7.5 mmol/l	**Elevated:** renal disease, dehydration, diabetes mellitus **Decreased:** nephrotic syndrome, liver failure

There are various preparations available for estimating GFR:

- **Inulin** is a solution that is considered to be the gold standard for measurement of GFR (Taylor 1994: 92). It is a polysaccharide, which is freely filtered by the glomerulus, and is not secreted or reabsorbed by the tubule. However, it is not routinely used in paediatric practice because it requires the administration of a bolus injection followed by a continuous infusion. A simultaneous urine collection is also required.

- **Inutest® 25%** is more commonly used for estimating GFR in children. This is an aqueous solution of a water soluble fructan called Sinistrin. It performs in a similar way to Inulin, but can be given as a bolus injection, and simultaneous urine collection is not required. This preparation has recently become more

Table 6.4 Normal GFR levels in childhood

Birth	30–50 ml/m²
1–3 years	80–110 ml/1.73/m²
Over 3 years	110–120 ml/1.73/m²

Source: Taylor CM (1994)

difficult to obtain, requiring the evaluation of other substances which may be used instead (see Iohexol)

■ **Cr-EDTA** is a radioactive tracer with a high energy, low radiation yield. This makes it suitable for use in older children and adults, but not in neonates or children under 3 years.

■ **Iohexol** is a non-radiolabelled (non-radioactive) alternative to Cr-EDTA, which has been used as an X-ray marker for many years. As Inutest® 25% is becoming more difficult to obtain, trials are currently underway to test Iohexol's efficacy as a single bolus injection.

Method for evaluating GFR

Children require thorough preparation for this investigation, as it involves the insertion of two cannulae – one for administering the tracer, and one for blood sampling. A leaflet or verbal explanation of the test should be provided in advance, so the parent and child have a full understanding of what will happen. If the child is too young to understand verbal explanations, the presence of a play specialist to help with distraction can make the procedure less traumatic.

Local anaesthetic should be applied prior to cannulation to reduce pain and anxiety. An experienced practitioner should perform the cannulation.

The tracer to be injected must be properly prescribed according to local protocols and signed for by the person administering it. If Inutest® 25% is used, there is a small risk of respiratory compromise, so oxygen and a ventolin nebuliser should be readily available.

The tracer is administered slowly, over two minutes. Blood samples are obtained at regular intervals thereafter, according to protocol. The samples should be taken to the laboratory as soon as possible after completion of the test.

If other blood tests or scans requiring intravenous injection are being planned, these should be carried out on the same day if possible. This will avoid subjecting the child to repeated episodes of needle insertion.

CASE STUDY

Steven

Steven is a 10-year-old boy who presented in clinic with day and night-time incontinence and recurrent urinary tract infections (UTIs).

Steven is the middle of three children, one older brother and a younger sister. Both his parents work full time. Steven attends a private school and is a high achiever. There is no family history of any medical problems and Steven is otherwise fit and well.

In clinic, his physical examination was normal, but a flow study and bladder scan showed an abnormal voiding pattern and incomplete bladder emptying. Steven's blood pressure was also slightly elevated at 115/70.

After discussion with Steven and his mother, it was agreed that he would undergo a full day bladder assessment with the nurse specialist with a formal renal and bladder ultrasound and routine full blood count and urea and electrolytes.

The bladder assessment revealed a reduced urinary flow rate and residual urine volumes of 50–100mls of urine despite two attempts at voiding on each occasion. Steven also found it difficult to drink adequate amounts of fluid because he was afraid of being incontinent. His mother admitted that this was also a problem at school, although she felt he drank well at home. He had never suffered from constipation, and his abdomen was soft on palpation.

The ultrasound showed Grade 3 vesico-ureteric reflux and incomplete bladder emptying. Steven's blood tests were all within normal limits except for his creatinine level which was elevated to 102 Ìmmol/l. These results suggested that Steven's impaired bladder function was having a detrimental effect on his renal function.

The results were discussed with Steven and his parents, and plans were made to proceed to videourodynamic studies, DMSA scan and

GFR estimation. Videourodynamics confirmed vesicoureteric reflux with high detrusor (bladder muscle) pressures on filling the bladder and on voiding. Steven's bladder capacity was normal (300 mls), but he had a residual urine volume of 100 mls. His GFR was estimated at 70 mls/1.73 m2/min. The DMSA scan showed renal scarring on the right with divided renal function of (Right) 30% (Left) 70%.

The treatment for Steven's condition is clean intermittent catheterisation to facilitate complete bladder emptying, and anticholinergic therapy to reduce bladder pressures.

Steven found the idea of urethral catheterisation unacceptable, so he had a Mitrofanoff stoma formed which he began to use three weeks after surgery. Steven's renal function will be assessed on a yearly basis to ensure no further deterioration.

Conclusion

There is a whole range of investigations which may be undertaken to identify bladder dysfunction and possible renal impairment in children. These range from the simple to the complex. Those which are invasive, or which involve subjecting a child to repeated doses of radiation, should be avoided unless absolutely necessary. So careful and thorough assessment by an experienced practitioner is essential for identifying which investigations are needed. In some cases, treatment can be started without the need for invasive investigations (Loening-Baucke 1997; Mattsson *et al.* 2003).

Appropriate information must always be given to children and their families about all investigations being proposed. This will ensure that where consent is given, it will be informed consent. It will also reduce the trauma of the investigations which are carried out, and encourage better concordance with treatment on the part of patients and their families.

References

Alon US, Ganapathy S (1999) Should renal ultrasonography be done routinely in children with first urinary tract infection? *Clinical Pediatrics*, 38(1): 21–5

Bankhead RW, Kropp BP, Cheng EY (2000) Evaluation and treatment of children with neurogenic bladders. *Journal of Child Neurology*, 15(3): 141–9

Carty HM (2002) Imaging. In: Thomas DFM, Rickwood AMK, Duffy PG (eds) *Essentials of Paediatric Urology*. London: Martin Dunitz

Durand E, Prigent A (2002) The basics of renal imaging and function studies. *The Quarterly Journal of Nuclear Medicine*, 46(4): 249–67

Fisher R, Frank D (2000) Detrusor instability: day and night-time wetting, urinary tract infections. *Archives of Disease in Childhood*, 8: 135–7

Frederickson M, Neitzel JJ, Miller EH, Reuter S, Graner T, Heller J (2000) The implementation of bedside bladder ultrasound technology: effects on patient and cost postoperative outcomes in tertiary care. *Orthopaedic Nursing*, 19(3): 79–87

Hoebeke P, Van Laecke E, Van Camp C, Raes A, Van De Walle J (2001) One thousand video-urodynamic studies in children with non-neurogenic bladder sphincter dysfunction. *British Journal of Urology International*, 87: 575–80

Hunter E (2002) Micturating cysto-urethrogram (MCUG). *Synergy*, Jan: 18–21

International Children's Continence Society (2005) The Standardisation of Terminology of Lower Urinary Tract Function in Children and Adolescents: Report from the Standardisation Committee of the ICCS

Issenman RM, Filmer RB, Gorski PA (1999) A review of bowel and bladder control development in children: how gastrointestinal and urologic conditions relate to problems in toilet training. *Pediatrics*, 103(6): 1346–52

Kaschak Newman D (1996) Urinary incontinence management in the USA: the role of the nurse. *British Journal of Nursing*, 5(2): 78–88

Loening-Baucke V (1997) Urinary incontinence and urinary tract infection and their resolution with treatment of chronic constipation of childhood. *Pediatrics*, 100(2): 228–32

Mattsson S, Gladh G (2003) Urethrovaginal reflux – a common cause of daytime incontinence in girls. *Pediatrics*, 111(1): 136–9

Norgaard JP, Van Gool JD, Hjalmas K, Djurhuus JC, Hellstrom A-L (1998) Standardization and definitions in lower urinary tract dysfunction in children. *British Journal of Urology*, 81 (suppl 3): 1–16

Rickwood AMK (2002) Urinary incontinence. In: Thomas DFM, Rickwood AMK, Duffy PG (eds) *Essentials of Paediatric Urology*. London: Martin Dunitz

Rickwood AMK, Malone PS (2002) Neuropathic Bladder. In: Thomas DFM, Rickwood AMK, Duffy PG (eds) *Essentials of Paediatric Urology*. London: Martin Dunitz

Ross J (1994) A Plan of Action – continence assessment. *Nursing Times*, 90(27): 65–6

Rossleigh MA (2002) Urinary tract infection and other pediatric considerations. *The Quarterly Journal of Nuclear Medicine*, 46(4): 304–10

Royal College of Physicians (2003) Incontinence management. www.eguidelines.co.uk

Silverstein DM (2004) Enuresis in children: diagnosis and management. *Clinical Pediatrics*, 43(3): 217–21

Smellie JM (1994) Management and investigations of children with urinary tract infection. In: Postlethwaite RJ (ed.) *Clinical Paediatric Nephrology* 2e. Oxford: Butterworth-Heinemann

Taylor CM (1994) Assessment of the glomerular filtration rate. In: Postlethwaite RJ (ed.) *Clinical Paediatric Nephrology* 2e. Oxford: Butterworth-Heinemann

Winder A (2001) Continence assessment in primary care: what is the next step? *British Journal of Community Nursing*, 6(10): 520–21, 524

7 Nocturnal enuresis

Jonathan Evans

Key Points

- Nocturnal enuresis is a common and often distressing problem for children and young people.

- Underlying abnormalities, including nocturnal polyuria and occult detrusor overactivity, are often present.

- Enuresis alarms are not suitable for all children, but they can lead to long-lasting benefit for some.

- Desmopressin is effective in suppressing wetting.

- Imipramine, although effective, has an unacceptably high incidence of adverse effects.

- Oxybutinin may be effective in children with underlying detrusor overactivity.

Nocturnal enuresis (NE) is now recognised to be the result of several different, interacting mechanisms including alterations of bladder function, nocturnal urine production and sleep-arousal mechanisms. Both genetic and environmental factors contribute to the development of wetting. With better understanding of the underlying causes of NE, the importance of a thorough patient evaluation is even greater as treatment can be more effectively targeted if the underlying cause of the enuresis is recognised.

There is strong evidence that enuresis alarms, dry bed training, desmopressin and imipramine are all effective treatments; but only alarm-based treatments have been proven to offer a persisting benefit. Imipramine is considered too toxic to advocate its use as a routine treatment. Oxybutinin combined with desmopressin may have a role in the management of refractory enuresis and enuresis associated with detrusor overactivity.

CASE STUDY

Evidence-based practice

Joe, a 10-year-old boy with nocturnal enuresis consults you. He wishes to be rid of his wetting permanently and says he 'will do anything' to get rid of it, but he also has a pressing need to be dry next week because he is sleeping in a tent for two nights. On further assessment you establish that Joe has primary, monosymptomatic NE, has no psychosocial problems and has supportive parents. A baseline record shows wetting on six nights a week and no daytime problems.

You review the evidence presented in this chapter and note that the evidence on the effectiveness of treatment comes from recently updated systematic reviews of randomised controlled trials in children with nocturnal enuresis. This evidence is therefore robust (Level 1 evidence) and directly applicable to this particular child.

The only treatment for which there is evidence of a long-lasting benefit is the enuresis alarm. This would therefore seem the best option for 'getting rid' of Joe's enuresis. The chances of him becoming permanently dry are better than 50%, because he has good prognostic factors such as absence of daytime wetting and psychosocial difficulties. The odds may be further improved by using 'overlearning' or 'dry bed training'.

Alarm treatment does not work quickly and is not practical in a tent so you consider alternative measures to cover the short-term need! Medication such as desmopressin or imipramine are both effective in monosymptomatic NE and work quickly. Imipramine has an unattractive incidence of adverse effects and is rejected by the boy. Desmopressin is very likely to improve the wetting but cannot be guaranteed to prevent wetting. You therefore advise Joe of this and suggest that he could consider additional precautions such as an absorbent pad or 'pull-ups'.

Definitions

The terminology used to describe children who wet at night is unfortunately confusing. Although the term 'bed-wetting' is fairly unambiguous, the definition of 'nocturnal enuresis' is more problematic. In common use, nocturnal enuresis refers to children who are of an age where they are not expected to wet the bed, who wet the bed regularly without any identifiable disease that might explain the wetting. As our understanding of nocturnal enuresis evolves, we are however finding more and more disorders that explain bed-wetting in these children that by this definition means they no longer have nocturnal enuresis but have bed-wetting due to an underlying disorder, for example detrusor overactivity or nocturnal polyuria. For epidemiological studies, rigid definitions are used that specify an age cut off (e.g. more than 5 years old) and frequency (e.g. one or more times week).

The International Children's Continence Society has defined nocturnal enuresis (NE) as intermittent urinary incontinence while asleep. This definition therefore encompasses a number of different conditions where the endpoint is intermittent incontinence while sleeping, and includes conditions such as over-active bladder (in which daytime wetting may also occur) or less commonly renal or urological disorders.

Prevalence

Nocturnal enuresis is a common disorder. Present day prevalence rates are hard to come by and reported prevalence varies between studies, probably due to different definitions and methodologies. It is clear that NE is a worldwide problem with broadly similar prevalence rates reported in the UK and other European Countries, the United States and in a number of countries in Asia and Africa. Typically, prevalence rates are 15–20 % of five-year-olds, 5 % of ten-year-olds and 1–2% of fifteen-year-olds. Historically, spontaneous remission rates were reported of around 15% of affected children per year.

Aetiology

There has been a lot of progress in our understanding of NE during the last 25 years and it is now clear that NE is not a single condition but the end point of a number of underlying disturbances or disorders of heredity, environment and physiology.

Predisposing factors

Many factors are known to be associated with the presence of or development of enuresis. Few of these links have been the subject of adequate scientific study to confirm whether the association is causal or incidental.

Genetic factors

It has long been recognised that there is a genetic predisposition to NE. up to 75% of affected children will have an affected first degree relative and there is a greater concordance for the presence of NE in monozygotic ('identical') compared to di-zygotic twins. A more recent groundbreaking study of families with NE has demonstrated a strong link between the development of NE and the inheritance of a particular locus on the short arm of Chromosome 13 confirming the strong genetic basis in these families (Eiberg *et al.* 1995). Other gene loci have subsequently been identified but the actual genes themselves and the mechanism by which they lead to enuresis is not yet known.

Early life

The hypothesis that early life events might adversely affect the acquisition of bladder control is an attractive one. There is an association between both low birth weight and not being breastfed and the development of NE. Stressful early life events in the first few years also increase the likelihood of NE.

Psychosocial

Perhaps the most confusing area is the relationship between NE and psychosocial factors. The interpretation of the literature is confounded by the tendency of earlier studies to include 'mixed' wetters, for example those with both day and night wetting or onset wetting. 'Stressful early life events' have been reported to be associated with primary NE, while psychosocial factors are often identified as a trigger for onset NE. NE is more common in lower social classes and more likely where there is paternal unemployment.

Even though all the aforementioned factors may in some way contribute to the development of NE, this is not evidence that NE is a psychological disorder. A strong body of literature has now accrued that shows that, while a minority of children with primary NE will have psychological, emotional and behavioural problems, the considerable majority do not; furthermore the proportion with these problems is probably little different to the general childhood population (Glazener and Evans 2006).

In contrast, the proportion of children with secondary onset NE, day and night wetting (particularly voiding dysfunction) and faecal soiling with behavioural and emotional disorders is far higher – indicating a much stronger causative link.

Pathology/physiology

Most parents will be aware that when their children become dry at night this is usually achieved by being able to last all night without needing the toilet. It is possible to infer from this that these children have a nocturnal bladder capacity greater than their urine output. It is also evident that older children and adults are clearly able to wake up when their bladder becomes full, something that children with NE do not do.

Detailed physiological studies have furthered our understanding of the factors that contribute to enuresis.

Nocturnal polyuria

Non-wetting children and young adults have a circadian rhythm to urine production regulated by vasopressin secretion. Typically, they produce urine overnight at less than half the daytime rate and can contain this within their normal bladder. For example, nocturnal urine production is less than the normal bladder capacity for age.

A substantial proportion of children with NE have nocturnal polyuria, producing more urine than their bladder can hold. This has been shown to be associated with a relative lack of nocturnal vasopressin secretion in some children even if their fluid intake is rigorously controlled (Norgaard et al. 1985). Furthermore, urine production is higher on wet nights than on dry nights. Not all polyuric children have abnormal vasopressin secretion and it has been postulated that in some it may be associated with excessive urinary sodium or calcium losses at night.

Bladder dysfunction

It has long been recognised that the presence of daytime wetting indicates the likelihood of bladder dysfunction, most commonly detrusor overactivity or dysfunctional voiding. In these children, the night time wetting may well be due to the same disorder. It is now evident that there is a significant minority of children with NE who have no daytime symptoms but have nocturnal detrusor overactivity (Medel *et al.* 1998). This is difficult to prove in clinical practice (researchers use overnight natural fill urodynamic studies) but may be recognised by multiple wettings per night, small wetting, waking with urge. Others may simply have a reduced functional bladder capacity which means that the 'normal' urine production is 'relative nocturnal polyuria'.

Sleep – arousal

It is still unclear whether the sleep of children with NE differs from others. They appear to have the same stages and depth of sleep in the same proportions. Wetting occurs when the children are asleep and is not confined to the deepest levels of sleep (Hunsballe *et al.* 1995). What is evident is that children do not awaken when their bladder empties although lightening of sleep may be seen (children may become restless prior to wetting). This problem with arousal can also be seen in most of the studies looking at the ability of children with NE to wake to noise.

Heath promotion

Despite the progress in our understanding and treatment of NE, there is very little known about measures that might prevent the development of NE. Some authorities have observed that the age children become 'potty trained' has increased during the last 30 years, inferring that the relaxed modern attitude to training and the advent of comfortable disposable nappies has lead to problems. Others however point out that earlier potty training was probably achieved simply by frequent use of the potty rather than any accelerated development of bladder control. Furthermore there is no evidence of an increasing prevalence of NE nowadays.

Despite the lack of high quality evidence, it is still possible to give some advice on health promotion measures for bladder control provided these measures are based on reasonable assumptions and are

Table 7.1 Measures aimed at promoting continence

	Measure	Rationale
Potty training	Potty training when individual child appears ready. Avoid 'punitive' approach	Punishment and conflict over potty training may become a stressful early life event that leads to NE
Fluids	Encourage a healthy intake of water/dilute squash throughout the day.	Prevent constipation, encourages development of a good bladder capacity, reduces need for evening drinking
Carbonated drinks	Avoid excessive amounts of carbonated and caffeine-containing drinks	Caffeine is a diuretic and may worsen urgency and wetting. Large amounts of these drinks are bad for general health
Diet	Adequate fruit vegetables and fibre	Prevent constipation, general health measure
Bowels	Avoid constipation through diet and fluid intake	Enuresis and urine infections are more common in constipated children
Toileting	Regular relaxed (unhurried) voiding	Avoid UTI, constipation and poor bladder habits that may lead to wetting

consistent with general child health advice. The measures indicated in Table 7.1 may well be valuable therefore.

Pathway and care

Nocturnal enuresis is an extremely common problem that can be managed without recourse to specialised investigation and therapy. The vast majority of children should therefore be managed within the community.

Self-help

Parents and children who wish to help themselves without involving their healthcare professionals should and can have access to information, advice and treatment with enuresis alarms (but not pre-scription medicines). It is beyond the remit of this book to provide an exhaustive list of reference materials but independent information is available from NHS Direct.

Primary care

The responsibility for providing continence services in the UK lies with the individual Primary Care Trusts. The precise services and arrange-ments will therefore differ from area to area. The Department of Health does provide guidance on the good practice. In general, health visitors, general practitioners and school nurses are the first point of contact and should all be able to provide first line advice. Some will also be able to provide further treatment including enuresis alarms and medication with support and supervision themselves. Others, depending on local NHS configuration, will refer on to enuresis services.

Enuresis clinics

Enuresis clinics are set up with the information, time, facilities and per-sonnel needed to support children and carers. Most clinics are based in the community and staffed by school nurses with or without the sup-port of a community paediatrician or specialist nurse. These clinics should be able to provide a range of different treatments. Because of the frequent co-existence of daytime wetting, bed-wetting and faecal soiling, there is an increasing trend towards providing integrated child-hood continence clinics.

Specialist services

A minority of children with refractory problems need assessment in more specialised services. Specialised continence services may involve hospital or community paediatrics or paediatric urology.

Assessment

The purpose of assessment is to gather sufficient information in order for you, the health professional, to give the correct opinion and advice to the child and carer. Assuming that 'bed-wetting' is the presenting complaint then one priority is to determine if there are underlying medical disorders that might be the cause of the problem and require assessment and management in their own right. If the problem appears to be enuresis then you can focus on gathering information that might influence your advice and treatment recommendation.

History

An elimination history should cover the nature, time-course and extent of the wetting and include important information such as bowel habits, diet, drinking pattern, difficulties over toileting and clues as to the cause of enuresis such as daytime urinary frequency, urgency and wetting.

Further history should include other past or present medical conditions (co-morbidity) as well as psychological, emotional and behavioural disorders. It is important to establish the importance of the wetting to both the child and other family members; how does the wetting affect the child, what is the parents response to wetting, how concerned are the child and parent and in what way are they concerned? It may be helpful to talk to the child and parent separately and questionnaires may also be of value.

Examination

The physical examination fulfils three purposes, to check the general health of the child, to help identify physical causes for the wetting and reassurance. The yield of abnormal findings is however very low, particularly if the child has nocturnal enuresis without any daytime symptoms.

A basic physical examination should probably include the following:

- Appraisal of general appearance and demeanour (signs of neglect/abuse and of skin rashes caused by wetting);

- Measurement of height, weight and blood pressure;

- Abdominal palpation;

- Inspection of lumbo-sacral spine;

- Eliciting of ankle reflexes.

Some medical authorities advocate more detailed examination including inspection of genitalia, eliciting the ano-cutaneous reflex and testing peri-anal sensation but this contributor uses such intrusive investigation very selectively in children where a neurogenic bladder or structural urinary tract anomalies appear likely from the history and other aspects of physical examination.

Frequency volume chart

Most people do not memorise details of their bladder and bowel function. A prospective record of these matters is therefore invaluable to supplement the information from the history. The most basic chart simply records wet and dry nights but a great deal more can be learned if information on extent and time of night wetting is included as well as daytime urinary frequency, voided volumes, wetting and urgency, bowel actions and fluid intake is recorded for a minimum of three days as well. If the child is using nappies or pull-ups, it is also quite easy to record overnight urine production to determine whether there is nocturnal polyuria.

Investigations

The incidence of structural disorders of the urinary tract is so low in children with monosymptomatic nocturnal enuresis that radiological imaging is unnecessary. In contrast urinary tract infections are relatively common, particularly in girls; all children should therefore be screened for infection. Children with daytime wetting are more likely to have UTI and the incidence of urinary tract anomalies is a little higher, therefore investigation with a bladder scan for post void residual or a renal tract ultrasound should be considered either at presentation or if initial treatment is not successful. Children with voiding dysfunction, severe daytime incontinence, recurrent UTI and physical signs suggesting underlying disease will need more extensive specialised investigations.

Urinalysis of a clean catch specimen of urine can test for protein, blood, glucose, leucocytes and nitrites and if all are normal this has almost ruled out UTI, diabetes mellitus and any major renal disease. If nitrite and leucocyte testing is not undertaken then simple urinalysis (blood, protein, glucose) and urine microscopy and culture are needed.

More detailed information about investigations is given in Chapter 6, by Rosie Kelly.

Treatment

Initial management should start by removing nappies and pull-ups as these give a conflicting message (pee in this while you're asleep!) to the objectives of treatment. All the measures outlined in Table 7.1 should be addressed prior to, or at the same time as, initiation of formal treatment. Occult constipation, in particular, is often missed (see Chapter 8 by Kenneth Wilkinson).

In a condition with a tendency to improve over time, in which the severity of wetting varies from week to week, it is easy to claim that treatments are successful. Only randomised controlled studies (RCTs) are capable of identifying with any certainty, which treatments are of value. In eight RCTs involving 185 children given a placebo as one arm of the study, the mean improvement in wet nights per week during placebo treatment was 0.9 (95% CI 0.7 to 1.0), i.e. an additional dry night every week.

Simple behavioural and physical interventions

These interventions include rewards such as star charts, lifting or waking the child at night to urinate, retention control training to enlarge bladder capacity and fluid restriction.

Star charts and rewards

There is evidence from three small controlled studies that star charts reduce wetting compared to no treatment (Glazener and Evans 2005a). It is probably not a highly effective treatment in that only 20% of children responded in one cohort study. It is however a useful initial therapy that can be used while collecting baseline information; can be continued if initial benefit is seen during the first few weeks; and may also be adapted to act as an adjunct to other treatments, such as alarms and medication, in order to encourage adherence with treatment.

Lifting and/or waking schedules

These have not been evaluated in controlled trials so their value is not proven. Lifting without waking is probably counter-productive as the manoeuvre is in effect training the child to void in their sleep. Lifting and waking on its own is of doubtful value in teaching children to become dry as it simply avoids the need for the child to recognise when the bladder is full. There may however be individuals where a lifting and waking programme is of value as an adjunct to other treatment, such as the dry bed training regimen.

Retention control

There is no reliable evidence that these training routines to increase bladder capacity are of benefit. In one small study enuresis alarms were more effective (Glazener and Evans 2005a).

Fluid restriction

Considering how widely used this manoeuvre is, there is remarkably little research. In one small RCT (Glazener and Evans 2005a), fluid restriction was markedly less effective than imipramine. Most experts consider fluid restriction to be ineffective as most families have already tried it. There is also a widely held view that many children drink insufficient fluid during the day and that a better strategy is to increase daytime fluids thus reducing the need for children to rehydrate themselves before bedtime. A pragmatic approach to fluid management is therefore to advocate healthy drinking in the day (1.5 to 2 litres of water per 24 hr with three quarters of this before 6 pm) and only restrict evening fluids if you have objective evidence that the child is drinking excessively in the evening despite an adequate daytime intake.

Enuresis alarms

Enuresis alarms consist of an alarm which is activated by micturition. The alarm may be a noise, vibration, light, a voice or any combination of these. The alarm is either bedside alarms with a urine sensor on the mattress, or a miniature body worn alarm with the sensor worn in the underwear. The exact mechanism by which alarms relieve wetting is still the subject of debate. It is usually described as a training programme designed to teach the child to 'wake up and hold on'. Three 'conditioning' processes have been proposed: Classical conditioning, where the alarm teaches the child to link the stimulus (full bladder) to the desired response (wake up and hold on), Aversive conditioning, where the alarm is the unpleasant response and operant

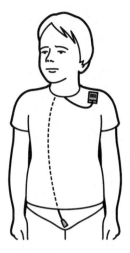

Figure 7.1 Example of an enuresis alarm (1)

conditioning, where the child responds to a reward for the desired response (wake up and hold on). At a physiological level children who become dry with alarm treatment do so through two mechanisms: Arousal – learning to wake up when necessary and suppression of the micturition reflex which enables the child to hold on to a greater volume of urine. It is well-known that the latter mechanism is the most common response.

The success rate of alarm treatment varies between clinical trials, depending on the population studied. Because the alarm is an intrusive and tiring treatment program, drop out rates are often high and treatment is less successful in children with behavioural and emotional problems and in situations of parental stress such as marital discord and intolerance to the child's wetting. It is possible that introducing

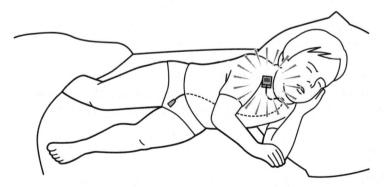

Figure 7.2 Example of an enuresis alarm (2)

alarm treatment into an already stressed household may actually worsen matters. Most research studies have therefore selected children/families that were perceived as 'suitable' for an alarm.

Alarms are clearly more effective than no treatment. In a meta-analysis of RCTs, children using an alarm fared better than those not treated; the relative risk of failure was less in the alarm groups of all the trials (98/304, 32% did not achieve 14 dry nights compared to 239/248, 96% in no-treatment controls, RR 0.36, 95% CI 0.31 to 0.43) (Glazener, Evans and Peto 2005a). Although some children relapsed after treatment was stopped, children were still less likely to be wet after the end of standard alarm treatment. Overall, 45/81 (55%) of the alarm treated and 80/81 (99%) of the control group (RR 0.56, 95% CI 0.46 to 0.68) remained wet or relapsed after stopping treatment. Overlearning, whereby the child, once dry, challenges their bladder by taking a large drink each night and continuing with the alarm and drink until dry again, may reduce the likelihood of relapse.

Alarm treatment has been combined with a number of behavioural measures such as waking routines and cleanliness training in 'dry bed training' to try to improve efficacy. The evidence from controlled studies suggests that this probably does improve success rates compared to the alarm alone but it is not widely used, probably because of the increased amount of training necessary (Glazener, Evans and Peto 2005b).

In another attempt to improve success rates, desmopressin has been used concurrently with the alarm during the first few weeks. The evidence supporting this strategy is not strong: one small controlled study showed a significantly better outcome – perhaps through reducing dropouts in the early weeks or by facilitating the arousal response to the alarm. However, a more recent, large RCT failed to confirm any benefit (Bradbury, Gibb *et al.* 2004).

Drugs

Medication can be used when the potential harm of the drug is less than the benefits of treatment. A large number of drugs have been used over the years but very few of these are of proven benefit.

Desmopressin

Desmopressin acetate is a synthetic analogue of human arginine vasopressin (anti-diuretic hormone). Its main pharmacological action is to reduce urine output through increasing water reabsorption in the renal collecting ducts by stimulating the V2 receptors. It has a duration of action of about 8–10 hours and can be taken intranasally or orally, the two routes of administration being equally effective although the dosage required for oral administration is tenfold higher. Adverse effects are uncommon but rare instances of water intoxication have been reported. The mechanism of action is thought to be through the reduction in nocturnal urine output after a night-time dose. Those with nocturnal polyuria respond better than those with small bladders. Desmopressin may interact with other drugs that alter urine production such as indomethacin, tricyclic antidepressants and carbamazepine.

There is good evidence that desmopressin is effective (Glazener and Evans 2005c). In a meta-analysis of RCTs that compared intranasal desmopressin (in doses of 10 to 60 micrograms) with placebo, desmopressin consistently reduced wetting by one to two wet nights per week more than placebo. For example, in 11 studies involving over 800 children and comparing desmopressin 20 mcg to placebo, the weighted mean difference (WMD) in wet nights was −1.34 (95% CI −1.57 to −1.11). Although significantly more children became dry during treatment than with placebo (RR for failure to achieve 14 consecutive dry nights with 20 mcg 0.84, 95% CI 0.79 to 0.91), it was notable that only 28 out of 146 (19%) who received desmopressin became dry.

There is strong evidence that short courses of desmopressin offer no persisting benefit, in that wetting recurs once treatment stops (Glazener and Evans 2005c). Some uncontrolled studies report a persisting benefit if used for 6 months or more (Hjalmus 1995). The drug can be taken long-term without any evidence of tolerance or alterations in innate regulation of urine concentration; the product licence does however recommend a short break from treatment every 3 months. The low frequency of adverse effects and its rapid onset of action make it ideal for short-term use to cover holidays or occasions where the child sleeps away from home.

Tricyclic antidepressants

Imipramine is the tricyclic antidepressant most often used for NE, though amitriptyline and nortriptyline are also used. How imipramine works in NE is not fully understood but it has a wide range of actions throughout the body, including central nervous system effects, anticholinergic effects and reducing urine output, which might contribute to its action.

Imipramine taken orally, has a very variable duration of action that makes it a difficult drug to use: the same dose may be ineffective for one patient and to high for another. This, combined with its wide range of actions is the reason that adverse effects are common. Gastrointestinal upset and CNS effects such as drowsiness, agitation and mood change are all common. In overdose its cardiotoxic effects (arrythmias) are potentially lethal. There is also a concern that it may cause arrythmias in therapeutic doses in susceptible individuals (Tingelstadt 1991).

There is good evidence that imipramine reduces wet nights by about one per week compared to placebo from 4 RCTs involving 443 patients (WMD –1.19, 95% CI –1.56 to –0.82). More children became dry when taking Imipramine compared to placebo (RR for failure 0.77, 95% CI 0.72 to 0.83), but this still only amounted to 86/400 (21%) (Glazener, Evans and Peto 2005c). As with desmopressin there is evidence that no benefit persists beyond the end of treatment.

Because imipramine is of limited effectiveness, has a high frequency of adverse effects and is particularly dangerous in overdose, most experts are reluctant to use it except in exceptional circumstances.

Anticholinergics

The recognition that occult detrusor overactivity is relatively common among children with NE has lead to renewed interest in the use of anticholinergic and bladder smooth muscle relaxants, such as oxybutinin. In two small placebo controlled studies of primary NE, oxybutinin was no more effective than placebo (Glazener, Evans and Peto 2005d). In one non-randomised study in children with bed-wetting associated with detrusor overactivity, the combination of oxybutinin and desmopressin was more effective than oxybutinin alone with approximately 70% 'responding' compared to 50% (Caione *et al.* 1997).

Whilst absolute proof that oxybutinin works is lacking, it is a relatively safe drug and it is reasonable to consider its use, in combination with desmopressin in children with NE associated with detrusor overactivity and in enuresis refractory to desmopressin on its own. A single night-time dose of 2.5 mg to 5 mg is a suitable starting dose.

Other drugs

Indomethacin, diclofenac, carbamazepine and diazepam have all been shown to reduce wetting compared to placebo but are not licensed for

Table 7.2 Treatments for continence problems: costs and benefits

Treatment	Patient Group	Benefits	Cost of treatment / risks to patient
Star Chart	All	Small percentage get dry Motivational tool	None
Alarm	All *except* when psychosocial difficulties within family or adverse circumstances (including a lack of motivation) preclude alarm usage and infrequent wetters	Of those undertaking treatment, 2/3 will get dry and 1/3 will get dry and remain dry after treatment stops. Success may be improved if combined with 'dry bed training' Overlearning may reduce relapse rate	£70 for a typical alarm (2007 prices) Drop-out rate high because it is hard work for child and carer
Desmopressin	Monosymptomatic NE most effective in those with nocturnal polyuric and normal bladder	Rapid response, 2/3 improve but a minority are completely dry and few stay dry when treatment stops. Prolonged use (over 6 months) *may* be associated with greater response	£92 (3 months) (£184 if on max dose) Adverse effects uncommon
Imipramine	All *except* those with medical contraindications to imipramine such as cardiac disease and epilepsy	2/3 improve, few get dry and very few stay dry	£3 (3 months) Adverse effects frequent and may be severe
Oxybutinin	Bladder dysfunction	Some evidence of improvement. Better if combined with desmopressin	£35 (3 months) Adverse effects frequent but minor

this indication and, the latter two drugs in particular are far too toxic to merit serious consideration (Glazener, Evans and Peto 2005d).

Complementary therapies

Hypnosis, psychotherapy, acupuncture, chiropractic, dietary manipulation, faradisation, homeopathy have all been evaluated in controlled trials (Glazener, Cheuk and Evans 2005). There is no strong evidence that they are effective, because of methodological weaknesses in the studies. Among the treatments, acupuncture and psychotherapy appeared most promising. Despite the fact that these treatments are widely used in practice, current evidence does not support their widespread use until proper randomised trials have demonstrated their effectiveness.

Conclusion

Nocturnal enuresis is one of the most common of childhood disorders. There are a range of established treatments that mean most children can be helped, either by effecting a cure through successful alarm treatment or by controlling or improving the wetting through medication. As the underlying causes of NE are identified it is now possible to target treatment more effectively accounting for both the pathology and the patient and carer needs and preferences.

References

Bradbury MG, Meadow SR (1995) Combined treatment with enuresis alarm and desmopressin for nocturnal enuresis. *Acta Paediatrica*, 84: 1014–18

Caione P, Arena F, Biraghi M, Cigna RM, Chendi D *et al.* (1997) Nocturnal enuresis and daytime wetting: a multicentric trial with oxybutinin and desmopressin. *European Urology*, 31: 459–63

Eiberg H, Berendt I, Mohr J (1995) Assignment of dominant inherited nocturnal enuresis (ENUR1) to chromosome 13q. *Nature Genetics*, 10: 354–6

Gibbs S, Nolan T, South M, Noad L, Bates G, Vidmar S (2004) Evidence against a synergistic effect of desmopressin with conditioning in the treatment of nocturnal enuresis. *Journal of Pediatrics*,144 (3): 351–7

Glazener CMA, Cheuk D, Evans JHC (2000) Complementary and miscellaneous interventions for nocturnal enuresis in children (Cochrane Review). *The Cochrane Library*, Chichester: John Wiley & Sons

Glazener CMA, Evans JHC (2005a) Simple behavioural and physical interventions for nocturnal enuresis in children (Cochrane Review). The Cochrane Library, Issue 1. Chichester: John Wiley & Sons

Glazener CMA, Evans JHC (2005b) Desmopressin for nocturnal enuresis in children (Cochrane Review). The Cochrane Library, Issue 1. Chichester: John Wiley & Sons

Glazener CMA, Evans JHC, Peto RE (2005a) *Alarm interventions for nocturnal enuresis in children (Cochrane Review)* The Cochrane Library, Issue 1. Chichester: John Wiley & Sons

Glazener CMA, Evans JHC, Peto RE (2005b) Complex behavioural and educational interventions for nocturnal enuresis in children (Cochrane Review). The Cochrane Library, Issue 1. Chichester: John Wiley & Sons

Glazener CMA, Evans JHC, Peto RE (2005c) Tricyclic and related drugs for nocturnal enuresis in children (Cochrane Review). The Cochrane Library, Issue 1. Chichester: John Wiley & Sons

Glazener CMA, Evans JHC, Peto RE (2005d) Drugs for nocturnal enuresis in children (other than desmopressin and tricyclics) (Cochrane Review). The Cochrane Library, Issue 1. Chichester: John Wiley & Sons

Hjalmas K (1995) SWEET, the Swedish enuresis trial. *Scandinavian Journal of Urology & Nephrology*, 173 (suppl): 89–93

Hunsballe JM, Rittig S, Djurhuus JC (1995) Sleep and arousal in adolescents and adults with nocturnal enuresis. *Scandinavian Journal of Urology & Nephrology*, 173 (suppl): 59–61

Medel R, Ruarte AC, Castera R, Podesta ML (1998) Primary enuresis: a urodynamic evaluation. *British Journal of Urology*, 81 (suppl 3): 50–52

Norgaard JP, Pedersen EB, Djurhuus JC (1985) Diurnal antidiuretic hormone levels in enuretics. *Journal of Urology*, 134: 1029–31

Norgaard JP, Van Gool JD, Hjalmas K, Djurhuus, Hellstrom AL (1998) Standardization and definitions in lower urinary tract dysfunction in children. *British Journal of Urology*, 81 (suppl 3): 1–16

Tingelstadt JB, (1991) The cardiotoxicity of tricyclics. *Journal of the American Academy of Child and Adolescent Psychiatry*, 30: 845–6

8 Faecal soiling in childhood

Kenneth Wilkinson

Key Points

- The subject of this chapter is soiling due to faecal overloading. Faecal overloading is often associated with constipation and is the most common cause of soiling in children.

- Treatment requires the rectum to be regularly emptied.

- Initial treatment is aimed at getting the lower bowel empty. Continence may come later. The family and child need close support at this stage.

- There is a progression in treatment from bowel emptying, to maintenance treatment, to resolution.

- Treatment will take months or years.

- Sometimes predictable incontinence may have to be an acceptable solution at least in the short term.

- Defecation in infancy occurs by a reflex act. This comes under voluntary (psychological) control with age.

Health promotion points

- Achieving continence is a process of achieving a pattern of behaviour. For all behaviours, wise parents reward good behaviour and not bad behaviour.

- For the bowels this system often breaks down due to a mixture of dietary, environmental and psychological factors. These are all amenable to health promotion.

Constipation is the most common cause of soiling. The chapter describes key questions useful for making the diagnosis and deciding on the most appropriate treatment. How to ensure compliance with treatment and making the switch from medical (drug) management to dietary and behaviour management is also discussed. For some children continence will not be attained and regulated incontinence may have to be the goal. Bowel activity involves an interplay between diet, psychology, environment and medical treatment. All four need to be adjusted or discussed at various stages to facilitate success. Techniques of approaching these areas and dealing with specific problems are described.

Promoting health

Nutrition

Breast milk produces soft stools whereas formula milks based on cows' milk often lead to hard stools, which may be painful. Breastfeeding should therefore be encouraged. Because of this problem with formula milks it is likely that more manufacturers will modify their milks for example by adding probiotic oligosaccharides. Weaning on to foods with increased fibre, fruit and vegetables may help. Reducing milk intake in the later stages of the weaning process also helps. Regular intermittent meals and not snacking are better able to produce a gastrocolic reflex and bowel emptying. Increased exercise facilitates bowel function. Many advocate increasing water drinks.

Health promotion and the home environment

As our homes become smarter and more sanitised, mistakes such as bowel leaks become far less acceptable – and a child's fear of an accident increases. This may lead to holding-on behaviour. The ease of disposable nappies reduces the effort that parents put into toilet training because of the immediate gains, the need for far less effort relative to having to wash and dry fabric nappies. Houses with children need to be child-friendly and tolerant of the accidents that occur during the learning of any new skill.

Health promotion and psychological health

The language of bowel control is not always useful. We would not, for instance, think too much about someone saying, 'He's filled his nappy – you have him.' Yet, as far as the child, is concerned the offending stool is his creation. So he and his creation are being rejected.

There are few – if any – pretty or encouraging words to describe bowel opening. The child cannot be blamed for concluding this is something not to be talked about. Factors such as this, plus an intrinsic tendency to diet-related constipation leads to painful defecation. We all try to avoid pain – why should a child be any different? If having the bowels opened causes physical or psychological pain, then of course the child will try not to do it again. Unfortunately this is not the solution: a cycle of pain, retention, more constipation and more pain can develop until the holding-on behaviour causes loss of bowel control. Loss of bowel control can in turn lead to disapproval, low self-worth and more psychological pain.

Definitions

This chapter concerns constipation and soiling. *Constipation* implies overloading the bowel. Overloading the lowest part of the bowel, the rectum, causes the anal sphincters to leak. *Soiling* is the involuntary passage of faeces at an inappropriate age, usually into the under-clothes. The condition is often called *encopresis* to make an analogy with enuresis. Some use the term *encopresis* to mean passage of normal stools from a normal bowel in inappropriate places, e.g. smearing. Parents cannot easily understand the term *encopresis*, although most understand the meaning of *soiling*. Furthermore, there is confusion in the use of the term *constipated*. Many parents see it as passing hard stools. Others see it as passing big stools and yet others as passing infrequent stools. Whichever definition of constipation is used, the breakdown of the control mechanism is due to *overloading*. This occurs when faeces accumulate to form a big lump, which may be hard or putty like. Soiling is the result of overloading and is therefore a symptom and not the cause. By not using the term 'constipation' but the term 'overloading' I find my ideas more quickly agree with those of the family. Many medical conditions at first described by a symptom (soiling) are later described by the cause (faecal overloading) as they become better understood.

Prevalence

Boys are more likely to be affected by this problems than girls. Blackwell, quoting Lukeman (1997), gives the following table.

Table 8.1 Guidelines for childhood soiling

Age in Years	Boys	Girls
3	11%	5.2%
5	3.5%	1%
7	2.4%	0.7%
10–12	1.2%	0.3%

Source: Blackwell C (2003) *A Guide to Encoporesis*, revised ed. Bristol: ERIC

The problem with all definitions of prevalence is how we define the cut-off points. The child who has an accidental skid mark once a year is not likely to come to attention other than to a parent. Is once a month often enough to make a diagnosis of soiling? If it is, for how many months must it occur?

Soiling is common. It damages lives and makes parents like their children less.

It makes children not want to go to school or do PE. It causes children to dislike themselves. It is associated with urinary infection and it can be the cause of both daytime and night-time wetting.

Aetiology

Not all soiling is due to faecal overload, but the majority is and that is what forms the subject of this chapter. The primary problem is over-filling of the lower bowel leading to loss of control by the anal sphincters and leakage. This overloading, with time, destroys the sensitivity and reflex responses of the control mechanism. It is the disruption of the normal physiology of the lower bowel that causes the problem. Diagrammatic representation of the structures involved can be found in Figures 5.1 and 5.2 in Chapter 5 on 'Anorectal anatomy and physiology' by Anton Emmanuel.

In the resting state there is a bend in the system due to the pubo-coccygeal sling. This and other bends of the sigmoid (bendy) colon slow down the descent of faeces just as 'S' bends slow down a car. The sphincters only have a secondary or safety role. Faeces are now in the anal canal and the sharp pubo-coccygeal bend is opened out.

Depending on the sensitivities of the child and family, I may use the analogy of a gun. The gun is safe in the normal resting state, the firing chamber below the internal anal sphincter is empty and the safety catch, in the form of the ano-coccygeal sling, is on. Once faeces are below the ano-coccygeal sling then a shell (or bullet) is now in the firing chamber, the safety catch is off, because the ano-coccygeal sling is now straightened out. From now on there are only three options:

1 Go to the toilet or potty and let it out.

2 Tighten up the external anal sphincter and nibble it back up until the next time.

3 Repeat action 2 to a point where the physiological limit is reached. This will lead to overloading and leakage.

The three options

If trying to let the faeces out, the child goes to an appropriate place, toilet or potty, leans forward to help straighten out the rectocolic angle at the pubo-coccygeal sling and perhaps grunts a bit by breathing against a closed glottis to increase intra abdominal pressure, then with descent of the stool into the anal canal there is a reflex peristaltic rush and success with the relief of any abdominal discomfort. Many can also initiate a defecation starting with an empty anal canal just by sitting, leaning forward and grunting thereby forcing a stool down into the anal canal and once the stool is in the 'firing chamber' this in turn initiates the peristaltic rush.

If the child goes for the second option, then he or she needs to tighten up the external anal sphincter and move the stool from the firing chamber back up above the ano-coccygeal sling. This in itself is not a bad thing to do; we all have to learn to put off defecation – or for that matter urination – if the situation demands it. This 'nibbling' process requires some skill and effort. If we find anything difficult, it is likely to show in our faces as an 'overflow of neuronal activity'. It is very difficult to tighten up the external anal sphincter while leaning forward, so to make it easier we stand erect and clench our buttocks. A child does the same. Mothers usually recognise the bottom clenching as holding-on behaviour, or do so after explanation. The child who bends backward and groans on the toilet is trying to hold on to a stool, what they are not trying to do is have their bowel opened. Children are well aware of this bottom nibbling behaviour; it is very difficult indeed to tighten up the anal sphincters if bending forward. Children seem to understand the term 'bottom nibbling'.

It is rare for the third option to be adopted through a deliberate act of will. Parents may think children who do this are wilful, but if you ask the children themselves whether they would like to be clean, unless there truly is some deep psychological problem it won't take them long to decide in the affirmative. What is usually happening is that option 2 has been tried, but the child is so full of faeces that the task of pushing it back up again is impossible. After a while the external sphincter tires and there is either a leak or a big lump slips out. Once this stage has been reached various vicious circles further increase the problem. The retained faecal mass is occasionally passed causing pain and leading to a wish never to pass a big stool again and hence further holding-on. The distended bowel becomes progressively less sensitive to further overloading. The overused external sphincter probably gets stronger and stronger at holding on causing further distension and loss of sensitivity. There is an occasional child who stays clean or keeps accidents to a minimum who has solved things by rushing to the toilet once the external sphincter is felt to dilate beyond the point of retrieval.

It should be emphasised that bottom nibbling is not wrong in itself. The problem is that it only works so many times. Eventually, such a large quantity if faeces will have accumulated and want to come out, that pushing or nibbling it back up will fail. Sometimes, by rewarding a child for being clean, parents are inadvertently rewarding him or her for the very activity which when continued causes soiling.

Assessment

This comprises history and examination. The history will be as for any child with a problem but will involve some questions specific to the condition. The history should be taken confidently and without embarrassment. The questions in themselves often lead to the family understanding the condition.

1 *Did (name of child) open his/her bowels in the first 48 hours after birth?*
   This question is specifically directed to try to exclude
   Hirschsprung's disease. Children with Hirschsprung's disease
   generally have trouble in passing meconium in the first 48 hours.

2 *Tell me about your child's early feeding and bowel activity*
   The breastfeeding period is usually uneventful. The average infant
   does not pass stools that can be rolled around, but several a day

that are soft and will mould to the bottom. Many parents think that a one-year-old who passes one stool a day that can roll off the nappy is normal and so need to know that three a day which are moulded to the bottom are more normal. Fully breastfed babies can be very variable in bowel frequency. They can also change bowel frequency from a small amount after every feed due to the gastro-colic reflex or several days between bowel actions.

3 *How long has this problem been going on?*
This may determine the severity of the problem and length of treatment needed.

4 *Describe the problem. What can you see?*
Ask about bleeding on or after the stool, pain, holding on behaviour. The parents may think going stiff-legged is trying to go – it is not!

5 *Does your child sometimes pass very big stools?*
This is a question to exclude Hirschsprung's disease – children with this condition do not pass big stools but children with holding on behaviour usually do. If the child *never* passes big stools then the diagnosis of soiling being due to holding on behaviour should be questioned. Hirschsprung's disease must be considered. The parents of a typical child who is retaining faeces often say that finally passing a giant stool sometimes blocks the toilet.

6 *Is your child well?*
Most children who soil are well unless they are grossly distended with a large abdominal mass.

7 *Does your child have wetting problems?*
Both daytime and night-time wetting can be associated with constipation because of pressure effects on the bladder. There may be shared control problems. Urine infections are also associated with constipation.

8 *Is there mucus or blood in the stool?*
If there is, it may suggest inflammatory bowel disease.

9 *Is there any family history of bowel problems?*
The family need to know you are thinking about bowel diseases. A diseased bowel works badly at what it is meant to do, that is removing food and water from the gut. The intestines of soiling children work too well!

10 *Where does your child go to open his or her bowels?*
Children often hide or go behind the settee or curtains, indicating
an awareness of rectal sensation. But some children show no
signs at all, often an indication of overflow soiling.

11 *How does the problem make you, as parents, feel?*
What about other relatives?
Bowel activity may be under psychological control.

12 *Does your child **ever** use the potty or toilet?*
The question, put like this, identifies the younger child who is not
yet toilet trained, but is also much less embarrassing for the older
child. This question is preferred to asking *when* the child uses the
potty or toilet, and gives encouragement if he does.

13 *Where does you child hide the dirty underwear?*
Children almost always do, and asking the question this way
round saves both time and embarrassment.

14 *What has been tried and what works best?*
This question stops you looking silly by revealing what the family
see as useless. It also tells you what the family are likely to accept.

15 *Does your child have tummy pain, and if so where?*
Be careful about dismissing abdominal pains that are not central
or midline. Waking at night with pain is not usual as the large
bowel tends to rest at night even when overloaded. Pain can
occur as a result of treatment, in which case this needs to be
given at a different time. The child may have pain from the
gastrocolic reflex. This pain is central and is colicky in nature,
worse on eating or shortly after. The child who gets this pain may
have learned to only take snacks. Many mothers say that their
child stops eating when they have not had their bowels open.
Explaining the condition explains the pain.

16 *How many sheets of paper are needed for bottom wiping?*
This is really a question about whether stool is stuck in the anal
canal. A big stool remains in the anal canal and pokes its nose
out. This results in perpetual bottom wiping but never getting
clean. Often one hears of the child who is fine but just 'lazy' and
is said not to wipe his bottom. Is this really true or is he a child
with retention?

Finally, a question to the child: Do you want to be clean?

If the answer is no then psychological help may be needed. The autistic child or child with learning difficulties should also be identified during these discussions.

A note on toys: My practice is not to have toys in clinic. The child needs to hear about his problem. The normal child doesn't want his mother to tell anyone – especially a stranger – about it. Toys are a distraction. The embarrassed (usual) child uses toys (especially noisy ones) to stop the clinic working effectively.

The response to treatment

If the diagnosis is correct, the response to treatment will be predictable. If it doesn't follow the expected pattern, re-question the diagnosis.

Examination

A general physical examination should be performed. It is important to record and plot height and weight. If weight is low for height, inflammatory bowel disease needs to be considered along with other causes of chronic illness. A high weight for height or growth slowing could point to hypothyroidism.

A neurological examination should be included specifically looking for a spinal anomaly, a flat bottom, a patulous anus or up-going plantar reflexes, all of which indicate a possible neurological cause of soiling.

Feeling the abdomen may reveal a mass of faeces, this may extend above the umbilicus from the pelvis. In most cases nothing abnormal is found.

Examine the anus. Does it look normal and is it in the correct place? If it is not, you need a surgical opinion.

I do not routinely do a rectal examination unless the history is atypical or response to treatment is not as expected. Specific consent must be obtained.

The classic retentive soiler will have a rectum with faeces in it. This may not be the case if they have just had a clear out. Examination of the bottom frequently shows soft faeces that have oozed out and you may see a faecal 'nose' on separating the buttocks. There may be anal dilatation on buttock separation revealing a 'nose' of faeces poking out. This dilatation has sometimes erroneously been ascribed to sexual abuse. Touching the perianal area with a blunt orange stick or split tongue depressor can be used to test sensation.

Investigations

These are usually not essential. Plain abdominal X-ray may help. However a child on a high fibre diet may also appear to have a loaded colon. The problem is also not necessarily one of an overloaded abdomen but an overloaded rectum. If looking for an overloaded colon you may be looking for something associated in many cases with the problem but not the actual site of the problem. Some centres measure bowel transit time in some patients using swallowed radio opaque markers.

Blood tests can exclude certain other conditions (such as hypothyroidism) but are not routine. They may be called for if the outcome of treatment is not as expected. (See also Chapter 6 on 'Investigations for bladder problems' by Rosie Kelly.)

Treatment

Co-operation in treatment is essential but, if it is to be achieved, the patient and family must first understand why the treatment is necessary. I use a length of tubilast and crème eggs, or tubilast and conkers, to demonstrate this laying it out as shown in Figure 8.1. Medical treatments are aimed at getting and keeping the anal canal empty. This is the opposite of what the child has been doing. Parents know that one can grunt a stool out, that one leans forward and pushes, they have usually just not thought why. The consequences of holding-on behaviour, loss of the pubo-coccygeal angle can be demonstrated. Why holding on always eventually fails can be demonstrated. The patient or parent can be invited to push two, three or four 'eggs' along the tube with one hand. With each extra egg it gets proportionately more difficult. The effect of having a large stool in the anal canal can also be shown (i.e. it holds the external anal sphincter ajar). The stool pushes at the 'back door' and the little runny stools leak out. These are sometimes known as *leakers*. Sometimes the bottom gets tired, the floodgates open and a large one is dropped. These are sometimes known as *sneakers* as the child is often unaware. This may well be true. The anal canal is a sensitive sampling chamber. It can (when working well) tell you if it is holding solids or gas. Regular over-distension causes loss of

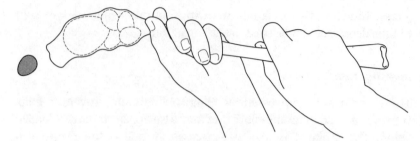

Figure 8.1 Using tubilast and chocolate eggs
to demonstrate the 'sneaker'

sensation. This is a common physiological mechanism, the faeces being the stimulus. The longer and stronger the stimulus is applied the less aware one becomes (e.g. loud noises became less loud; bright lights less bright; new sheets or clothes only feel new for a short time). The cause of soiling with holding on behaviour is the holding on behaviour. Just as a bladder can only hold so much urine, or a child carry only so many cups, a bowel can only hold so much faeces. The holding-on behaviour itself may have dietary, environmental or psychological causes. Holding on itself is not 'naughtiness'. We all do it. We all have to learn to do it. It is when it is practised to excess that, instead of causing cleanliness, it causes soiling.

Dietary intervention

Parents often want to know what they did wrong. The answer is likely to be nothing, but you may have to discuss diet. The digestive system starts with the teeth, the smaller something is cut up or chewed the easier it is for the digestive juices to get to work and digest it. What goes into the mouth starts on the farm or in the sea, but usually passes through a food processor or supermarket. On the way it is often ground up (e.g. to make flour). This grinding is in to much smaller pieces than our teeth would do. The child doesn't need teeth to eat cake. In the past, food was unprocessed and grinding it was hard (hence the expression 'the daily grind'). Cooking also makes things more digestible. We could eat raw vegetables but mostly we choose not to. We could eat uncooked potatoes. We could eat boiled whole wheat for breakfast as I did as a child but now I eat porridge. Grinding and cooking processes aid digestion but it all makes it too easy for our guts. In just a few generations we have gone from a rough to a refined diet. The gut digests the food and absorbs the water. With such effective digestion there is little to hold the water in the bowel, resulting in hard stools.

There is little to be gained by telling mothers all this, however, for what can they do? They think that they give their child a healthy diet, and they probably do. But it may well not be the diet our guts need, and is certainly not what was eaten a few generations ago. The problems of a soiling child will not usually be solved just by a dietary change. Such a change may soften the stools but if there is still an anal lump it will just make the leaking worse. The occasional family will succeed by giving prune juice every day. Dietary adjustments are useful in prevention and recovery and are also discussed under 'Promoting health' and 'Recovery to discharge'.

Psychological factors

If the family have understood the physiology, then they can understand that overloading is the problem. They will also be able to understand that holding on is part of what we all do or need to learn, but that trying too hard may lead to a disaster. They need to accept that mistakes happen while a skill is being learned. The child who soils only at home is the child who feels safer at home and is not trying to irritate the family. The child who hides his dirty pants just wants to run away from his problems in the same way that adults might hide a bill. Once the child experiences pain on defecation, a vicious circle sets in. Fortunately most parents, at least in clinic, can act in a supportive way.

Having one's bowels open is something that most children learn to regulate at the age of around 2 years. It is the anal stage of development, during which the child learns control over whether or not to produce a stool. If the stool is greeted with disgust, then the child may decide not to produce one. If pain occurs, then the pain tells the child not to do this again. Normal psychology can so easily be turned to the child's disadvantage. Externalisation is a technique used to help separate the thinking of 'the poo problem' and the child, i.e. 'the poo' can be seen as the common enemy and the child and parents can be united in overcoming it. (See also Chapter 12 on 'Psychological issues of incontinence' by Melinda Edwards.)

Medical treatment

Medical treatments are aimed at getting and keeping the anal canal empty. The first phase is sometimes called 'the disimpaction phase', this is the opposite of what the child has been doing. This can be achieved by enema, by suppository or by stimulant laxatives given by mouth. Enemas and suppositories work quickly and are more predictable, but generally less acceptable, than stimulant laxatives given by mouth. If oral stimulant laxatives have failed, the parents or child may welcome suppositories or enemas. For the child with learning difficulties, mobility problems or autism, it may sometimes be better to start with predictable incontinence on treatment and progress from there; this may require rectally administered treatments.

Manual evacuation may occasionally be needed in a child who has a greatly distended bowel, for example with a faecal lump which is palpable up to the umbilicus or where faecal impaction interferes with breathing or bladder emptying.

Movicol paediatric (a macrogol) is a relatively new product (2004) on the UK market but not in the USA. The drug data sheet indicates how to use it. It works by retaining fluid in the gut but, unlike lactulose, seems to be able to break down large lumps and is sufficiently potent to be useful for disimpaction. The object of disimpaction is to empty the rectum and the worst thing one can do is fail to empty the rectum. Unless the rectum is emptied, the child may be more leaky than before. The remaining rectal lump of faeces will hold the external anal sphincter open. In this situation, treatment – especially with stool softeners – will cause the faeces above the obstruction to become softer and more leaky. This will make the situation worse. Macrogols are very effective, but compared with stimulant laxatives are less predictable in terms of when a bowel action will occur. This is because macrogols have an action that persists within the bowel. The stimulant laxatives reach a crescendo of activity which then wanes. For the individual child with imperfect bowel control, finding this peak will allow life to be lived around the medication more easily than with a macrogol. If the rectum is empty, frequent soiling should be replaced by infrequent soiling. This is because, once the rectum is empty, it will act as a reservoir filling up between dosages of medication.

Follow-up needs to be arranged within days after an enema, or within a week or two of starting treatment to ensure that continual soiling has stopped. If not, rectal examination may be needed.

Following the disimpaction phase, the next stage is the maintenance phase. This is likely to involve the continuing use of stimulant laxatives by mouth.

Dosages of stimulant laxatives to be given by mouth

The dosages needed are much higher than previously used. The Royal College of Paediatrics and Child Health gives guidance in *the British National Formulary for Children (BNFC)*. Formerly known as *Medicines for Children*, this publication includes expected time for each medicine to take effect.

For stimulant laxatives the purpose of treatment is to cause the bowel to contract sufficiently vigorously to empty the lower bowel. An insufficient dose will just cause pain and this in turn may lead the family to reduce the dose. A lower dose will continue to be ineffective. The younger the child the more difficult it is to overcome holding-on behaviour by talking therapies. Higher doses than those recommended in the British National Formulary for Children (RCPCH 2006) are needed. According to Clayden *et al.* (2005), the dose suggested for all children over one is the same (see Tables 8.2 and 8.3). This reflects the reality of my practice: the table gives the range of dosage which parents tell me is effective. Personal communication with the BNFC reveals that this is an area under discussion. There may well be a gap between the licensed and the 'real' doses. Alternatively there may be a gap between what works in primary and secondary care.

Table 8.2 Prescribing advice: Senna

Dosage of Senna 7.5 mg /5ml		
RCPCH 2006	**Clayden et al. (2005)**	**Parents' views**
1 month–2 years: 0.5 ml/Kg max 2.5 ml daily	**Aged over 1 year:** 2.5 ml increasing to a maximum of 25 mls (from Clayden's flow sheet)	Insufficient data
2–6 years: 2.5–5 ml daily in morning		7–10 mls at night
6–12 years: 5–10 ml daily night or morning		10–15mls at night
12–18 years: 10–20 mls daily usually bed time		Insufficient data

Table 8.3 Prescribing advice: Sodium picosulfate

Dosage of Sodium picosulfate 1 mg = 1 ml		
RCPCH 2006	**Clayden et al. (2005)**	**Parents' views**
2–4 years: 250 ĺg/kg, max 5 mg at night	**Above 1 year:** 5–10 mls*	5–10 mls
4–10 years: 2.5–5 mg at night		7.5–10 mls
10–18 years: 5–10 mg at night Text indicates recommended doses may be exceeded on specialist advice.		Insufficient data

*In his text Clayden states sodium picosulfate can be exchanged for forms of senna in the flow sheet.

Timing of dosing

Through the night most children with soiling due to retained stool are clean because the external anal sphincter tightens up. The analogy of a bird's feet tightening on the branch when it is asleep may be used. It is rare for stimulant laxatives given at bed time to work until the next day. For both reasons stimulant laxatives are best given at bed time. The peak time for normal bowel activity is around breakfast time. This is the time when the child should be encouraged to try to go to the toilet or use the potty. If the time when toileting is induced is inconvenient (for example the medication works at midday when the child is at school and doesn't like to use the toilet), then my advice would be to move the time of administration forward. Do not move it too far forward or the medication may try to work during the night and will have lost its effect by morning. If the above plan does not work, or if the child gets pain in the night, then I would move treatment to breakfast time with the hope of a bowel action between coming home from school and going to bed.

Dosing frequency

This depends partly on what the agreed objective happens to be. A child may come to clinic because of school refusal due to regular soiling. For this child it may be best to give stimulant laxatives on Friday and Saturday nights with the hope of good bowel evacuations on the following days, with a further dose on Tuesday night and a day off school on Wednesday. During the holidays, daily dosing may be best. Emptying the bowel once a day achieves regularity and gives plenty of opportunities to practise skills.

With an autistic child, the initial target may be predictable incontinence with later plans for predictable continence. The big advantage of predictable incontinence is that it gives the family some social freedoms for holidays and school trips. Being clean at the Mosque can be most important. It may be that only one parent can cope with the incontinence and it can be timed accordingly. For some other children, the aim of immediate continence may not be achieved and good predictable emptying of the lower bowel, with predictable continence at other times, gives the parents and child a break. If predictable incontinence is the aim, less than daily dosing is used. The child could then be expected to stay clean on days following no medication. Predictable but infrequent, even if it is every four days, is preferable to frequent and unpredictable.

It may be that the child manages to achieve continence with daily medication, but only has a bowel action every other day. If this happens, there is probably no point in giving stimulant laxatives on a daily basis as medication is likely to be wasted or cause abdominal cramps. The reason why the medication may not work every day is a physiological one. The more distended the bowel, the more likely it is to contract – it is the stretching of the bowel that causes it to contract. This reflex occurs even in the less sensitive stretched bowel. It may be that, at first, the stretched bowel will only respond infrequently. This phenomenon explains why the dosages needed for maintenance are as high – or higher – than those needed for disimpaction. The parents need to know this, or they will reduce the dose with the likely result that the child will fill up again. I advise the parents to ring me first if they plan to reduce the dose. If the child suffers pain but does not open his bowels then the muscles are squeezing hard enough to cause pain but not to empty the bowel. Increase the dose or reduce medication frequency. What is *not* needed at this stage is a family who keep trying to stop the stimulant laxatives. This will cause the child pain and reintroduce the original problem of 'holding on'. Keeping the lower bowel regularly empty, either with stimulant oral laxatives or suppositories, usually leads to improvement even if continence is not at first achieved. Occasionally stimulant laxatives may fail because of the time of day when they are given as discussed above under 'Timing of dosing'.

Which laxative to use?

Any medication that empties the lower bowel is suitable. Sodium pico-sulfate has a faster effect but shorter duration of activity than senna and is, in most cases, my starter choice. Other professionals may be more familiar with other medications. The medication has to be one that the child will take. Some children will refuse to take certain medi-cines, for example if they don't like the taste. A change of medication is reasonable. What is not permitted is not taking any medication.

My choice is to avoid using stool softeners in children with holding-on behaviour; the thinking behind this being that stool softeners make it easy to go, but they do not make you go. They are also likely not to cause the abdominal feelings that remind the child of the need to go to the toilet. Lactulose at this stage often seems to give a rectal lump a leaky sugary coating and make matters worse. While some profession-als argue that stool softeners should be used to reduce pain, they will not (apart from Movicol) break up an established mass. Stimulant lax-atives alone can move the faeces on before they become hard. Giving one medicine only is easier for everyone to understand and comply with.

What if the child gets pain?

Contractions in a loaded bowel will cause pain. Once the bowel is empty the pain goes. If there is pain and no bowel action then either the dose should be increased or a different stimulant laxative used (e.g. a change from senna to sodium picosulfate). If the pain is followed shortly by profuse diarrhoea, then the dose should be reduced. If, how-ever, you reduce the dose too much to produce a 'normal' stool you run the danger of returning to an overloaded state.

Persuading the child to use a toilet or potty

In my experience, many children in the 3–6 year age range with soiling have difficulty giving up nappies even though they may be skilful at using the toilet for bladder function. These children may think that the nappy is the right place. Others may only allow their bowels to open behind the settee or curtains. This is not that unusual behaviour in the sense that we adults do not feel comfortable in having our bowels open in public. A process called backward chaining can be used in this situ-ation. The child is only put in the nappy in the bathroom and then once this is achieved he is encouraged to open the bowels with the nappy on while sitting on the toilet. The nappy can then be put on loosely or put in the toilet or even used with a hole in it. For the child who insists on hiding behind the settee, the potty can be put there.

Young children exhibit animistic behaviour. One of the characteristics of this is to ascribe life to lifeless things. Thomas the Tank Engine certainly has feelings to a child. 'Poos' also have feelings. Since the child 'creates' them, he has a duty to look after them: he should not keep them in when they want to come out, and let them do what they want to do. Children can be persuaded that poos like to dive and swim and be with the mummy and daddy poos. This animistic approach in my work is very useful in helping turn the child from holding on to letting go. Although the parent is important in terms of following advice, it is the child who has to change. Talking to parents is discussed in Chapter 2 by Ruth Emery.

Recovery to discharge

This is the third stage and follows the maintenance period. The family should be left in no doubt that it is a 'long journey'. Buchanan and Clayden's (1992) book *Children who Soil* (see pages 133–4) indicates that months or years will be needed. As a rule of thumb, it takes about as long to treat as the condition has lasted for. The exact duration depends a lot on changing the behaviour of the child. If the child still shows signs of holding on, then treatment – as for maintenance – needs to continue. When the child is always clean and happy to use the toilet regularly then one can consider withdrawing stimulant laxatives. During the recovery phase the physiology of the lower bowel has recovered to the extent that the child can feel when a stool has entered the anal canal and wants to be let out. At this stage, the use of lactulose or Fybogel and diet comes to the forefront. There is a school of thought that milk allergy causes constipation. Our ancestors certainly knew that the casein in milk made a good glue and one observes this if you let milk bottles dry out. The question as to whether milk causes problems by its constituents or because of allergy has not been answered. I recommend a maximum intake of not above a pint or 500 mls of milk in total a day. While drinks are good at maintaining hydration and can stimulate the gastrocolic reflex, sugar containing drinks provide energy but no fibre. High fibre diet is recommended in the recovery to discharge phase. There are many high fibre foods on the market which children will not eat, but they will usually eat Weetabix.

Some families use skimmed milk on Weetabix, which makes it soggy and unpalatable while denying children the fat soluble vitamins A and D. Most children will eat beans and peas, and many snack on sultanas and raisins. A lot of children will eat fruit. Changing the diet in this way makes the bowel less likely to become constipated. The child needs to go to the toilet after breakfast and, if not successful, after other meals as well. The child needs to know that they do not have to wait until they need a bowel action. They can go to the toilet after meals, sit on the toilet, lean forward to straighten the bowel and grunt out a 'poo'. A child who manages this is probably all right, but needs to be advised to revert back temporarily to stimulant laxatives should the need arise.

Information for patients and carers

The family should get a copy of the clinic letter. They need to have a contact number to ring if they think they need to change treatment or have other concerns. Otherwise the discussions are very much as outlined above. Many parents want you to treat their child so that he or she becomes continent instantly, producing solid stools just like an adult. The child who has experienced weeks of pain will not suddenly change. He or she will continue to try to hold on but your medication will gradually overcome that behaviour. The most important person to talk to is the patient. The person least likely to listen at least until there is some success, is the patient. It is important to develop skills to make that communication possible. If the clinic is set up like a toyshop it can be very distracting and the child is likely to be very noisy in an attempt to stop the family disclosing what, until then, has often been kept secret. Picture books for children that show how your insides work can help your communication and be a positive distraction.

Conclusion

Soiling in children is a common problem causing great distress and anger. Treatment of the established case takes months or years. Avoiding pain of a physical or psychological nature at and before the time of toileting is likely to be a wise investment. It is often a very secret condition. Those not involved in the management of these children can easily ignore it as a problem and make fun of those who are affected by it. This is no help to anybody.

References

Blackwell CL (2003) *A Guide to Encopresis,* revised ed. Bristol: ERIC

Buchanan A, Clayden G (1992) *Children Who Soil.* Chichester: John Wiley & Sons.

Candy DCA, Edwards D (2003) The management of chronic constipation. *Current Paediatrics,* 13: 101–106.

Clayden GS, Keshtgar AS, Carani-Rathwell I, Abhyankar A (2005) The Management of Chronic Constipation and Related Faecal Incontinence in Childhood. *Archives of Disease in Childhood: Education and Practice,* 90: ep58–ep67

ERIC (2001) Childhood Soiling: *Minimum standards of practice for treatment and service delivery – benchmarking guidelines.* Bristol: ERIC

Royal College of Paediatrics and Child Health (updated annually) *BNF for Children.* London: RCPCH (also available online from www.rcpch.ac.uk/publications)

9 Urinary tract infection in childhood

Jim Beattie

Key points

- Clinical features of urinary tract infection (UTI) are often non-specific and every young child with an unexplained fever should have a urine culture.

- A negative combination urine dipstix analysis does not exclude UTI, particularly in infants.

- All children should have a urinary tract ultrasound scan after a first proven UTI. Subsequent investigation should be dictated by age, presenting symptoms and family history.

- Vesico-ureteric reflux (VUR) is found in up to 30% of children with a history of UTI but renal scarring may occur in the absence of VUR.

- The pathogenesis of renal scarring in association with VUR is gender specific with prenatal dysplasia being predominant in boys and post infective scarring in girls.

- The long-term risk of hypertension in patients with unilateral renal scarring is very small but patients with bilateral renal scarring require lifelong review.

Health promotion points

- Encourage the child to help him or herself by the following measures:
  - adequate fluid intake;
  - good hygiene;
  - appropriate choice of clothes.

- Ensure the child understands the principles of double voiding and why it is helpful.

Controversy has never been far away from the subject of bacterial infection of the urinary tract (UTI), despite the numerous contributions in the scientific literature ranging from the pre-antibiotic era to the present day. The main areas of ongoing controversy are the pathogenesis of infection and the relationship to renal scarring, the management of vesico-ureteric reflux (VUR), the optimal investigative/imaging strategy and the long-term consequences.

Epidemiology

UTI is one of the most common bacterial diseases in children. A study of 7-year-old school entrants from Sweden (Hellstrom *et al.* 1991) showed that 8% of girls and 2% of boys had had a symptomatic UTI confirmed by urine culture and in half of these children the UTI was associated with fever. Serial epidemiological data from Sweden have consistently shown the incidence of first UTI is highest in the first year of life in both boys and girls reflecting the high level of awareness in primary and community care in that country. Unfortunately this epidemiological pattern has not been replicated in the UK where the peak incidence of referral of children with apparent first UTI is 2–5 years (Christian *et al.* 2000).

The overall prevalence of UTI is around 5% in febrile children aged 0–2 years but varies with race and gender. Caucasian children have a two to fourfold higher prevalence compared with African-American children, and females have a similarly higher prevalence than circumcised males. Caucasian females aged 0–2 years with a fever of $\geq 39°C$ will have a prevalence of UTI of 16% (Shaw *et al.* 1998). Finally the recurrence rate is around 50% in girls and 15% in boys.

Clinical presentation

Symptoms such as unexplained fever, poor feeding, anorexia, failure to thrive and irritability are more likely in the 0–2 year age group. In older children specific symptoms such as dysuria, increased urinary frequency, urgency, loin pain, wetting and frank haematuria are more likely. Other indications for urine culture are unexplained vomiting and/or abdominal pain, prolonged neonatal jaundice, hypertension and suspected sexual abuse.

It is helpful to distinguish 'upper tract' or acute pyelonephritic (APN) symptoms such as fever, lethargy, general malaise, vomiting and loin pain from 'lower tract' symptoms consistent with cystourethritis, such as non-specific abdominal pain, urgency, increased urinary frequency, wetting and frank haematuria. The risk of renal parenchymal abnormalities is higher with a history of 'upper tract' symptoms (Christian *et al.* 2000).

Diagnosis

Urine sampling

When a diagnosis of UTI is suspected the first step is to obtain a suitable urine specimen in order to confirm the diagnosis and identify the causative organism. In the continent child a mid-stream specimen of urine (MSSU) is the ideal, whereas in infants and toddlers an alternative method is necessary. With all the alternative techniques, the perineum in girls and the glans penis in boys should be cleaned with sterile water and no antiseptic solutions used.

In practice the clinical situation, in particular the necessity for immediate introduction of therapy, dictates the technique used. In the ill infant a suprapubic bladder aspirate (SPA), clean catch (CCU) or urethral catheter specimen (CSU) have sufficiently low contamination rates to allow treatment to be started immediately after the specimen has been obtained.

SPA, preferably under ultrasound guidance, is still regarded as the gold standard technique but is the most invasive of the three techniques. A CCU requires the carer to hold the child over a sterile container until he or she micturates. It is more time-consuming and requires a little patience but has the advantage over SPA and CSU techniques in being non-invasive. Some centres prefer to use CSU as an alternative to either SPA or CCU but, although more convenient, it is invasive and there is concern about trauma to the urethra – particularly in boys.

If for some reason none of the above techniques are possible *and* if it is deemed safe that treatment can be deferred, a sterile bag specimen or pad specimen can be used. The main disadvantage of both these techniques is the unacceptably high contamination rate and a positive result must be confirmed by an SPA, CCU or CSU specimen.

Definition of significant bacteriuria

The diagnosis of UTI is confirmed by microbiological methods, specifically the number of bacterial colony-forming units (CFU) in the inoculated urine specimen. The traditional criteria of $\geq 10^5$ CFU/ml was based on studies of adult women with a clinical diagnosis of either acute pyelonephritis or cystitis in whom 95% of the study group had $\geq 10^5$ CFU/ml in a clean voided urine specimen.

In infants and children, the probability of UTI using the above criteria is 80% if demonstrated on one clean voided and 95% if demonstrated on three specimens. If urine is obtained by SPA, any gram negative bacterial growth or $\geq 500-1000$ CFU/ml of gram positive bacteria is consistent with infection. The probability of infection in a CSU specimen is 95% if the colony count is $\geq 10^5$/ml, likely if 10^4-10^5, equivocal if 10^3-10^4, and unlikely if $< 10^3$.

Combination dipstix urinalysis and urine microscopy

The use of urine dipstix analysis for detecting a white blood cell enzyme, leucocyte esterase (LE) in combination with urinary nitrite, the latter based on the ability of most urinary pathogens to reduce dietary derived nitrate to nitrite, has become popular over recent years.

The main advantage for both the clinician and laboratory is that dipstix is more rapid and less expensive than urine microscopy. The sensitivity of the LE/nitrite combination in the child over the age of 2 years in whom symptoms are more reliable, is sufficiently high (around 80%) for the clinician to be confident that a negative result to both eliminates the need for a urine culture.

In the younger child the sensitivity of the above combination is lower, perhaps related to the increased frequency of bladder emptying and the low colony counts per positive culture if an SPA or CSU specimen is taken. In practice a lower threshold should always be applied for the use of urine culture in this age group (Gorelick and Shaw 1999).

Urine microscopy is routinely carried out in most microbiology laboratories, and the use of phase contrast microscopy and gram staining ensures a higher diagnostic sensitivity than combination dipstix urinalysis (Gorelick and Shaw 1999).

Urine transport

If a universal container is used and not immediately transported to the laboratory, the specimen should be stored at 4°C (domestic fridge temperature) to reduce the risk of multiplication of contaminating organisms.

Boric acid containers are popular in primary care because of the long shelf-life. Boric acid inhibits bacterial growth until the specimen is inoculated onto growth medium and it is important to ensure that the container is filled to the appropriate level to ensure that the concentration of boric acid is not too high.

The advantages of Dipslide containers that have a culture plate incorporated are increased rapidity of results as well as the ability to send the specimen from home through the postal system.

Asymptomatic bacteriuria

The prevalence of covert or asymptomatic bacteriuria (ASB) is 3% in infants and preschool children. The relevance is that identification of ASB merely indicates a possible 'at risk' patient group in that on investigation of school children with ASB, 30% have a history of symptomatic infection, 25% have VUR, and 15% have renal scarring (Aggarawal *et al.* 1991). However there is no evidence that screening for ASB prevents subsequent episodes of symptomatic infection or renal scarring.

Microbiology

The main offending organism in community-acquired bacterial UTI in childhood and the organism that has been subject to most study is *Escherichia coli* (*E coli*) that accounts for up to 75% of cases. The remaining 25% are caused by infection with *Enterococci*, *Klebsiella*, *Proteus*, *Serratia* and *Pseudomonas* species. Non-bacterial causes of UTI are relatively rare and include fungal (*Candida*) and viral (adenovirus, BK virus).

Treatment

The main aim, apart from resuscitative measures on presentation, is to initiate appropriate antibiotic therapy after a satisfactory urine culture has been obtained.

The 'best guess' oral antibiotics are trimethoprim, co-amoxiclav and cephradine but in the child who is systematically unwell, the young infant and those who are unable to tolerate oral therapy, an intravenous third generation cephalosporin or a combination of gentamicin and ampicillin should be used. If there is no response within 24–48 hours the initial antibiotic should be changed (see Figure 9.1).

The duration of therapy in the child with 'upper tract' infection should be 7–10 days and oral antibiotics are as effective as the intra-

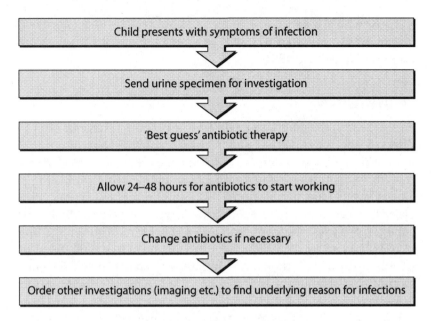

Figure 9.1 Treatment pathway

venous antibiotics with the important caveat that compliance with oral therapy is satisfactory (Craig and Hodson 2004). In the child with a 'lower tract' infection, a 2–4 day course is as effective as a 7–10 day course (Michael *et al.* 2002).

Prophylactic antibiotic therapy

Low dose antibiotic prophylaxis has been an accepted clinical practice for several years particularly in children who have a higher risk of recurrent infection and/or renal scarring. The antibiotics commonly used are trimethoprim (1–2 mg/kg), nitrofurantoin (1 mg/kg) and co-amoxiclav (0–1yr: 2.5ml, 1–6yrs:5ml of 125/31 solution; 6–12yrs: 5–10mls of 250/62 solution), given as a single dose at night. However, a recent evaluation of the literature highlighted that the evidence base for the effectiveness of this intervention is limited (Le Saux *et al.* 2000).

Pathogenesis of UTI

It is generally assumed that almost all bacterial UTI occurs via the ascending route, the organisms originating in the gastrointestinal tract. As with any infection, complex and not yet fully understood biological events underpin UTI and both bacterial and host factors are important in pathogenesis.

Bacterial factors

E coli has been the main subject in the study of uropathogenic mechanisms. A number of mechanisms have been examined but the one that has received most attention has been that of adherence characteristics that are frequently associated with pili or fimbrae, which are hair-like extensions of the bacterial cell wall that recognise specific uro-epithelial receptors. There are two main types of fimbrae, firstly the common or Type 1 that is of low virulence in terms of the production of APN but may be significant in the production of scarring. Type 2 or p-fimbrae have been shown in a number of reports to be associated with APN, particularly in the absence of VUR. A major criticism of this work has been based on the fact that organisms have been studied after sub-culture and it is recognised that sub-culture techniques can alter the expression of adherence characteristics such as fimbrae. However there is little doubt that bacterial virulence factors are important in the production of APN and these factors may be less relevant in the presence of VUR or obstruction (Johnson 2003).

Host factors

Any degree of urinary stasis either as a result of anatomical obstruction that is uncommon, or more frequently functional stasis (e.g. low fluid intake, infrequent voiding, incomplete bladder emptying and chronic constipation) will increase the risk of UTI. Other susceptibility factors, such as peri-urethral colonisation with uropathogenic bacteria and/or impairment of lower urinary tract defence mechanisms, predispose children to UTI and differ in importance in children of different age and gender.

At birth all mammals are germ free, and heavy peri-urethral colonisation with *E coli* and enteroccocci normally becomes established in both sexes shortly after birth. It progressively diminishes throughout the first year of life and normally becomes light after the age of 5 years. However, *E coli* continues to be the dominant gram negative species in the peri-urethral flora in girls of all ages.

In contrast to healthy children, susceptible children frequently show heavy gram negative peri-urethral colonisation in the days preceding a UTI and serotyping of the dominant *E coli* confirms that peri-urethral colonising strains are responsible for the infection. In boys the foreskin is important in determining the peri-urethral flora and circumcised boys have a lower incidence of UTI than uncircumcised boys. This is consistent with the data that suggests that the peri-urethral carriage of *Proteus* is higher in uncircumcised boys.

The use of antibiotics has a significant effect on peri-urethral colonisation by replacing normal with antibiotic resistant flora and there are experimental data showing that ampicillin increases heavy and persistent vaginal colonisation. Uro-epithelial cell surface structures that serve as receptors for bacterial adhesion have been identified at all levels of the urinary tract and inhibition of binding can be demonstrated in experimental animal models.

Although uro-epithelial mucus has been shown to be an important antibacterial mechanism in animal models there is no evidence for a disturbance in this or the specific immune system in humans with recurrent UTI.

Vesico-ureteric reflux

VUR, which is present in up to 40% of children with UTI (compared with an incidence of 1% in normal neonates), has been recognised as a potential risk factor for both infection and renal scarring over many years and has generated a significant degree of controversy. VUR defined as a retrograde flow of urine into the ureter, sometimes extending into the renal pelvis, calyces and collecting ducts, may occur as a primary abnormality or secondary to urethral obstruction, neuropathic bladder dysfunction or severe non-neuropathic dysfunctional voiding. Sometimes the distinction between primary and secondary is difficult to make in practice. The ability of the vesico-ureteric junction to prevent reflux of bladder urine is determined by the length of the submucosal ureter that is genetically determined. In patients with primary VUR the length of the submucosal ureter is proportional to the grade of VUR based on contrast micturating cystography (MCUG) (see Figure 9.2). The submucosal ureter increases in length throughout childhood perhaps explaining the high natural remission rate (International Reflux Committee 1981; Elder *et al.* 1997).

The main consequences of VUR are urinary stasis of refluxed urine and enhanced delivery of bacteria and bladder pressures to the upper urinary tract. In view of this it has been assumed that VUR predisposes to recurrent UTI, APN and infection-related renal scarring. These

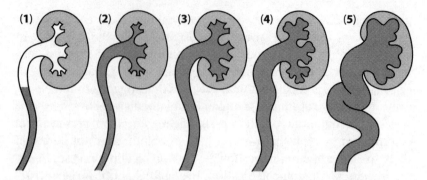

Figure 9.2 Development of vesico-ureteric reflux (VUR)

assumptions have led to the widespread use of antibiotic propylaxis as well as anti-reflux surgery. However review of the literature does not support many of the roles attributed to VUR (Garin *et al.* 1998) and although low-dose antibiotic prophylaxis is the commonest intervention used to prevent UTI, as previously stated, this intervention has not been appropriately studied in patients with VUR (Le Saux *et al.* 2000).

It is likely that the inheritance of VUR is autosomal dominant with variable penetrance. Approximately one third of siblings of index patients with VUR also have VUR, in the great majority of a mild degree, although most (75%) do not have a history of UTI. The overall risk of renal scarring in association with VUR in siblings is around 3% (Hollowell and Greenfield 2002). There is no consensus on screening for VUR in the presence of a family history but, in practice, if the index case has significant VUR and renal scarring, selective imaging of siblings or offspring should be discussed and a low threshold stressed for investigation of febrile illness.

Pathogenesis of renal scarring

Coarse renal cortical scarring is found in about 10% of children with a history of UTI. Recognised risk factors are early (within the first 3 years of life), repeated and inadequately treated febrile infection and anatomical obstruction. High grade VUR (≥ 4 as shown in Figure 9.2) is also a major risk factor but clear gender-specific differences have been established with global renal parenchymal loss occurring more often in boys with high grade VUR and focal scarring in girls with low grade or absent VUR particularly after a history of recurrent febrile UTI (Wennerstrom *et al.* 2000b). These findings support the contention that high grade VUR is associated with renal dysplasia that occurs during fetal life with UTI as a risk factor for postnatal scarring and renal functional decline. Other relevant factors particularly in patients who have no demonstrable VUR, are dysfunctional voiding, bacterial virulence and the host inflammatory response.

The frequency of renal scarring in children presenting with a first proven UTI does not vary with age (Christian *et al.* 2000). This may be explained by scarring having occurred at the time of a previously undiagnosed UTI or alternatively that age-related susceptibility is relative. The incidence of new scarring however is relatively rare and usually in specific circumstances e.g. obstruction, neuropathic bladder dysfunction or dysfunctional voiding.

Management

The management of the child with a history of UTI should firstly address the basic measures designed to reduce the recurrence of UTI and identify those who have or who are at risk of renal damage irrespective of whether there are potential risk factors such as VUR identified. It is also important to ensure full parental explanation of the treatment and investigation and this is enhanced with the use of written information (Table 9.1). In addition we have found that a dedicated, nurse-led UTI service enables rationalisation of the referral process with initial imaging on the same day as the outpatient appointment, standardisation of initial and subsequent investigation and more consistent advice on preventive measures.

Clinical experience suggests simple measures like increasing fluid intake, ensuring a satisfactory voiding frequency, management of voiding dysfunction, treatment of constipation and avoidance of perineal irritants are helpful in the prevention of recurrence. Patients with a history of recurrent UTI and a normal urinary tract should in addition be offered a 6–12 month period of antibiotic prophylaxis.

As VUR is a recognised risk factor for renal scarring, the ideal management (i.e. prevention of recurrence of infection and new or progressive scarring) has been, and continues to be, the subject of intense debate that has focused on the relative value of 'medical' therapy, meaning prophylactic antibiotics over surgical correction of VUR. Fortunately, a substantial amount of data are now available from randomised controlled trials of these interventions to inform individual clinical decisions.

Table 9.1 Information for parents of children with UTI

WHEN?	**When to suspect urinary tract infection in a child or a baby**
	Your child or baby may have infected urine without having the fishy smell and burning pain on passing urine that occurs in adults with cystitis. In a baby or toddler you should think of urine infection if he/she is unwell and/or has a high temperature, unless there is clear evidence of some other explanation. You should also think of it in a baby who as repeated bouts of fever, vomiting, jaundice or poor weight gain and, of course in any child who does have symptoms related to passing urine.
WHAT?	**What to do if you think your child may have a urine infection**
	It is important to treat urinary tract infection quickly, particularly in the very young child because prolonged infection may make them quite ill and delay in treatment may damage the kidney. You should contact your doctor as soon as you suspect infection and ask for an urgent appointment and urine culture.
HOW?	**How to diagnose urinary tract infection**
	Urinary infection can only be diagnosed with certainty if a clean catch specimen is collected in a sterile container and sent without delay to the laboratory for examination. A urinary infection cannot be demonstrated reliably on a dipstix test of the urine. A full result should be available after 48 hours. The ideal method in babies and toddlers is the catch specimen which has been demonstrated to you in hospital. However if an adhesive plastic bag is used and shows a positive result, this should be confirmed by a clean sample.
TREATMENT	**Treatment**
	In babies and toddlers who are unwell and any child with distressing symptoms, it is likely that treatment will be given before the laboratory results are available. The most common antibiotics prescribed are trimethoprim, augmentin, nitrofurantoin and cephradine. It may be necessary to change the antibiotic after 48 hours if your child is not obviously better. In this case the laboratory result will probably show that the term causing the infection is not sensitive to the antibiotic chosen and will also indicate what other antibiotics to choose. Full treatment should be continued for 7–10 days and after that all children should continue to take a small regular dose of antibiotic until the kidneys and bladder have been checked by scans.

Table 9.1 (*continued*)

THEN?	What to expect after treatment
	It is now accepted that all children who have had a urinary tract infection should have at least one scan to check the kidneys and bladder are normal. For children that test should include an ultrasound scan of the kidneys (like the scan used to measure the baby during pregnancy). Further scans will be necessary in the young child and if the ultrasound scan is abnormal. Other children who have recurrent infections may also need further tests. However when the further tests have been completed make sure you understand the results and the reasons why further tests and treatment may be necessary.
LATER?	**What may happen in the future**
	Boys rarely get further infections and if they do it usually happens quite soon after the first one. Girls however often get further infections. It does not necessarily mean that something is wrong, but it might be an indication for further tests and perhaps long-term treatment. Long-term treatment may be necessary, particularly in the young child and in those children who have an abnormality of the bladder or kidney. Ensure you ask enough questions and that you understand the reasons for your child's need for prolonged treatment.

General measures to reduce the risk of recurrent infection

1 Encourage regular and complete bladder emptying, at least twice in the morning, at least twice in the afternoon and twice before going to bed.

2 Watch out for constipation and if not responding to diet some mild laxative treatment may be necessary.

3 Ensure regular bathing and avoid highly scented soap and bubble bath. It is preferable to avoid shampooing the child's hair while he/she is in the bath.

4 Ensure that following a trip to the toilet the bottom is wiped clean from front to back, using soft absorbent toilet paper.

5 Enquire about access to satisfactory toilets at school – this should be easy for the child.

The data shows no clear benefit of anti-reflux surgery over medical treatment in overall UTI recurrence risk. Although anti-reflux surgery does reduce the risk of a febrile UTI recurrence, there is no difference in renal function or new or progressive scar formation (Wheeler *et al.* 2004).

In practice, the patient with VUR is offered prophylaxis as a first line intervention. The ideal duration is unclear but should continue at least throughout the high-risk period of the first three years of life and until continence is achieved. The absence of serial changes in renal imaging, and the knowledge of the high natural remission rate, should also inform the timing of discontinuation of prophylaxis.

Breakthrough infections can result from either non-compliance with medication, which may be relevant in as many as 50% of patients, or true bacterial resistance. Non-compliance or incomplete compliance should be suspected if the infecting organism is sensitive to the prophylactic agent. If breakthrough infections continue despite medical management, some centres recommend circumcision as the next step in boys as the risk of UTI in circumcised male infants is significantly lower than in those who are uncircumcised.

The main indications for anti-reflux surgery are ongoing breakthrough infection, particularly where there is concern over compliance with prophylactic antibiotics, and/or new or progressive scarring on serial imaging.

Two forms of anti-reflux surgery are available and equally effective. The first is the endoscopic injection of a biodegradable material into suburothelial space at the level of the ureteric orifice. The success rate is around 70% and may be used for all grades of VUR. The procedure can be undertaken as a day case, is easily repeated and appears to have minimal morbidity. The potential local or distant migration of the injected material is of concern but there have been no reports in humans of this occurrence so far.

The second and more traditional form is open surgical re-implantation, which has a higher initial success rate but carries the disadvantages of a prolonged inpatient stay, a surgical scar and the potential for post-operative ureteric obstruction (although this is relatively rare).

Long-term outlook

It is now over 40 years since the original studies (Smellie *et al.* 1964) demonstrated the link between VUR and renal scarring, the term 'chronic pyelonephritis' being used to describe the parenchymal lesion. Later the term 'reflux nephropathy' (RN) became popular to describe the triad of UTI, VUR and renal scarring, however this diagnostic category inevitably contains patients with renal dysplasia in addition to those with post-infective renal scarring.

Renal function and blood pressure

The most serious complication associated with renal scarring is renal impairment and from the original description until relatively recently the risk of renal dysfunction was perceived to be significant based on small selected series and on registry data. In the UK Renal registry the diagnosis of RN was applied to 7% of children with established or end-stage renal failure (ERF or ESRF). In the Australia and New Zealand ESRF registry, 13% of patients between the age of 5 and 44 years had a diagnosis of RN between 1971 and 1988 with no clear trend of change throughout this time frame. These investigators concluded that treatment to prevent UTI in the context of VUR had not been associated with a decrease in ESRF and suggest that patients with RN who develop ESRF may represent a sub-group with congenital dysplasia/hypoplasia that is not amenable to postnatal intervention. In contrast, data from the Swedish ESRF registry has shown a reduction in the incidence of RN as a cause of ESRF in childhood from 6% between 1978–1985 to zero between 1986–1994. This suggests that the known high diagnostic rate for UTI is associated with a reduction in the long-term consequences (Esborjner 1997). A more recent cohort study from Sweden of 57 patients with renal scarring and an age and sex matched control group evaluated 16–26 years after presentation with UTI showed no difference in glomerular filtration rate (GFR) between the two groups. However, patients with bilateral renal scarring had a small but significant drop in GFR on follow up evaluation (Wennerstrom *et al.* 2000c).

The incidence of hypertension was also evaluated in the above cohort and no difference was found in ambulatory profiles between the two groups (Wennerstrom *et al.* 2000a). Further follow up of this and other cohorts are necessary but these data tend to contradict the previously widely held belief that renal scarring carries a substantially increased risk of hypertension and chronic renal failure.

Pregnancy-related complications

Pregnant women have an increased risk of UTI if they have had VUR as a child and this risk is not reduced if they have undergone anti-reflux surgery. Renal scarring significantly increases the risk of pregnancy-related hypertension, pre-eclampsia and pre-term delivery, particularly if associated with pre-existing hypertension (North *et al.* 2000).

Investigations

Imaging techniques

Whenever imaging of the urinary tract is considered, the least invasive technique should always be chosen. In addition, algorithms are particularly useful since they require agreement between clinicians and radiologists as well as ensuring rational use of imaging resources. Ultrasound(US) imaging is non-invasive with no radiation burden and provides excellent anatomical detail of the urinary tract and will demonstrate dilatation/obstruction but has a relatively low sensitivity for the detection of VUR and renal scarring. Renal cortical scintigraphy with 99m Tc DMSA is the most sensitive technique for the detection of renal parenchymal damage associated with UTI/VUR and allows an accurate evaluation of differential function but is unable to distinguish dysplasia from post-infective scarring. Dynamic radioisotope scanning with 99m DTPA or MAG3 is mainly indicated for the further evaluation of pelvic and/or ureteric dilatation demonstrated on ultrasound and has a lower radiation dose than DMSA scanning. Dynamic radioisotope scanning can also be used as a non-invasive assessment of VUR (indirect cystography) in the child who is continent and co-operative but is less sensitive than direct cystography. Micturating cystourethrography (MCUG) is still regarded as the definitive method for assessing bladder and urethral anatomy and for the demonstration of VUR. Radioisotope cystography (99m Tc pertechnetate) requires urethral catheterisation but has a higher sensitivity than MCUG for the detection of VUR and a very low radiation dose. The main disadvantage is that no comment can be made on the urethral or bladder anatomy. However it may be used to detect VUR initially in girls and for follow-up evaluation in both sexes.

The advantage of the *plain radiograph* is in the detection of calculi that may be overlooked on ultrasound scanning and visualisation of the lumbosacral spine if neuropathic bladder dysfunction is suspected. Requests for *Intravenous Urography* should be tailored to specific situations in order to limit the number of radiographs and the radiation dose and should be seen as a second line investigation.

Imaging guidelines

Despite the frequency of UTI in childhood and the numerous contributions on the subject in the literature, there is surprisingly little consensus on urinary tract imaging requirements, perhaps reflecting the relative paucity of high quality intervention studies and data on long-term outcome.

Diagnostic imaging following UTI in childhood has been accepted practice since the original studies in the early 1960s showed a high prevalence of abnormalities and specifically a link between renal scarring and VUR. Inherent in this strategy was the assumption that identification of these abnormalities and intervention would influence outcome. Our understanding of long-term outcome has developed in the intervening decades and we now know that the great majority of children with UTI have an excellent prognosis, although more long-term follow-up studies would be helpful, it appears that the risk of renal functional impairment and/or hypertension is much lower than previously thought and likely to be limited to those patients with renal dysplasia. In addition, there is no clear indication that investigation/intervention influences outcome and it is within this context that imaging guidelines should be seen.

Initial imaging guidelines for febrile children up to the age of 2 years by the American Academy of Pediatrics (1999), involve a combination of US, MCUG or isotope cystography. UK guidelines (RCP 1991) are similar for the infant and young child but also include renal cortical scintigraphy with DMSA. Guidelines for the older child reflect differing professional opinion, predominantly on the need for scintigraphy. In the light of the increasing use of prenatal anomaly scanning, some authors have suggested that if a child presenting with UTI has had a normal late prenatal ultrasound scan, further US scanning should be limited to those who have a complicated course and MCUG should be used as the sole screening test. However, apart from the invasive nature of MCUG and the reluctance of many radiologists to undertake this study beyond infancy, this protocol is predicated on the unproven assumption of the value of prophylaxis in patients with VUR. In addition, VUR is of low grade in the majority of patients and associated with a low risk of parenchymal scarring.

Despite the availability and recognised high sensitivity of renal cortical scintigraphy, the use of this modality in imaging practice is variable. Some authors advocate DMSA scanning as a first line investigation in lieu of ultrasound because of the greater sensitivity in identifying APN, but it is difficult to justify this approach unless confirmation of APN is shown to alter initial management and subsequent outcome. There is nevertheless some logic in adopting an imaging strategy beyond the acute phase that defines the presence or absence of renal scarring and/or dysplasia as this is associated with

Table 9.2 Initial urinary tract imaging guidelines

0–1 years	**Urinary tract ultrasound** 99m Tc DMSA scan The DMSA scan should be carried out 4–6 months after infection. MCUG should be performed when the urine is sterile and should be undertaken urgently if there is gross dilatation of the collecting system(s) and/or obstructive uropathy is suspected on ultrasound.
1–4 years	**Urinary tract ultrasound** If there is a history of recurrent UTI or an episode of UTI with 'upper tract' symptoms or a family history of VUR/reflux nephropathy, a 99m Tc DMSA scan should be carried out. If an abnormality on either of these two imaging studies is found, a reflux study will depend on the degree of continence of the child. In the pre-continent child, MCUG or a direct radionuclide cystogram (see below) should be carried out In the child who is continent and cooperative, indirect radionuclide cystography using 99m Tc DTPA or MAG3 should be used.
5 years	**Urinary tract ultrasound** If there is a history of recurrent UTI or a history of UTI with 'upper tract' symptoms or a family history of VUR/reflux nephropathy, a 99m Tc DMSA scan should be carried out. If an abnormality is detected on either of these two imaging studies, a 99M Tc DTPA or MAG3 indirect radionuclide cystogram should be considered.

long-term risk, albeit small. However, as renal scintigraphy is invasive there is a need for a controlled application dictated by factors such as age, recurrence and the presence of fever/systemic upset (Christian *et al.* 2000), accepting that some of the abnormalities found may have no long-term significance (Table 9.2).

One must exercise some caution before dispensing with ultrasound in the child with uncomplicated UTI. Prenatal anomaly scanning is by no means universal in the UK and, for maximum sensitivity for the detection of a dilated fetal urinary tract, the scan would have to be undertaken at or greater than 20 weeks gestation. In addition, ultrasound is of value in demonstrating bladder wall morphology and voiding efficiency in the older child with UTI and daytime wetting. Finally, in view of the link between referral from primary care and imaging, one would have to ensure that other important aspects of the consultation, particularly simple preventive advice, are not lost merely because imaging may be considered unnecessary.

Conclusion

UTI in childhood is a relatively common disease predominantly encountered by primary healthcare professionals and the management and investigation of these children consumes considerable healthcare resources in secondary care.

Fortunately the great majority of children with UTI have an excellent prognosis and the long-term consequences are much less significant than previously thought. There remain a number of unanswered questions about the relationship between UTI, VUR and renal scarring but the recent encouraging data should inform the ongoing debate on optimal imaging protocols. However, debates over imaging strategy should not be allowed to overshadow the importance of early, accurate diagnosis and treatment of UTI as the greatest potential for prevention of renal damage lies in increased awareness of these aspects of management in primary care.

References

Aggarawal VK, Verrier Jones K, Asscher AW, Evans C, Williams LA (1991) Covert bacteriuria: Long-term follow-up. *Archives of Disease in Childhood*, 66: 1284–6

American Academy of Pediatrics (1999) Committee on Quality Improvement, Subcommittee on Urinary Tract Infection. Practice Parameter: The diagnosis, treatment and evaluation of the initial urinary tract infection in febrile infants and young children. *Pediatrics*, 103: 843–52 [Erratum, 103:1052]

Christian MT, McColl JH, MacKenzie JR, Beattie TJ (2000) Risk assessment of renal cortical scarring with urinary tract infection by clinical features and ultrasonography. *Archives of Disease in Childhood*, 82: 376–80

Craig JC, Hodson EM (2004) Treatment of acute pyelonephritis in children. *British Medical Journal*, 328: 179–80

Elder JS, Peters CA, Arant BS Jr, Ewalt DH, Hawtrey CE, Hurwitz RS, Parrott TS, Snyder HM 3rd, Woolf SH, Hasselblad V (1997) Pediatric Vesicoureteral Reflux Guidelines Panel: Summary report on the management of pediatric vesicoureteral reflux in children. *Journal of Urology*, 157: 1846–51

Esborjner E (1997) Epidemiology of chronic renal failure in children: a report from Sweden 1986–1994. *Pediatric Nephrology*, 11: 438–42

Garin EH, Campos A, Homsy Y (1998) Primary vesicoureteral reflux: review of current concepts. *Pediatric Nephrology*, 12: 249–56

Gorelick MH, Shaw KN (1999) Screening tests for urinary tract infection in children: A meta-analysis. *Pediatrics*, 104 (5): e54

Hellstrom A, Hanson E, Hansson S, Hjalmas K, Jodal U (1991) Association between urinary symptoms at 7 years of age and previous urinary tract infection. *Archives of Disease in Childhood*, 66: 232–4

Hollowell JG, Greenfield SP (2002) Screening siblings for vesico-ureteral reflux. *Journal of Urology*, 168: 2138–41

International Reflux Committee (1981) Medical versus surgical treatment of primary vesicoureteral reflux. *Pediatrics*, 67: 392–400

Johnson JR (2003) Microbial virulence determinants and the pathogenesis of urinary tract infection. *Infectious Disease Clinics of North America*, 17 (2): 261–78

Le Saux N, Pham B, Moher D (2000) Evaluating the benefits of antimicrobial efficacy of low dose prophylactic antibiotics to prevent urinary tract infections in children: a systematic review. *CMAJ*,163: 523–9

Michael M, Hodson EM, Craig JC, Martin S, Moyer VA (2002) Short compared with standard duration of antibiotic treatment for urinary tract infection: a systematic review of randomised controlled trials. *Archives of Disease in Childhood*, 87: 118–23

North RA, Taylor RS, Gunn TR (2000) Pregnancy outcome in women with reflux nephropathy and the inheritance of vesico-ureteric reflux. *Australia and New Zealand Journal of Obstetrics and Gynaecology*, 40: 280–85

Royal College of Physicians (1991) Report of a Working Group of the Research Unit: Guidelines for the management of acute urinary tract infection in childhood. *Journal of the Royal College of Physicians of London*, 25: 36–42

Shaw KN, Gorelick MH, McGowan KL, McDaniel Yakscoe, Schwartz JS (1998) Prevalence of urinary tract infection in young febrile children in the emergency department. *Pediatrics*, 102: e16

Smellie JM, Hodson CJ, Edwards D, Normand ICS (1964) Clinical and radiological features of urinary tract infection in childhood. *British Medical Journal*, 2: 122–6

Wennerstrom M, Hansson S, Hedner T, Himmelmann A, Jodal U (2000a) Ambulatory blood pressure 16–26 years after the first urinary tract infection in childhood. *Journal of Hypertension*,18: 485–91

Wennerstrom M, Hansson S, Jodal U, Stokland E (2000b) Primary and acquired renal scarring in boys and girls with urinary tract infection. *Journal of Pediatrics*,136: 30–34

Wennerstrom M, Hansson S, Jodal U, Sixt R, Stokland E (2000c) Renal function 16–26 years after the first urinary tract infection in childhood. *Archives of Pediatric and Adolescent Medicine*, 154: 339–45

Wheeler DM, Vimalachandra D, Hodson EM, Roy CP, Craig JC (2004) Interventions for primary vesico-ureteric reflux. Cochrane Database Systematic Reviews, 3: CD001532

10

Surgical assessment and management of urinary continence in children with neuropathic bladder

Su-Anna Boddy, Sue Affleck and Stella Snell

Key points

- All children presenting in the outpatient clinic for continence problems will need a full assessment to determine whether or not they have neurological impairment.

- If this is not present, they have a good chance of being cured by a structured programme of bladder and bowel training.

- The majority of children who have neurological impairment of the bladder and/or bowel still have well-functioning kidneys. This means they can usually be made socially continent using clean intermittent catheterisation (CIC) while maintaining good renal function with appropriate medication.

- There will, however, be some children who require major surgery.

- All children with neurological impairment of the bladder or bowel, whether or not they have surgery, will need to be monitored for the rest of their lives.

Continence in children with no neurological impairment

In order to be continent of urine a child requires:

- An adequate reservoir for urine, i.e. a low pressure bladder of adequate capacity with an effective sphincter to prevent leakage;

- Ability to empty the bladder – which presupposes the ability to understand the sensation of fullness, the acquisition of voluntary control and ability to empty completely.

The expected functional bladder capacity in millilitres for 1–12-year-olds is calculated by the formula: age (yrs) x 30 + 30 (Koff 1983).

Assessment

The following points need to be established.

1 **Has there ever been any dry period?**
   The severity of the problem is unchanged but any dry period
   excludes an ectopic ureter where urine drips all the time. If the
   ureter *is* ectopic (i.e. if it opens outside the bladder below the
   sphincter) then the problem will require removal of the ureter
   along with a portion of the kidney.

2 **Is the problem diurnal enuresis (daytime urgency,
   frequency and urinary leakage)?**
   In an ideal world, such a child should be managed in the primary
   care setting with appropriate referral to a secondary care
   paediatrician with a specific interest. If there are insufficient
   resources in primary care, referral to a continence nurse specialist
   or a paediatric urologist with an interest in neuropathic bladders is
   appropriate, as a problem like this should not be left without
   specialist attention.

3 **What type of fluids is the child drinking?**
   Tea, coffee, blackcurrant and fizzy caffeinated drinks (such as cola)
   are known to stimulate the bladder. Because of this, they should be
   avoided. If constipation is a problem excess milk should be avoided.

4 **Is the child's fluid intake adequate?**
   If a child restricts his or her fluid intake in order to stay dry, the
   bladder will not be stretched adequately. A child should be
   drinking 5–6 'mugs' of water-based fluid (containing 100–200
   mls each, i.e. 1000–1200 mls total) a day, depending on age.

5 **How often does the child go to the toilet?**
   Holding on to urine over-stretches the bladder and decreases the
   sensation of the need to empty the bladder, and the ability actually
   to empty it. This can be exacerbated by poor school toilets (Cooper
   et al 2003) as some children deliberately withhold drinks in order
   to avoid using the toilet.

6 **Does the child show signs of Vincent's curtsey
   or urge/giggle incontinence?**
   Vincent's curtsey describes the position in which girls crouch
   down, placing the heel of their foot in their perineum to stop a
   posterior urethral leak. This can be treated with ephedrine to

tighten the bladder neck, but only *after* bladder and bowel training have been tried and urodynamics performed. Problems relating to urge/giggle incontinence could be treated with anticholinergics to relax the detrusor muscle again *after* bladder and bowel training.

7 *Is there a family history of continence problems?*
If there is a family history of diurnal or nocturnal enuresis, the child may find it takes longer to gain urinary control, but may still be successful.

8 *What are the child's stools like?*
It is important to assess faecal loading and the type of stools passed. The Bristol Stool Form Scale (Heaton 2000) is a useful tool here. If the stool is large and splashes in the toilet, the child's urinary dysfunction may be a secondary problem resulting from faecal loading.

9 *Does the child have a problem with wetting?*
Many parents change their child's clothes just before coming into clinic, but no youngster who walks into clinic in tight white trousers is likely to have a problem with incontinence. Children who do have problems with wetting are much more likely to try and conceal it by wearing dark baggy trousers.

In addition, a number of physical checks need to be carried out. These are as follows:

1 *Abdominal examination*
This is to confirm that the child's anatomy is normal and to asses the degree of faecal loading. A distended rectum with faecaloma (revealed by X-ray), or a colon that is palpable throughout the abdomen may indicate bowel dysfunction, with urinary dysfunction as a secondary problem. If this is the case, a Bowel Training Programme is likely to be necessary, with the support of a stimulant laxative eg sodium picosulfate to help promote a regular bowel action and regain rectal tone.

2 *Assessment of spine and natal cleft*
Look particularly for sacral agenesis or a hairy patch, which may be indicative of underlying spinal dysraphism (De Gennaro *et al.* 1991).

3 *Check the ano-cutaneous reflex*
Does the anal sphincter 'wink' (positive) when the perianal skin is

sharply (but not painfully) stimulated? Negative reflex may be due to severe constipation rather than neurological abnormality.

4   *Check for spina bifida occulta if an abdominal X-ray has been taken to assess faecal loading*
Spina bifida occulta (failure of fusion of the 5th lumbar and/or 1st sacral vertebral arches) alone is a radiological normal variant that occurs in 10 per cent of the population. It is not associated with an underlying neurological abnormality but, in our experience, it will take longer for the child to gain urinary control (Samuel and Boddy 2004).

The next steps

After a full assessment and consultation, it may be apparent that the child needs disposable or reusable products to help support their bladder and bowel training programme. The child may also benefit from a Paediatric Clinical Psychologist to help restore their self-esteem (see Chapter 12 on Psychological Aspects, by Melinda Edwards). The family may be able to apply for Disability Living Allowance (DLA) to offset the cost of ruined clothing and excess washing because of the child's incontinence.

The next step (before urodynamics is considered) is usually starting on a bladder and bowel training programme.

The training programme

Bowel if faecal loading is a problem

- It is important that the child is given a high fibre diet, avoiding bananas (Graham Claydon, personal communication), excess milk and white bread.

- Use gastro-colic reflex for timing of defaecation – i.e. 20 minutes after meals. Encourage the child to sit in the correct position on the toilet. This should be a comfortable, with feet resting on a platform if they do not reach the ground (see Figure 10.1).

- Use stimulant laxatives to empty colon and regain rectal tone (e.g. sodium picosulfate elixir, 2.5 mg sodium picosulfate in

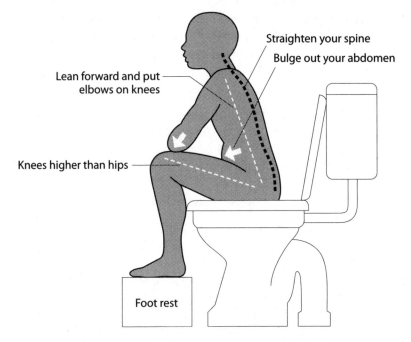

Straighten your spine

Bulge out your abdomen

Lean forward and put elbows on knees

Knees higher than hips

Foot rest

Figure 10.1 Correct position for sitting on the toilet

perle formation, bisacodyl) or macrogol/polyethylene glycol (Movicol paediatric plain). These need to be maintained for a long time, often well over a year.

Bladder

- Avoid giving the child drinks containing caffeine and blackcurrant.

- Ensure the child drinks 5–6 'mugs' of fluid (containing 100–200 mls each), every day.

- Encourage the child to empty his or her bladder at the same time, five or six times a day. This could be on waking, mid-morning, lunchtime, end of school, tea or supper time, with a final wee without a drink before bed.

- Teach the child to perform 'double micturition' at least twice a day. This involves sitting or standing to wee, wipe/waggle (girls front to back), finish and wash hands. Then return to toilet and try to wee out some more. If more urine is voided then the first bladder emptying was incomplete and the residual urine left in the bladder could have lead to bladder mucosal irritation and 'infection/contamination'. If more urine is obtained on second micturition longer time should be spent performing normal bladder emptying.

■ Care is needed to ensure that wiping is done properly. Make sure that girls *do* wipe from front to back so that they will not contaminate the urethra with bacteria from the anus. A fishy smell suggests contaminated urine (usually from poor emptying). It is often best to give the child a short course of prophylactic antibiotics, usually trimethoprim or nitrofurantoin.

Success of the Bladder and Bowel Training Programme is followed up optimally in the Continence Nurse Specialist Clinics, if available, or else by Primary or Secondary Care physician with a specific interest. If the programme is adhered to but not totally successful, it can be supported after 3–6 months by anticholinergics (Oxybutynin, Detrunorm or Detrusitol) in collaboration with the GP, supported by Care Pathway Guidelines. Urodynamics (see pages 90–93) are only performed if complete dryness cannot be attained, or if the child cannot be weaned off the anticholinergics, or long-term follow-up to ensure anticholinergics prescribed post urodynamics have been successful.

Newborns with neuropathic bladder

These are infants with spina bifida, sacral agenesis, posterior urethral valves or, occasionally, bladder neuropathy as a result of Hirsch-prung's disease or anorectal malformation.

All babies with any of these conditions will need to have renal tract ultrasound scans and blood tests (creatinine and electrolytes including bicarbonate, to assess kidney function) at 2 and 6 weeks of life. Values should be within the normal ranges:

creatinine	60–110 μmol/litre
urea	2.5–8.0 mmol/litre
bicarbonate	22–28 mmol/litre
sodium	135–145 mmol/litre
potassium	3.5–4.7 mmol/litre

Such babies will also need DMSA and ultrasounds scans at 6 months (see Chapter 6 on 'Investigations for bladder problems' by Rosie Kelly).

Newborns and infants diagnosed with spina bifida may need clean intermittent catheterisation plus anticholinergic medication by the age of one year (see below). They will also need to have their glomerular filtration rate (GFR) measured and urodynamics performed at 18–24 months and 3 years. This will enable monitoring of the need for or effectiveness of anticholinergic drugs, and ephedrine, and the effect of surgical changes 6 months after bladder augmentation or the insertion of an artificial urinary sphincter (AUS). These measures should be repeated annually for follow-up.

Figure 10.2 Evolution of the management of incontinence

1966 Guttmann
Introduction of STERILE Intermittent Catheterisation

1971 Lapides
Introduction of CLEAN Intermittent Catheterisation. (CIC)
Lapides was an American Urologist. He had a female patient requiring Guttmann's prescribed sterile intermittent catheterisation, who travelled to France and dropped her catheter on the floor of a French toilet. Having no other catheter available she picked up the catheter, washed it and used it with no adverse effects of infection. Lapides (1971) commented on the 'lack of sterility' of the above and hence conceived the concept of Clean Intermittent Catheterisation or CIC.

1971 Scott
Introduction of Artificial Urinary Sphincter (AUS)

1970s Urodynamics
Urodynamics involve the understanding of the need for a low pressure Reservoir

1980 Mitrofanoff
Introduction of continent vesicostomy

1980s Anticholinergic medication
Introduction of oxybutynin for uncontrolled bladder muscle contractions

1990 Malone
Antegrade continence enema (ACE)

Clean intermittent catheterisation (CIC)

(See also Chapter 14 on 'Managing clean intermittent catheterisation' by Rosie Kelly).

Most paediatric urologists caring for children with spina bifida now believe that CIC should be started in the first year of the child's life. This ensures complete bladder emptying and, in conjunction with prophylactic trimethoprim, should prevent infections. If the child and family become accustomed to CIC at an early age then the procedure is more easily accepted. A calm, expert and confident Continence Nurse Specialist (CNS) can go a long way towards allaying a family's fears that they may not be able to perform CIC on their child, or that they may harm the child.

CIC is taught in the home or school environment, and the concept is introduced with aid of teaching equipment such as a doll or anatomical model and demonstration of catheters. Both home and school carers can be taught, along with children themselves if they are of a suitable age. Even boys with normal sensation can be taught.

Sometimes the CNS and the consultant have to stand back and let the child attain the procedure of CIC at his or her own rate. Play support and child psychology are an essential part of this teaching procedure, and no child should ever feel they have failed themselves or their team who are trying to support them. This can all be achieved, sometimes very quickly, but that depends on the family and the child's willingness to learn. Home deliveries of equipment and repeat prescriptions or alternative catheters can be arranged in collaboration with the GP.

Surgical intervention

There are now three different anticholinergic drugs which can be used to counteract detrusor overactivity (uncontrolled bladder wall muscle contractions) or treat a non-compliant (stiff, non-yielding) bladder wall. CIC timing and technique can be fine-tuned so that, with the appropriate anticholinergic, the child has an adequate capacity bladder of safe low pressure (below 40 cm H_2O as demonstrated on urodynamics) to prevent upper renal tract dilatation and kidney damage. A bonus effect is that this will also make the child socially acceptably dry.

If the above cannot be achieved, then bladder augmentation is planned, with or without Mitrofanoff (a continent, catheterisable channel for draining the bladder). Preoperative assessment determines whether the augmentation needs combining with a bladder neck procedure because of sphincter incompetence and an antegrade continence enema (ACE) for bowel continence. The surgeon and continence nurse should have detailed discussions with the child and family, both in clinic and at home. Clear and appropriate information about the operative procedure should be given, and the parents and child should have the opportunity to meet with other families similar to themselves whose children have had the operation.

What happens?

The child is admitted two days prior to surgery, for bladder and bowel preparation. This involves clear liquid diet (oral sodium picosulfate with magnesium citrate in the form of Picolax) with enemas and rectal washouts if necessary.

Enterocystoplasty is the principal means of bladder augmentation. Small bowel (ileum) is currently favoured. Large bowel has excess mucous production which blocks catheters and causes stones and infection. Using the stomach is not a practical alternative as it causes haematuria and systemic alkalosis (Mahan et al. 1994). Just removing the detrusor muscle (autoaugmentation) does not have encouraging long-term results in terms of increased capacity and reduction of overactivity. It is only in rare cases that there is a non-functioning kidney which can be removed and the dilated ureter used as a ureterocystoplasty. Reimplantation of the ureters to prevent vesicoureteric reflux is rarely necessary, as the reflux usually resolves once the bladder has been augmented sufficiently to keep the pressure within it low.

In our unit, the operation for bladder augmentation involves making a Pflanensteil incision, through which 20 cms of small bowel are isolated on a mesentery (i.e. with its own blood supply), and bowel continuity restored. The small bowel augment is opened on the opposite side to the mesenteric border and then one side is sutured from the midpoint to the ends to construct an augment of 'witch's hat' configuration (see Figure 10.3). The bladder is opened in the sagittal plane from the trigone posteriorly to the bladder neck anteriorly (unless a Pippe Salle bladder neck procedure is being performed when a 2 cm wide, 7 cm long strip is cut from the anterior bladder wall based on the bladder neck – see below).

Mitrofanoff (1980) devised the principle of a continent catheterisable conduit for draining the bladder for patients in whom urethral CIC

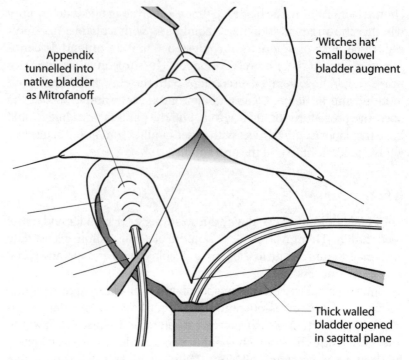

Appendix
tunnelled into
native bladder
as Mitrofanoff

'Witches hat'
Small bowel
bladder augment

Thick walled
bladder opened
in sagittal plane

Figure 10.3 Neuropathic bladder opened in sagittal plane incised down
to trigone posteriorly to create 'clam' configuration. Appendix Mitrofanoff
tunnelled into right flap of 'clam' (catheter in situ). Small bowel
augmentation detubularised and sutured in a 'witches' hat' configuration
in postion for suturing onto bladder

is impracticable. It is also an ideal safety second mechanism for draining an augmented bladder. The Mitrofanoff channel is formed from the
appendix or a small bowel Monti tube (an appendix equivalent – see
Monti *et al.* 1997), which is tunnelled, on its mesentery, into the lateral
wall of the native bladder. In this position, it will be occluded by
mucosal compression as the bladder fills, but the bladder can be
drained by passing a catheter down the appendix or Monti tube. On the
abdominal wall the VQ skin incision makes the Mitrofanoff look just
like another belly button. Our preferred practice is not to use the actual
belly button to site the Mitrofanoff because of an increased risk of
stenosis. However, the new 'belly button sites'/neustomas should be
marked with care postoperatively with consideration given to fashion,
body shape, whether the stoma can be seen by the child while sitting,
and the dexterity and hand dominance of the child. For example, if a
body brace is worn, can the Mitrofanoff be accessed without it being

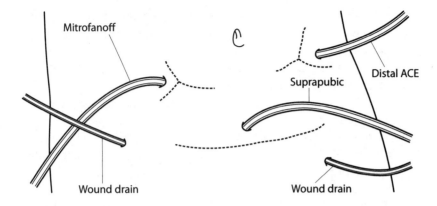

Figure 10.4 Immediate post-operative Augment 'Troff and ACE' showing closed Pflanensteil incision, Foley catheters in Mitrofanoff (patient's right), Distal ACE (patient's left), suprapubic catheter and 2 wound drains

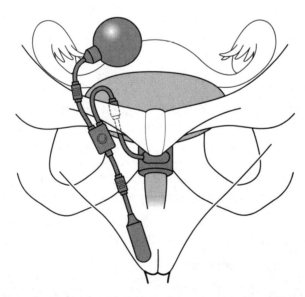

Figure 10.5 AMS 800 artificial urinary sphincter with cuff implanted around urethra at bladder neck in female patient, the pump which is implanted into the labia and the pressure regulating balloon which is sited in a plane between the peritoneum and the abdominal wall musculature (Reproduced with permission from American Medical Systems UK Ltd, Hanwell, Middlesex, UK)

removed? The small bowel augment is then sutured onto the opened bladder (Figure 10.3) with a 10/12F silastic Foley catheter down the Mitrofanoff channel, and a 12/16F Foley suprapubic catheter, both of which are left on free drainage post-operatively. (Figure 10.4 shows this, along with a distal ACE in the same patient.)

The child will then spend 48 hours in the paediatric intensive care unit, and a minimum of two further weeks in hospital. After one week, bladder washouts to remove mucus are started with 50 mls of 0.9% sodium chloride, increased over the next week to 100 mls twice a day routinely, more often if mucus is excessive. Prior to discharge, having ensured that the augmented bladder can be freely drained via the Mitrofanoff catheter, the suprapubic catheter is usually removed (although it will occasionally be left in place for up to six weeks). The Mitrofanoff catheter is then closed using a catheter valve for half an hour and then released. The length of timing for closing is gradually increased but the bladder is on free drainage overnight until urodynamic testing six months post-operatively prove the augmented capacity to be adequate.

By six weeks post-operatively, a child who can manage two-and-a-half hours of close and release while catheters remain in place will be brought back to hospital as a day case. The Mitrofanoff catheter will be removed by the continence nurse specialist and the child and carers taught how to recatheterise the channel. Follow-up renal tract ultrasound and blood tests are done at the same time. The ACE catheter will be removed and the child and carers taught how to recatheterise the channel on the same day case admission, if appropriate. The antibiotic is now changed from treatment dose (e.g. trimethoprim 4 mg/kg twice a day), to a prophylactic dose (e.g. trimethoprim 2 mg/kg at night). Older children performing self-intermittent catheterisation do not necessarily need prophylactic antibiotics (Clarke, Samuel and Boddy 2002).

Bladder neck incompetence

If the child's ano-cutaneous reflex is negative, it is likely that he or she will also suffer from bladder neck incompetence. Provided that urodynamics do not show up detrusor overactivity, ephedrine (an alpha stimulant) can be prescribed. This is usually very successful, especially in children without neurological impairment but for whom bladder and bowel training has had limited success. Surgery may need to be

considered, however, for children with neurogenic bladders whose urinary leakage fails to respond to a combination of anticholinergics, CIC
and ephedrine. Lack of urinary leakage, especially in a child who uses
a wheelchair, may be attained by bladder augmentation with CIC,
(which may or may not be combined with ephedrine), which will create adequate capacity in a low-pressure bladder that can be emptied
successfully.

Surgical techniques

Neither peri-urethral injections, nor bladder neck slings are favoured
for children. Surgical bladder neck closure involves the simultaneous
creation of a Mitrofanoff Channel. This should be carried out as a last
resort because it leaves just one (limited) avenue for endoscopic access
to the bladder. The Pippe Salle procedure – urethral lengthening at the
time of bladder augmentation – has between a 50% and an 80%
success rate. This procedure makes urethral catheterisation post-
operatively difficult: the child should be catheterised per-urethrally
only in cases of dire emergency. It does not rule out the option of urethral endoscopy, however.

The insertion of an artificial urinary sphincter (AUS 800) is an
excellent method of achieving urinary continence in selected patients
(Samuel, Madden and Boddy 2002). AUS can be inserted around the
bladder neck in children of both sexes, or around the bulbar urethra in
boys. The control button is in the labia or scrotum and the pressure
regulating balloon lies in a plane between the peritoneal cavity and the
abdominal wall musculature and can be seen as a 'cyst/opacity' on
plain X-ray. By pumping the control button the patient empties the
fluid from the cuff that occludes the bladder neck and so can empty the
bladder spontaneously or more usually with a catheter. The pressure-
regulating balloon then automatically refills the cuff after a short time
interval at the correct predetermined pressure.

The AUS (Figure 10.5) is an expensive mechanical device that can
break or become infected. The cuff can erode through the urethra, but
in the correctly chosen pubertal/just pre-pubertal children – those who
are motivated, old enough to perform self CIC, with good personal
hygiene and family support, and where urodynamics show no detrusor
overactivity and an incompetent bladder neck that fails to respond to
medication – it offers dryness to more than 80% (Samuel, Madden and
Boddy 2002).

Postoperative complications

The most common postoperative complications are as follows:

- An augmented bladder will require daily washouts to remove mucus.

- An augmented bladder can rupture if it is not emptied.

- The Mitrofanoff channel may become tight and difficult to catheterise. Leaving a catheter *in situ* for two weeks may correct the problem. The child may have to be admitted for endoscopy of the channel under general anaesthetic, or (on rare occasions) the VQ skin flap may need revision.

- An artificial urinary sphincter (AUS) may become deactivated. Reactivation requires a very firm push of the control button which is usually best performed under general anaesthesia.

- The artificial sphincter may need replacing later on; certainly lifelong follow-up is needed.

- The children sometimes find it difficult to adapt to being continent for the first time in their lives, and wish to continue using a 'safety' continence pad – 'just in case'. In our experience, some boys prefer the option of urethral catheterisation as they feel that they lose their sexuality if they do not use their penis.

Follow-up

After the intensive immediate post-operative period following bladder augmentation or AUS insertion, the urodynamics and glomerular filtration rate are checked at six months and one year. Once they are stable, the child will need a renal tract ultrasound at least once a year. Measurement of GFR and urodynamics need to be repeated at puberty prior to handover to a consultant urologist with a specific interest in the long-term following of patients with neuropathic bladders. There is an accepted morbidity inherent in the prolonged exposure of intestinal epithelium (the lining of the bowel used to enlarge the bladder) to urine which includes metaplasia and/or malignancy (Mahan *et al.* 1994). Current practice is to examine the augmented bladder endoscopically, five years post-operatively and then every two years. The risk of malignancy developing in small bowel placed on the bladder has been recorded but, in that particular case, the child was at risk of renal failure in the long term without bladder augmentation. The incidence of malignancy is actually extremely low, but long-term surveillance is nevertheless imperative.

Temporising cutaneous vesicostomy (opening the bladder onto the abdominal wall) is occasionally needed to reverse upper renal tract problems in young children. Urinary diversion into an ileal conduit is really an operation of the past. The future may be tissue culture of bladder cells to be used as bladder augmentation, thus avoiding potential complications of enterocystoplasty (bladder augmentation with small bowel).

Conclusion

Most of the children who have daytime urinary incontinence without associated neurological impairment are cured within a year or two by bladder and bowel training. This can involve stimulant laxatives, regular drinking and micturition ensuring complete bladder emptying. Some children need the support of prophylactic antibiotics and an anticholinergic, while a very small number also need urodynamic investigation. These children usually succeed in becoming clean and dry, and are able to discontinue taking medication.

The majority of children who have neurological impairment of the bladder (and/or bowel) still have kidneys that work properly. This means that they can usually be made socially continent, safely and successfully, with CIC or anticholinergics, with or without ephedrine. A few children need major surgery in the form of bladder augmentation with the Mitrofanoff procedure (to ensure they are able to empty the bladder). These procedures can be combined with bladder neck procedure and/or AUS. All of these children, whether or not they have surgery, will need lifelong surveillance of their urinary tracts.

References

Clarke SA, Samuel M, Boddy S-AM (2005) Are prophylactic antibiotics necessary with clean intermittent catheterization? A randomized controlled trial. *Journal of Paediatric Surgery*, 40(3); 568–7

Cooper CS, Abousally CT, Austin C, *et al.* (2003) Do public schools teach voiding dysfunction? Results of an elementary school teacher survey. *Journal of Urology*, 170: 956–8

De Gennaro M, Lais A, Fariello G, *et al*. (1991)Early diagnosis and treatment of spinal dysraphism to prevent urinary incontinence. *European Urology*, 20: 140–5

Heaton KW (2000) *The Bristol Stool Form Scale*. Harefield: Norgine Ltd

Koff SA (1983) Estimating bladder capacity in children. *Urology*, 21(3): 248

Lapides S (1971) Clean intermittent self-catheterisation in the treatment of urinary tract disease. *Trans-American Association for Genitourinary Surgery*, 63: 92

Mahan JD, Menster MI, Koff SA (1994) Complications of intestinal augmentation and substitution cystoplasty. *Paediatric Nephrology*, 8 (4): 505–7

Mitrofanoff P (1980) Cystomie continente trans appendiclaire dans le traîtement des vessies neurologiques. *Chirurgie Pediatrique*, 21: 297–305.

Monti PR, Lara RC, Dutra MA, Rezende de Carvalho J (1997) New techniques for construction of efferent conduits based on the Mitrofanoff principle. *Urology*, 49: 112–15

Samuel M, Boddy S-AM (2004) Is spina bifida occulta associated with lower urinary tract dysfunction in children? *Journal of Urology*, 171 (6 part 2): 2664–6

Samuel M, Madden NP, Boddy S-AM (2002) Factors that determine long-term outcome of artificial sphincters in children. *British Journal of Urology International* [in press] (Presented BAPS International Congress, Cambridge, July 2002)

11

A surgical perspective on intractable faecal incontinence

Edward Kiely

Key points

- Children whose faecal incontinence is a consequence of severe structural or functional disorders should be referred to a surgeon.

- Anatomical malformations or lack of nerve supply may make continence impossible. In such cases, management is best achieved by a 'washout' regime.

- The family will need plenty of support, preferably provided by a specialist nurse.

Health promotion points

- Bowel washouts can be the best way of managing a difficult situation, but support and teaching will be needed.

Faecal incontinence is defined as the involuntary discharge of faeces at inappropriate times and in inappropriate places.

Prevalence

Faecal incontinence is uncommon in healthy children without congenital malformations. Those children who are born with structural anorectal problems or with spinal dysraphism are much more likely to have trouble with bowel control. In children with large meningomyelocoeles, for example, faecal incontinence is almost universal, while more than 50% of children born with major anorectal malformations will have some degree of faecal soiling. Different figures are published for children affected by Hirschsprung's disease, but up to a quarter will have episodes of incontinence during childhood (Mishalany and Woolley 1987).

Aetiology

Bowel control implies the ability to sense the need for defecation, the ability to distinguish gas from liquid or solid stool and the ability to defer evacuation until the appropriate time. The mechanisms which underlie faecal continence are not clearly understood. On the sensory side, information from sensory receptors is fed to the spinal cord and to the brain, which in turn exert control over the muscles which are the motor side of continence. In the absence of either sensory or motor aspects, bowel control will be deficient.

Sensory receptors are located in the rectal wall, anal canal and the muscles of the pelvic floor. The manner in which these receptors function is not understood.

The motor side of continence comprises two sets of muscles – smooth and striated. The smooth muscle component is the internal anal sphincter. This is a thickening of the circular muscle of the bowel at the distal end of the rectum and it is an involuntary muscle. The external anal sphincter and levator ani (pelvic floor) are striated voluntary muscles which enclose rectum and anus on three sides – laterally and posteriorly. These two muscles coalesce around the rectum and anus and work together in a co-ordinated fashion. They maintain tonic contraction, which relaxes only at the time of defecation.

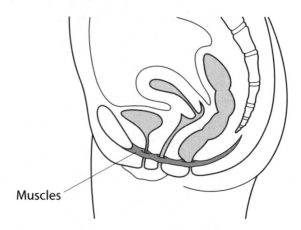

Muscles

Figure 11.1 The muscles of the pelvic floor, anus and rectum

Of all of these structures, the most important in terms of both sensation and motor control is the puborectalis, the caudal component of the levator ani. Damage to this structure or to its nerve supply will make normal bowel control impossible.

The sensory side of bowel control is often deficient in children born with anorectal malformations. In addition, the surgical correction of these malformations may further compromise sensory function. Surgical trauma may also be a factor when incontinence occurs after pull-through operations for Hirschsprung's disease. When such surgery is repeated after failure of the initial operation, the risk of damage to sensory and motor aspects of bowel control increases.

Severe constipation, which results in a megarectum, is associated with absence of any sensation of rectal fullness and often with continuous soiling. The rectal wall may become thickened and atonic and does not work normally as a result. If substantial structural change has occurred in the rectal wall, the process may not be reversible. For most however, successful treatment of the constipation will result in restitution of normal bowel control.

In children with congenital or acquired lesions of the spinal cord, sensory and motor aspects of bowel control are damaged to a varying degree. Faecal incontinence is the rule when the distal part of the spinal cord is affected.

Finally, in most of the children in the groups mentioned above, colonic motility is also abnormal. In those with a tendency to constipation and incontinence, reduced colonic motility will exacerbate these problems.

Assessment

From the history, it is usually clear if a child has any rectal sensation. Straining at stool is an automatic response to rectal distension in an infant. Absence of straining, for instance after surgical correction of an anorectal malformation, is in this author's experience a poor prognostic sign. On the other hand, an infant who strains and is aware of an impending stool will be continent.

When physical examination reveals a shortened sacrum, bulging perineum or patulous anus, sensory input and muscle function are deficient. Incontinence is then very likely.

The area in the spinal cord that exerts control over anorectal function also controls bladder function. In the presence of severe spinal malformations, a neuropathic bladder will result – often manifest by dribbling urinary incontinence with or without bladder distension. A child with a neuropathic bladder is unlikely to develop satisfactory bowel control in later life.

Investigation

A standard history and physical examination (including rectal examination) are usually sufficient to indicate the nature and extent of the problem.

In those who have undergone corrective anorectal surgery, more detailed examination under anaesthetic may be required. In some children rectal biopsy may also be necessary. Imaging is occasionally required. Contrast studies may show abnormal intestinal anatomy, such as severe megarectum and megacolon, and such findings will affect management.

Cross sectional imaging (MRI) gives more detailed information on internal anatomy. This may be required to evaluate the accuracy of corrective surgery or to delineate the extent of spinal cord anomalies.

Treatment

Faecal incontinence may prevent a child from attending nursery school and will affect placement at primary school later on. However, children under the age of five years have no interest in the means by which continence is maintained. At this age children ignore the problem – it seems to be the young child's way of dealing with a problem over which they have no control. After the age of five years, they take more interest in what is happening but are usually unwilling to co-operate with invasive forms of management until after the age of seven years or more. The difficulties this creates for a child in school can be imagined.

Once the assessment and investigations have been completed, initial treatment is directed toward correctable aspects of the problem. In other words, if there is pronounced constipation this should be addressed, usually with the aid of stimulant laxatives such as senokot or polyethylene glycol (Candy *et al.* 2006).

Should the problem persist despite adequate treatment of constipation and faecal loading, then treatment is aimed at emptying the rectum at appropriate times in order to provide a period of hours free from soiling. This may be accomplished by the use of suppositories or mini enemas, used in the morning to try and evacuate the distal intestine and thereby allow the child to concentrate on school work rather than possible continence problems.

For those whose incontinence is a consequence of intestinal hurry, with liquid stools, the use of loperamide may be very helpful. For those in whom an inadequate continence mechanism is the cause of the problem, we have had little success with dietary manipulation or with the use of drugs. In addition, we have not found biofeedback methods to be very helpful. As a result, we have used more invasive forms of management, including enemas, together with retrograde or antegrade washouts. Large volume retrograde washouts, designed to clean the entire colon have proved effective in managing children with spinal abnormalities (Shandling and Gilmour 1987). However, as the child is unable to do this unaided it creates a problem with the approach of adult life.

Antegrade washouts delivered through the appendix, a colonic conduit or button device are successful in the great majority (Squire *et al.* 1993). Clinical experience shows that children under the age of seven have neither the discipline nor motivation to establish a successful washout regime. As a general rule, the older the child the more successful this intervention.

The main prerequisite for successful use of antegrade washouts, or indeed any other regimen, is the availability of an experienced nurse who can work with the child and family to achieve a good outcome (Pena *et al.* 1998). Frequent adjustments to the regimen to define what suits the child is a job best done by a nurse. It is necessary to vary the type and quantity of washout fluid to find what works. In some children, the fluid used needs to be altered with the passage of time. The majority use some form of active ingredient (usually phosphate or bisacodyl) together with saline both to dilute the active ingredient and to achieve more efficient evacuation. Care is needed in regard to phosphate enemas, as severe hypocalcaemia has been reported after phosphate enemas in children and adults (Sotos *et al.* 1977). For the 7–10-year-old age group, 30 mls of a phosphate enema is usually sufficient, while a full enema is likely to be necessary by the mid teens. The volume of saline used is usually 100–500 mls at a time.

In almost all families the washout is done at night to allow for some fluid leakage overnight. The great majority perform the washouts on an alternate day basis and for most the entire procedure is finished within 45 minutes. In our patients, who are mainly incontinent as a consequence of anorectal malformations, the success rate for this form of management is about 90%.

In a small number of children who have disabling incontinence and for whom the antegrade washouts are ineffective or unacceptable, an alternative form of management is necessary. This usually takes the form of a colostomy.

When stomas are formed in young children there is a reasonable expectation that the stoma can be reversed in the teenage years. Stomas performed for faecal incontinence after this age are unlikely ever to be reversed.

Conclusion

Faecal incontinence is a distressing problem for children and their families. For those with no structural malformation, management is primarily by use of altered diet and medication.

Invasive forms of management are usually required for those with structural or anatomical problems. The antegrade washout has been the most reliable intervention under these circumstances.

A small group of children exists where none of these treatments is applicable. For these children, a stoma is a reliable method of removing the problem and improving their quality of life.

References

Candy DC, Edwards D, Geraint M (2006) Treatment of faecal impaction with polyethylene glycol and electrolytes (PGE+E) followed by a double blind trial comparison of PGE+E versus lactulose as maintenance therapy. *Journal of Pediatric Gastroenterology and Nutrition*, 43: 65–70

Mishalany HG, Woolley MM (1987) Postoperative functional and manometric evaluation of patients with Hirschsprung's disease. *Journal of Pediatric Surgery*, 22: 443–6

Pena A, Guardino K, Tovilla JM *et al.* (1998) Bowel management for fecal incontinence in patients with anorectal malformations. *Journal of Pediatric Surgery*, 33: 133–7

Shandling B, Gilmour RF (1987) The enema continence catheter in spina bifida: successful bowel management. *Journal of Pediatric Surgery*, 22: 271–3

Sotos JF, Cutier EA, Finkel MA, Doody D (1977) Hypocalcemic coma following two pediatric phosphate enemas. *Pediatrics*, 60: 305–7

Squire R, Kiely EM, Carr B *et al.* (1993) The clinical application of the Malone antegrade continence enema. *Journal of Pediatric Surgery*, 28: 1012–15

12 | Psychological issues of incontinence
Melinda Edwards

Key points

- Incontinence is likely to distress the children who suffer from it, as well as providing a challenge to their carers.

- The importance of comprehensive assessment cannot be over-emphasised.

- Appropriate psychological strategies can help morale, motivation and concordance with management plans.

Health promotion points

- Children need to be helped to see that incontinence is a problem to be managed, not a defining part of who they are.

- Parents may need help and guidance on how to communicate with their child about continence issues in such a way that it is clear the incontinence, and not the child, is the problem.

Although incontinence is a familiar problem, it can be very distressing for children and their families, and prove extremely challenging and frustrating to manage effectively. A comprehensive assessment is required to enable a good understanding of the problem and develop the most effective management strategy. This should include taking a careful medical and developmental history; detailed assessment of presenting difficulties, including evaluation of strategies already tried and current practice; and assessment of psychological factors relating to the child and family. In this chapter, we will look in more detail at psychological factors associated with incontinence, considering the meaning and impact of incontinence on the lives of children and families, psychological strategies for engaging, motivating and supporting children with treatment programmes, and helping children adapt and cope with enduring continence difficulties.

Throughout this chapter, 'parent' will refer to parent and/or carer, and 'child' will cover children of all ages, including adolescents.

Developmental factors

It is helpful to have an understanding of the normal developmental trends in acquiring continence as this can provide reassuring information for children and their families. For parents, it can lead to more realistic expectations of their child and help to alleviate pressure and increase tolerance of their child's problems (Butler and Price 2001). For children, it may be helpful for them to know that they are not alone, that other children of their age – or even older – are also experiencing difficulties with continence.

The age at which children generally acquire urinary and bowel control is variable, with studies indicating a steadily decreasing prevalence of incontinence with increasing age. Children generally acquire urinary control during the daytime before they achieve it at night, with bed-wetting being common even in later childhood (Butler, Golding and Heron 2005). A recent study conducted as part of the ALSPAC survey (Butler, Golding and Northstone 2005) has indicated that 15.5% of children at 7½ years wet the bed (with most wetting once or less than once a week). A higher prevalence was reported in boys than girls. Within this large cohort study, 3.3% of children had both daytime and night wetting. Epidemiological studies suggest that around 1–2% of children are still bed-wetting in the later teenage years (Verhulst et al.1985).

In terms of bowel control, around 10% of three-year-olds are still soiling at least once a month. Generally, 4 years is considered a diagnostic cut-off for encopresis. By 4 years, the rate has dropped to less than 5%, and by 7 years, the figure is nearer 1.5%. At age 10–12 years, soiling at a frequency of at least once a month affects 1.3% of boys and 0.3% of girls (Clayden et al. 2002).

Psychological impact

To be able to help children most effectively, and successfully engage them in a treatment programme, it is important to understand the social and psychological impact of incontinence on their lives. It is also important to understand how children might experience the whole process of coming to see a professional for help and the practical impact of implementing treatment strategies.

Clearly there are also children for whom incontinence may be an enduring problem alongside other medical challenges (Butler and Price 2001). In these instances the emphasis may be on supporting the child in adapting to the difficulties arising from incontinence by enhancing self-esteem and independence, in addition to addressing practical strategies for day-to-day management of incontinence within the wider context of illness or disability (Edwards and Davis 1988).

Incontinence can be extremely distressing, and anxiety provoking for children of all ages. Ollendick and colleagues (1989) found that school children rated 'wetting in class' as the third most stressful event possible (only behind 'losing a parent' and 'going blind'). In another study comparing young people with nocturnal enuresis with a control group, bed-wetting was ranked as the second most stressful life event by adolescents although it was only of minimal concern for the control group (Van Tijen *et al.* 1997). It is recognised that stress and anxiety may be related to a child's experience of shame, embarrassment and fear of their problem being discovered by others. Restrictions to social activities, such as staying with friends, or going on school trips are not uncommon, and children may avoid developing close personal relationships or go to extreme lengths to avoid being 'found out' (Butler 1998).

Many children with incontinence have lower than average self-esteem and low self-confidence as a result (Hagglof *et al.* 1997). It may not necessarily be apparent that children in this position hold negative views of themselves; indeed, some may come across as feeling very ambivalent or even completely disinterested in the whole subject. When children feel totally helpless and undermined by a problem that appears to them to be overwhelming, denial and dissociation can be a means of coping. Children may give the impression of not caring that they are wet or have been avoided by other children because they smell. One child reported that he just sought out the 'smelliest' boy in the class to stand next to, so that his own problems of soiling and smell ceased to be so evident! Some children have even 'given up' on all aspects of self-hygiene or using the toilet as they perceive it does not help them (Hagglof *et al.* 1997).

Unsurprisingly, such attitudes do not endear these children to others (such as teachers or carers) who might be totally exasperated by this apparent 'laziness' and resistance to any attempts to help them.

Children may also 'test out' the commitment and relationship with the professional helping them, as they may find it hard to be confident that someone will actually help them with their problem. Professionals may feel inclined to discontinue work with a child who appears unmotivated to change. In reality, however, the child's low emotional state may be obstructing him or her from engaging and cooperating in any programme. Further assessment of the child's emotional state may be indicated.

Children's low esteem and confidence can be further undermined by the reactions of relatives or others to their incontinence. For example, the child (rather than the incontinence) may be identified by the family as being the problem. This makes it difficult for children with continence problems to see themselves as anything other than dirty, naughty, or a nuisance, with other aspects of their life being overshadowed by this. Clearly, helping children feel better about themselves will require helping them to see that their problem with incontinence is only one aspect of their lives, and not the thing that defines who they are.

It cannot be overestimated how challenging and stressful incontinence can be for families. It is almost inevitable that this will have some impact on how family members respond to the child and make him or her feel. For example, in one family, the older brothers were constantly angry and hostile towards their sibling, refusing to let him come into their bedroom or sit on particular chairs in the living room as he 'makes everything wet and smelly'. They also blamed him for the fact they were too embarrassed to invite their friends around to visit them at home. It is also not unusual for children to have experienced rather punitive management strategies, which is often a reflection of how desperate and intolerant family members have become towards the problem.

In addition to poor self-esteem, children may have limited hope or confidence in their abilities to do anything to improve their situation. They may even have seen other professionals in the past, tried any number of treatments, and built up a belief that either the treatments do not help, or that they themselves are not good or clever enough to be successful. Children may feel very hopeless about any new treatment. They may feel so sure it will not work that they actually sabotage attempts to bring about change. Fear of failure can cause an unwillingness to try something new, or discourage the child from giving a new management programme a chance to succeed (for example by failing to try it for long enough, or giving up at the first difficulty). Consistent, clear and continuing support from health professionals

Figure 12.1 Helpful resources for children

- T Black and Williams I. *Poo Go Home*. Northumberland Mental Health NHS Trust, 1988

- T Black and Williams I. *Sneaky Poo*. Northumberland Mental Health NHS Trust, 1988

- R Butler. *Eric's Wet To Dry Bedtime Book. A Self-help Manual for Children Who Wet The Bed*. Nottingham Rehab, 1989

- ERIC, *All About Nocturnal Enuresis*. (An interactive CD ROM for children and their parents, available from ERIC, see Appendix 1)

- J Hindley and C King. *How Your Body Works*. Usborne Publishing, 1992

- J Mills and R Crowley. *Sammy the Elephant and Mr Camel. A story to help children overcome bed-wetting*. Magination Press, 1988

- K Williams (2002) *Fact File for Children: 'All about Poo'.* Queen's Medical Centre NHS Trust, Nottingham, 2002

and carers is crucial if setbacks like these are to be overcome. Figure 12.1 Gives a list of printed resources that children may find helpful.

Psychological aspects of treatment

Psychological strategies are an integral part of any good management or treatment plan. They should include engaging children, and facilitating their fullest co-operation by working collaboratively, motivating and empowering them in carrying out their agreed plan, at the same time as providing them with appropriate emotional and problem solving support.

Engaging children

Engaging children and developing a trusting relationship with them is an important prerequisite in helping them deal with their problems. Integral to achieving this is listening carefully to children, conveying that you are interested in them, respectful of how they are feeling and genuine both in wanting to understand their experiences and to help them.

A general principle for working effectively with children is to be child-focused within the treatment plan. Although the professional needs to be well informed and guided by treatment strategies, it is important to focus on the child's unique experience of incontinence, the meaning it has for the child, as well as the impact that carrying out any proposed treatment might have on daily life. It is also important to gain a good understanding of the positive outcomes that the child expects or hopes improved continence will bring. For one child, the goal being worked towards may be wearing prettier underwear, whereas for another child it may be the freedom to have a sleepover with a friend, or to go on a school trip with greater confidence. Without this consideration, it is easy to overlook particular obstacles the child is likely to face while carrying out a treatment plan, or to miss subtle opportunities for increasing motivation.

Gaining trust

It is important to recognise how uncomfortable some children may feel in being brought to a professional for help. Children may have developed very negative expectations of being seen, fearing they may be told off, humiliated or have their problems belittled. Very few children will have initiated seeking help; they are more likely to have been encouraged, persuaded, or even brought along unwillingly. It may be helpful to ask children how they felt about coming along to see you, and even praise them for coming to discuss such a difficult problem with you. This may also be a good time to reassure the child that you see many young people with similar difficulties and to make a comment about how some of them described feeling at the start ... and how they felt more comfortable over time. This can be very reassuring, both in terms of the child realising he or she is not alone in having a problem, but also in terms of knowing you are in a good position to help with their difficulties.

A primary aim of the appointment with you is to help children feel as comfortable and relaxed as possible. It can be useful to check with children what name (or nickname) they prefer to be called by, as often we are far more formal with a child than is necessary, and may unwittingly be calling them by the name only used when they are in trouble! It is also important to introduce yourself and your role and start to explain a little about what will be happening in the meeting. For example, whether you are just going to be talking, or if you will be physically examining the child following your conversation. In some situations, children may be anxiously awaiting 'something' to happen, if they do not know what to expect.

It may be helpful to talk initially about neutral topics such as family, school, or any particular activities or interests the child may have. It is also useful to try and engage children in a conversation about something they enjoy and feel positive about, or believe themselves to be good at or valued for. If children feel you have some positive knowledge or feelings towards them, it will make it easier for them to trust you and reveal information they are more concerned with or feel negative about. It also helps confirm for children that you are interested in them and not just in their problem. It may also be helpful to engage children in a conversation about their achievements, particularly those they have had to work hard for, such as learning to ride a bike, or finding their way to the next level of the latest computer game. This can prove a useful way in to talking about the rewards of keeping going in order to achieve your goal.

Children may not always be able to tell you when they feel distressed or uncomfortable in the room with you. It is important, therefore, to be attentive to non-verbal cues of distress and sensitive to the child's needs for reassurance or support while they are with you. A child may show distress by appearing very distracted or preoccupied by a thought or part of their body: they may fidget, or ask to leave the room to use the toilet for example. A child who is uncomfortable with you is far less likely to be able to listen and take in any information, and a child who has found the whole experience of coming to talk about their incontinence too stressful, may chose not to come back to any further appointments and drop out of treatment. Commenting on what you see, acknowledging unease and asking if there is anything you can do to help them feel more comfortable can be useful.

When children feel uneasy during a conversation, they may choose to engage in another activity while talking to you. This can be a distraction from feelings of discomfort, as well as giving them an excuse to avoid eye contact with you. It can therefore be helpful to have some small (and quiet) toys or objects around for the child to look at or handle. Children can often look very engaged in their play but be very attentive to the conversation at the same time! It might be helpful to explicitly offer children the opportunity to explore play items in the room, as parents may otherwise feel their child is being rude by seemingly not fully attending to you, the professional. (However, some professionals would actively discourage this approach – see, for example, Chapter 8 on 'Faecal soiling in childhood' by Kenneth Wilkinson.)

The wider family

Although the focus of this chapter is on the child's experience, it is of equal importance that parents are well engaged in the helping process, and that a careful assessment of their views, experiences and coping resources is made. Clearly, in most instances, families will provide the greatest emotional and practical support in dealing with continence problems and carrying out treatment plans. The relationship between the child and parent, as well as attitudes held by parents about the child's incontinence and their efforts to deal with it, will require careful exploration. If parents are extremely negative and punitive in their response to the child, some work may be needed to address this prior to embarking on a treatment programme, which may otherwise only put further pressure on the parent and child relationship. The challenge can be in hearing and acknowledging the parents' perspective, without parents speaking for their child and taking all the reponsibility for the management of the problem away from the child.

Exploring the child's experience

Exploration of the child's history, symptoms and the impact of their continence difficulties should be paced in such a way that it meets the child's needs. It is important to be sensitive to verbal and non-verbal responses to questions. You may also find it helpful to remind children that you meet many young people with this or similar difficulties to develop their confidence that you will not be shocked, overwhelmed or disgusted at what they might have to tell you, and to introduce some very positive accounts of how creative or successful young people can be in dealing with their difficulties.

It may also be important to monitor the impact of parents' presentation and history of the problem on the child, especially if either party is conveying a great deal of frustration, anger and negative emotion. It is important to acknowledge parents' distress and the challenges they have experienced in trying to manage their child's incontinence. It is also helpful to be aware that parents may have felt extremely undermined by not being able to sort out their child's problems themselves, and to reassure them that many parents have expressed similar feelings. It may be necessary to help parents understand more about how

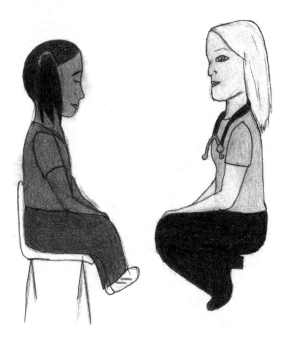

Figure 12.2 A child's drawing of herself with a health professional. In (**a**) she is unhappy, in (**b**) she is happy and confident

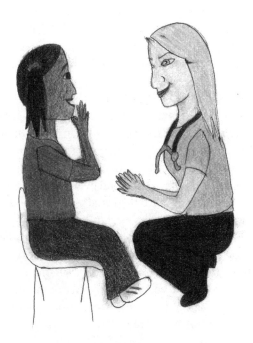

difficult their child's experience may be when hearing others talk negatively about their problems, and to help parent's reframe the challenges they are facing more appropriately. There may be an opportunity at this point to show your appreciation that the parent has been sufficiently concerned to make the commitment to bring along the child for the appointment, and to reinforce how important it has been for the child to come along in order to get some help to sort this problem out.

Assessment

Once the child is comfortable with you, a more in-depth exploration of their continence difficulties is possible. It can be interesting to ask children not only what the problem is, but also about their ideas or theories as to why it is happening. If children know, they will often tell you! Their answers may also reveal a great deal about what they have heard other people saying about them, in addition to indicating any misperceptions they have about their own body or the problem itself.

A careful assessment of the current situation is needed, to note the frequency and severity of the problem as well as current practice in dealing with it. This baseline information can be reviewed in all further appointments to monitor very openly with the child any progress that is made. It is also important to ask about all treatments previously tried, and to establish whether there were any aspects of these that helped at all or which proved just too difficult to carry out.

A comprehensive assessment of the history and presenting difficulties will help establish the type of incontinence and possible aetiology which will clearly be necessary to inform the most appropriate treatment. For example, whether faecal incontinence has arisen from associations with pain due to anal fissures; or fear, from aversion to the toilet; or some overly rigid, punitive or even absent toilet-training. Also whether any pattern of continence had ever been reliably established, and if so, what factors may have triggered or disrupted this routine.

Careful monitoring using diaries can be extremely helpful to gain an understanding of current practice with micturition or soiling. In a study reported by Rhodes (2000), in which diary recording of current bladder function and fluid intake was part of the assessment, some children were found to not be using the toilet at all during the school day (possibly due to lack of privacy or poor condition of school toilets) and an appropriate intervention involving regular toileting was indicated. For those children assessed to be passing urine frequently (suggestive of some degree of bladder instability) a different intervention was clearly indicated.

It can also be very informative to ask children who in their family has the greatest worries or problems about their incontinence, and how they know this (i.e. what the family member says or does to show their concern) and to keep following this line to establish where the child places him or herself in the worry picture. It can then be helpful to pursue what impact the wetting or soiling has on the child's life. Asking children what would be different for them if they were dry or clean may reveal useful information, both about the current situation and also about what goals a particular child may be motivated to work towards.

It can be very hard for some children simply to imagine how different life might be for them; one helpful strategy might be to suggest a scenario for a child to structure in their imagination (Weiner *et al.* 2000). For example, you might suggest to a child to imagine that overnight something very 'magical' happened which meant that the problem was helped a little bit. Then, ask what the first sign of this might be to the child him or herself, then to other people, and finally what might be said or done differently as a result. It may also be necessary to ask children what the best things might be about being continent but also to check what (if any) the drawbacks or negative aspects of this might be. For example, when asking children about the positive aspects and drawbacks of being able to self-catheterise, and take some independence in managing continence, many children reported the positive aspects being the privacy and control this gave them. However a number of younger children reported that they would miss out the special time and attention they had been getting from their mother in doing this (Edwards *et al.* 2004).

Another line of enquiry may be to ask who in the family or outside the family is aware of the problem. Given our awareness of the secrecy and shame that surrounds many young people with continence difficulties, very few people are likely to know. It may be that certain family members, close friends and important adults such as the child's teacher at school will *not* know. Although, clearly, not everyone has a need to know, it is helpful to explore who could be in a position to provide support or practical assistance. It can be an idea to suggest to the child that they can help choose their own 'team' of people to help with this problem. Children interested in football or netball teams can often be easily engaged with idea, and even choose to give their team a name

('Amy's Angels' for example), and draw or write out everyone chosen for the team. It can then be possible to identify what support role each individual and chosen team player might take. For example, a school teacher may be someone in the team who prompts or praises the child for using the toilet, or develops a special code of communication so that the child can easily leave the class to use the toilet; the classroom assistant may be the team player who can help with arrangements for the child to change clothes which are wet or soiled and an older sister might be another member of the team who helps by commenting positively on the successes of the child when at home.

Although some children may find talking about their incontinence very difficult, they may be more able or willing to draw something of their experience. Even asking children to draw a picture of themselves or their family can reveal a considerable amount about their self-image. If children enjoy drawing, you might also ask them to draw what it is like when they are wet or have soiled, and then draw what it would be like if they were clean and dry. These pictures can then be used as a concrete and visual reminder of the child's goals for treatment.

Formulating and carrying out a treatment plan

Any plan of treatment is more likely to be adhered to if it has been put together with the child. A good assessment will provide the basis and direction for all subsequent treatment plans, so it is vital you take as much time as necessary to complete a good assessment – engaging the child (and parent) in the process as fully as possible. This will give the best possible chance of a positive outcome.

Ideally, the assessment process itself will give children (and their parents) a sense of being supported. Certainly, it may help them to feel confident their continence problems are being understood and taken seriously, and that real efforts are being made to improve their situation. The management strategies employed will depend in part on the child's age, the identified problem, the child's own motivation and how much support is available. A range of psychological strategies can be implemented, and these will be reviewed briefly here. The evidence base for studies for the most effective interventions will then be examined.

In addition to an agreed treatment plan, strategies need to be explored to make the current situation more bearable. These might include using protective coverings for the mattress and pillow, taking clean clothes to change into at school, or using deodorising spray to both feel and smell fresh. For children experiencing a high degree of urgency when using the toilet, a special card (bearing the words 'I just can't wait') is available from Incontact (see Appendix 1) and can be presented to shop assistants and/or staff when out and about to gain quick and easy access to toilets. This may alleviate some of the anxiety a child may have about going out.

It is always best to work as collaboratively as possible with a child, jointly agreeing the steps of the treatment programme and working out a way of monitoring progress and celebrating (or reinforcing) success. To be effective, the treatment plan will need to be manageable within the context of normal daily demands and activities for the child (and parent); so appropriate discussion with families will be necessary to ensure the plan is not only good on paper, but can be carried out in practical terms.

Clearly, children who feel they have 'ownership' of a plan are likely to feel more committed to carrying it out. Working in partnership with children can also serve to empower them and raise their self-esteem as they feel more in control of what is happening to them. This is particularly important when one considers how out of control their body may seem to them because of their lack of continence.

It is also important to be valuing and positive about the child's own goals and reasons to be successful. For example, an adult may want the child to be dry so they do not get infections or wet their clothing and smell, whereas a child may just be interested in being able to choose more attractive underwear. All goals need to be valued.

Specific strategies

Education

Helping children understand how their urinary system or bowels work can be effective in demystifying what may have been experienced as an incomprehensible and uncontrollable body process. Informing children can empower and enable them to be actively involved in devising a plan, rather than carrying out instructions without understanding why.

Effective information giving requires establishing what children already know or understand, providing clear, well structured information, and then checking carefully with children what meaning and sense they have derived from this, before adding further or more complex information.

Developing regular routines

If the child has experienced problems with continence over a long period of time, it is likely that any normal or regular toileting regime has never been successfully established or has been lost along the way. Part of any effective management plan is to re-educate about regular toileting and re-establish an appropriate pattern of using the toilet.

It can also be helpful to look at any way of incorporating other parts of the treatment plan within daily routines, as this can make it easier to remember. For example, tablets might be taken with a drink at breakfast time. One young girl decided this was the best way of trying to remember to take her tablets and even made sticky labels for her cereal packets to prompt her to do this!

Setting realistic goals

While being respectful of the child's overall goals, it is important to help set realistic and achievable steps to achieving those goals. It would clearly be very unhelpful and extremely demoralising for children if they had set themselves a goal that is too advanced or too complex for them to achieve. It can sometimes be helpful to liken the whole process of overcoming the problem with climbing a very high mountain: it is hard work, and you have to set yourselves little 'resting places' where you take a few minutes to rest and congratulate yourself for your achievements before taking on the next stage of the mountain. The aim is always to set achievable targets, which enable the child to experience success and grow in confidence throughout the course of the treatment (see Figure 12.3). Each step is decided jointly with the child with the next step agreed at each subsequent meeting.

Behavioural and cognitive-behavioural techniques

The most common behavioural approach is operant conditioning with rewards for appropriate behaviour. Positive reinforcement is provided to reinforce and shape behaviour often by means of reward or star charts. Stars can be a reward, for example, for removing soiled or wet clothes to the laundry basket, sitting on the toilet, or any other desired action. Star charts can also be an effective way of monitoring and showing the child explicitly how successful they have been, with the 'stars' being intrinsically reinforcing as well as currency for a reward that has been negotiated between parent and child (Weiner *et al.*

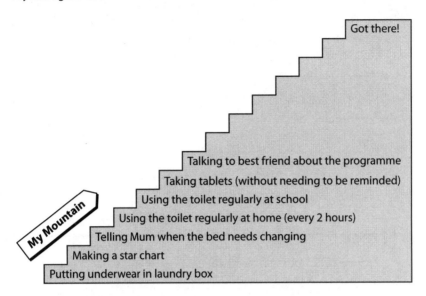

Figure 12.3 'My mountain' step chart

2000). For example a set number of stars can be exchanged for a treat such as time on the computer or a toy the child would like. It can be very helpful for children to be involved in developing their own star charts, using pictures or stickers that they find appealing (see Figures 12.4 and 12.5). Children may enjoy decorating their star charts with drawings or importing images from their computer. Involving children in this way can help engage them and empower their role in their treatment plan. There are also a number of excellent websites offering a

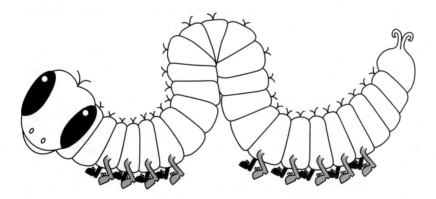

Figure 12.4 Caterpillar star chart for young children

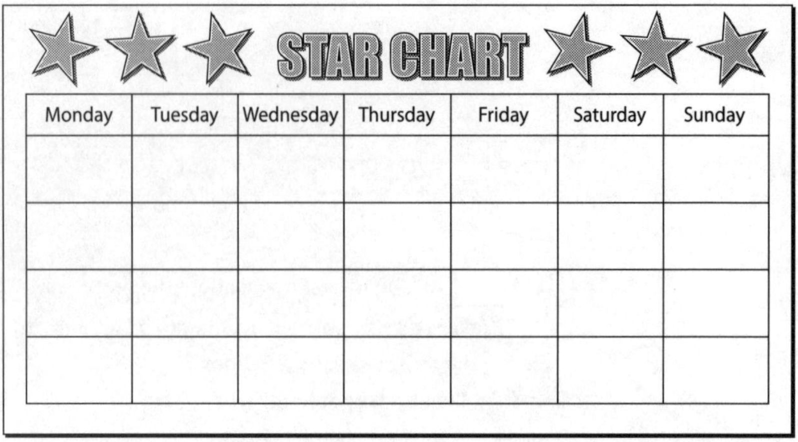

Figure 12.5 Computer-generated star chart for older children

range of reward and star charts which are referenced at the end of the chapter.

Any task which enables children to take an active part in developing their treatment plan, measuring their progress, or sharing problem-solving ideas to address practical problems they encounter, can help them to feel they are taking an active role in changing their problem, which can lead to more confidence, positive self-esteem and greater belief in themselves. The psycho-educational component of treatment will help children develop knowledge about their continence difficulties, and help challenge unhelpful misperceptions they might have, such as it being their fault that they have problems, or that nothing will work and they will always soil or be wet. Changing the way children feel about themselves and creating hope and possibilities for change are all integral psychological aspects to treatment.

Using contracts

Contracts are a way of engaging the child more fully with the treatment plan, with explicit goals and agreement regarding the part the child will play and the role of others. The contract can be used to specify the rewards or incentives for the child keeping to their plan, and therefore the consequences (agreed by the child) of not doing so. Some children may enjoy the explicit and formal nature of a contract that they can sign themselves, alongside parents and professionals.

Externalising the problem

At the simplest level, externalising involves seeing the child as *having* a problem with incontinence rather than *being* an incontinent child. The manner in which you relate to the child and show interest in the whole child, not just the problem, will reflect this.

Therapeutically, much work has been carried out using externalising (see White 1989), taking the problem outside the child, and enabling the problem to be tackled more collaboratively by the child with the family and professional rather than the child feeling the focus of the problem and treatment. The idea of 'sneaky poo' being an entity itself and looking at the impact this has on the child and family has become a popular way of working with faecal incontinence, with some books for children developing these ideas further (see Black and Williams 1988, also Chapter 8 by Kenneth Wilkinson). Clinically it is possible to look at situations when it is more likely to come and when not and then to work out a plan to battle 'sneaky poo', to tell 'sneaky poo' to go away.

Encouraging responsibility

Much of what has already been discussed will support the treatment aim of encouraging the child to take on appropriate responsibility for their continence problems. It is not unusual for parents to have adopted an increased level of responsibility to compensate for a child who is very ambivalent or overwhelmed by their problem. As the child is encouraged to take 'ownership' and responsibility in a supported manner, this will hopefully increase motivation and co-operation with the treatment plan. The role of parents can become one of support rather than a more intrusive or even oppressive 'taking on' of the child's problems or being seen as someone continually 'nagging' the child.

The level of responsibility taken on will be dependent on the child's cognitive and emotional maturity. Responsibility can range from helping to devise or fill out diaries or charts, to informing their parent when clothing is wet and helping to change soiled bedclothes. Negotiating appropriate responsibility with the child (and parent) can be very effective and serve to really involve and empower the child.

Making the programmes fun

Children and parents can have some very good ideas as to how to make the treatment programme as fun as possible for them, and it can be very helpful to listen to these ideas. One boy planned out a most imaginative scene with soldiers around the bathroom to make the time spent sitting on the toilet less tedious for him, and one parent shared her trick of placing a brightly coloured table tennis ball in the toilet, so that her son could make a game of 'aiming' and 'firing' at the ball to increase his motivation and fun with a regular toileting routine.

Enuresis alarms

These are discussed more fully in Chapter 7 by Jonathan Evans, and are clearly the most effective treatment for enuresis as shown by a comprehensive review of the literature (Carr 2000). However, the child's motivation plays a central part in any success with this technique, which can be hard work. Successful implementation requires active involvement from parents (to ensure the child takes him or herself off to the toilet, rather than just switching off the alarm) as well as emotional support. Effective programmes have also included a psycho-educational component, retention control training and over learning of the procedure of waking and responding to a full bladder by using the toilet. Long-term success (and tackling possible relapses) will require a continuing support system to be in place.

Psychological support during treatment

Ideally, the face-to-face discussion you have already had with the child and parent will have resulted in a treatment plan that can be implemented practically into daily life, anticipating and finding solutions for a range of possible obstacles and challenges that may arise. Clearly it is not possible to anticipate everything and any programme that requires time and commitment is always potentially vulnerable when families are under any stress, however well motivated they might be at the outset. It is always important, therefore, to build in a support strategy to help maintain the programme.

One aspect of this support strategy might be to prepare the child and family for the reality that all plans have 'off days' and that progress does not necessarily follow a smooth, straight path. Although setbacks are frustrating and disappointing, preparing for such difficulties and talking through strategies for dealing with them can help you provide a structured response.

It is also important to consider with the family what support they may require from others, including wider family members or school staff, and what they might require from you, particularly how often it might be helpful to meet, and what access they have to you between appointments. Although time consuming, a 'prompt letter' reminding the child of their goals and plan, and wishing them luck, or regular phone calls to talk about how things are going can provide a powerful means of support and reinforcement for the child's efforts.

Even after the child has experienced success with the programme, it is important to put in place some low level support system, to ensure this is maintained. Relapses are not uncommon, and are particularly associated with a change of routine such as during holidays or significant family events. They can often be managed by talking through what may have triggered them, or retracing and repeating steps of the treatment programme as a 'booster' session.

Incontinence as a symptom of emotional distress

Tackling the incontinence itself may resolve some emotional or behavioural difficulties, and certainly help many children feel better about this aspect of their lives, and themselves. However, incontinence can be both a cause and a symptom of emotional distress. Through the assessment process it may become apparent that emotional difficulties are so severe as to undermine any attempts to resolve the continence problems. It may also be revealed or suspected that the incontinence has been triggered by emotional trauma and opportunities should be provided for the child to be able to talk about this safely. In these instances referral on to a child mental health specialist is indicated.

Children with enduring continence problems

For those children with enduring problems, particularly those in the context of other medical conditions, it is equally important to understand and explore the distress caused by incontinence, and not make assumptions about what is particularly challenging for them. Children who have obvious physical disabilities may feel comfortable that their mobility or sensory needs are well recognised, understood and supported by others. However, difficulties with continence are less visible and may be felt to be unacceptable to others. This may result in children feeling it is not possible to be open about these difficulties, or request help with them. A study of children with spina bifida (Lie *et al.* 1991), found that urinary and faecal incontinence were rated among the most stressful aspects of the condition, and rated more highly in this regard than impaired motor function.

Sadly, many children who catheterise or use an ACE stoma for bowel management (see Chapter 14 by Rosie Kelly) still feel they must keep this 'shameful secret' from their peers. This can place a considerable burden on children, to the extent that some children refuse to co-operate with catheterising outside of the home, and in particular places such as school where they most fear being discovered. Even when special toilets are provided, some children are unwilling to use these to self-catheterise, as they feel simply going to a different toilet will bring unwanted attention and questions from others. One young boy at school described how he spent most of his breaktimes keeping watch on the corridor in which his toilet was situated, and feeling he could only enter and leave the toilet when no-one else was around. Following several breaktimes feeling 'trapped' inside the toilet and missing break altogether, he was highly resistant to using the toilet at all.

It is not surprising that some children become resentful and unco-operative with their self-care regimes when it impacts so intrusively on their social activities, such as this young boy at school, or children who need laxatives and then find themselves unable to feel confident to leave the house in case of an accident. Children may find it hard to accept their toileting needs are (and may always be) different from those of their peers. Alternatively, they may just get fed up with always *having* to do this self-care. Typically, adolescence is a time when issues around conforming and the transition of taking increasing responsibility for self-care may occur. However, the emotional distress of needing to carry out these techniques can occur at any age. Keeping an open dialogue with children about how they are getting on and managing their continence difficulties can make access to help with difficulties as they arise easier to provide. Providing opportunities to meet others in a similar situation can be extremely helpful if this is possible. Informing families about ERIC (see Appendix 1), and inviting children to explore their website or read their publications can also be greatly effective.

One rarely discussed area of concern for teenagers may involve their sexual function and an opportunity to talk about this privately should be provided. It is important to be mindful of the number of professionals in the room when giving this opportunity and to offer them time without their parents (or others in the room) if appropriate. Advice may be requested on what to say to a potential sexual partner or how to cope with practical issues of incontinence within the context of an intimate physical relationship.

Children may require the assistance of adult carers, both within and outside their family to support, supervise or even carry out personal aspects of self-care, including ACE stoma care and catheterisation. Psychological support may be needed to enable children to be able to communicate effectively and assertively with carers so that their physical needs can be addressed with respect, privacy and dignity.

Summary

Incontinence is a common but distressing condition in children. It is important to assess psychological factors in terms of aetiology and maintaining factors of the problem and to be able to effectively engage, support and motivate the child in any treatment programme. General principles for any management programme include involving the child fully in the development of the treatment programme, taking in to account the impact and meaning incontinence has on the child's life, and valuing and working towards the treatment goals prioritised by the child. Careful monitoring, and consistent and continuing support is required throughout the treatment plan and after-care.

References

Black T, Williams I (1988) *Poo Go Home*. Newcastle: Northumberland Mental Health NHS Trust
Black T, Williams I (1988) *Sneaky Poo*. Newcastle: Northumberland Mental Health NHS Trust
Butler R J (1998) Annotation: night wetting in children – psychological aspects. *Journal of Child Psychology and Psychiatry*, 39: 453–8
Butler RJ, Golding J, Heron J, ALSPAC Study Team (2005) Nocturnal enuresis: a survey of parental coping strategies at 7½ years. *Child: Health Care and Development*, 31: 659–67
Butler RJ, Golding J, Northstone K, ALSPAC Study Team (2005) Nocturnal eneuresis at 7½ years: prevalence and analysis of clinical signs. *British Journal of Urology International*, 96: 404–10

Butler U, Price K (2001) Bowel and bladder management in children with
disabilities. *Current Paediatrics*, 11:143–8

Carr A (2000) *What Works with Children and Adolescents? A Critical Review of
Psychological Interventions with Children, Adolescents and their Families*. New
York: Routledge

Clayden G, Taylor EA, Loader P, Borzyskowski M, Edwards M (2004) Wetting and
soiling. In: Rutter M, Taylor E (eds) *Child and Adolescent Psychiatry* 4e. Oxford:
Blackwell Publishing

Edwards M, Borzsykowski M, Cox A, Badcock J (2004) Neuropathic bladder and
intermittent catheterisation; social and psychological impact on children and
adolescents. *Developmental Medicine and Child Neurology*, 46: 168–77

Edwards M, Davis H (1988) *Counselling Children with Chronic Medical Conditions*.
London: BPS Books

Hagglof B, Andren O, Berstrom E, Marklund L, Wendelius M (1997) Self-esteem
before and after treatment in children with nocturnal enuresis and urinary
incontinence. *Scandinavian Journal of Urology and Nephrology*, 31: 79–82

Lie HR, Lagergren J, Rasmussen F, Lagerkvist B, Hagelsteen J, Börjeson M-C,
Muttilainen M, Taudorf K (1991) Bowel and bladder control of children with
myelomeningocele: a Nordic study. *Developmental Medicine and Child
Neurology*, 33: 1053–61

Ollendick TH, King NJ, Frary RB (1989) Fears in children and adolescence:
reliability and generalizability across gender, age and nationality. *Behaviour
Research and Therapy*, 27: 19–26

Rhodes C (2000) Effective management of daytime wetting. *Paediatric Nursing*,
12 (2): 14–17

Verhulst FC, van der Lee JH, Akkerhuis GW, Sanders-Woudstra JA, Timmer FC,
Donkhorst ID (1985) The prevalence of nocturnal enuresis. Do DSM 111
criteria need to be changed? *Journal of Child Psychology and Psychiatry*, 26:
989–93

Van Tijen NM, Messer AP, Namdar Z (1997) Perceived stress of nocturnal
enuresis in childhood. *British Journal of Urology*, 181 (Suppl 3): 98–9

Weiner J, Scales MT, Hampton J, *et al.* (2000) Long-term efficacy of simple
behavioural therapy for day-time wetting in children. *Journal of Urology*,
164 (3): 786–90

White M (1989) The externalising of the problem and the re-authoring of lives
and relationships. *Adelaide Dulwich Centre Newsletter*, Summer

Websites for reward charts and parent information

www.patient.co.uk (a site with a good search facility)

www.rewardcharts.com

www.rewardboad.co.uk

www.surgerydoor.co.uk/medcons/print.asp?Recno=23068691

Holistic assessment for adaptations, equipment and product needs

Julie Vickerman and Debra Evans

Key points

- Promoting independence in all areas of daily life can also promote quality of life for both the child and his or her family.

- It is important to choose the right piece of equipment or product for any given child – it may not be the same as the appropriate piece of equipment or product for another child.

- Multi-professional working is crucial for the success of treatment and management strategies.

Toileting is a very personal area of life and is the one activity in which most people wish to regain or maintain independence. This is often the case with children who are either striving to remain independent despite failing health or function, or are keen to develop skills to allow more independence and freedom from relying on others (Carvet 1998). An assessment of the child, their home and school environment and family needs is often carried out by an occupational therapist (OT) at any point during their life span and takes into account current, emerging and future needs of the child (Vickerman 2002). This holistic practice is one where all aspects of a person's circumstances are considered simultaneously.

Most health trusts and social service departments will supply equipment although the range will vary and may be limited in some areas. Disabled Living Centres generally offer an independent assessment service and have a range of products to see or try. Local Authorities offer a range of grants, which are available for housing adaptations. The amount available and eligibility criteria does also vary.

General principles of assessment

When assessing a family for adaptations and equipment needs, it is important to have clear aims at the outset (Vickerman 2002). You need to begin by asking questions that can help you define the situation:

- Who uses the toilet?

- Who are you designing the toilet for? For example, is this a toilet for one child, or for a number of children – as in a school environment? Is it a toilet for a child with special needs? Or for a family, one of whom has special needs?

- Are the child's needs expected to change within the lifetime of any proposed adaptation?

- Does the child actually *need* to access the toilet or bathroom, or are toileting needs being met in other ways?

For any child to be able to use the toilet and bathroom, whether with help or independently, safe and easy access is crucial. Adequate space is important for every family, but is especially so for families who have a child with special needs or a disability (Chester *et al.* 2001).

Risk assessment

When assessing the suitability of the environment (home, school, college, family support network) in meeting the toileting needs of the child, it is useful to apply the same principles as found in any standard risk assessment:

- What are the risks for the child?

- What are the risks for the carer?

- How can the environment be adapted to minimise these risks?

It is also worth remembering that the duty of care for both the child and carer must extend beyond the terms of the assessed risk and the situation. The assessment must take into account the developing child and his or her changing needs. It must allow individual children to develop to their full potential but also for the changing needs of carers – ageing parents, for example (Mandlestam 1997).

To ensure that you cover all aspects of a risk assessment, it may be useful to use the acronym **TILE** as a reminder of all the different aspects to include:

T *is for task*

What is the **task** you are assessing? The task is to enable the child to achieve the skill of continence, that is to be able to empty his or her bladder and/or bowels at a socially acceptable time and place, whether that is in a potty, toilet, commode, urinal or into a pad (Norton 1996).

What are the important aspects of achieving this task? It may be useful to carry out an activity analysis before starting the assessment. An activity analysis involves a thorough breakdown of the component aspects of an activity into the skills and attributes that are required to carry out this activity.

I *is for individual*

In this situation the individual is the **carer**. What does the carer need to do to help the child? Is the carer able to do what is needed? Assessment of the child's ability will help to identify the level of support that is required. In this aspect of the assessment, there are a number of variables which will need to be considered:

- The number of carers – does this vary from situation to situation?
- The ages of the carers – this will vary from situation to situation and through time;
- The physical ability of the carers;
- The carers' cognitive ability – their ability to learn new information, read the written word, etc.;
- The carers' relationship with the child.

L *is for load*

In this situation, the 'load' is the **child**. When assessing the child, there are an infinite number of variables. The more of these variables that can be identified and covered, the more successful and appropriate the assessment will be. Some examples of the variables to be considered include:

- Continence in relation to age and any information on previous toilet training, regardless of whether or not it was successful;
- Functional abilities in relation to age;
- Medical diagnosis and prognosis;
- Restrictions to physical development;
- Cognitive abilities in relation to age;
- Developmental milestones achieved and when;
- Coping skills already developed (child or carer);
- Patterns of challenging behaviour;
- Size and weight in relation to age;
- Mobility and transferring abilities;
- Sitting and standing balance;
- Medication and any adverse effects;
- Manual dexterity skills in relation to age.

E *is for environment and equipment*

A good general knowledge about what sort of **equipment** is available is a prerequisite for effective assessment. You should also be able to make detailed searches following the assessment. It is not always possible to know the finer details of exactly what will be required until after the child and carer have been assessed.

More information about equipment is given later in this chapter.

Environmental assessment

The fundamental question to be answered is whether the environment supports or promotes the acquisition of continence and toileting skills. Matching the child, carer and equipment to the environment is always a challenge (Vickerman 2002).

There are a number of essential aspects to an environmental assessment.

Accessibility issues

- This should include access to the building and access to the toilet area. How much space is there? Can it be increased? In some instances, the only option may be to build something new.

- Entrances and doorways are another area of concern. Are doorways sufficiently wide enough to allow the child to pass easily, along with any mobility equipment and/or a carer? A door that is to be used by a wheelchair user should have a minimum of 900 mm clear opening (more if possible). The approach area or hall should also be large enough to allow easy access for the child and the rest of the family. Space should allow for a turning circle for a wheelchair or hoist if used (or likely to be used in the future). Try to allow for space for developments you cannot foresee (involving both the child and the carer). A good rule of thumb is, the more dependent the child, the more space will be needed.

- Raised thresholds and sills, especially of UPVC doors, can also hinder wheelchair access. Different types of UPVC frames (for example, using compression material) are now readily available.

The toilet and bathroom areas

Toilet and bathroom areas should be large enough to allow a child, wheelchair and carer to manoeuvre in safety. If building a new toilet is being considered, allow space for any specialist equipment that may be needed, now or in the future. This may include a changing table, a hoist, sani chairs and disposal units. The following points also need consideration:

- The toilet should allow the child dignity and privacy. It should be possible to shut the door properly, and the child should have the option of using a lock. Mechanisms are available which can be opened from the outside if necessary.

- It may be helpful to consider using a door that opens outwards.

- Toilets are available in varying heights, but the needs of the growing child must be considered, as must the needs of other family members. If any equipment or adaptations are fitted to the toilet, it should be possible to remove and/or re-fit them easily. Toilets can be raised on plinths to use with a sani chair or 'clos-o-mat' style toilet (wash and dry facility).

■ The child should feel comfortable and secure on the toilet, and sufficiently well supported to relax.

■ The toilet roll needs to be positioned within easy reach, but not so close that the child is tempted to use it as a rail to pull on or lever against.

■ Floor covering in the bathroom must be non-slip. It is not easy to use wheelchairs in carpeted areas such as hallway entrances to bathrooms. Wooden flooring, tiles or cork could be considered as alternatives.

■ Light switches should be positioned where the child can reach them easily.

■ Different styles of light switch are available, for example rocker switches, touch-sensitive panels, pull cords and movement-sensitive sensors.

■ If a ceiling track hoist is thought necessary, it is important to check the direction and strength of joists.

■ Wash hand basins should be set at an appropriate height to allow the child to use them independently wherever possible. Height adjustable models are available for use with the growing child and other family members. Different styles and designs of controls for adjusting height are available, as are different kinds of tap. Some alternatives are electric powered, sensor or foot operated.

■ Stainless steel sinks and toilets are available, and may be particularly appropriate for a child whose challenging behaviour has resulted in damage to the toilet fittings.

Provision of equipment

A number of general points must be considered before taking decisions about the provision or purchase of any piece of equipment. These are outlined below.

Suitability

The use to which the purchase will be put, and its benefit to the child should be the first considerations. The equipment should be appropriate to the child's stage of development, and must not hinder developmental progress (Chester *et al.* 2001).

It is also advisable to consider how easily the item can be adapted:

- Is there a sufficient range of adaptation to accommodate the child's needs for a realistic period of time?

- How easy is the equipment to adjust, and will any adjustments be secure and tamper-proof?

- Do adjustments have to be carried out by a specialist or can the family do this?

Acceptability

Equipment is only useful if the child is prepared to use it, and no child will make proper use of equipment he or she does not find acceptable. The equipment should appear as standard as possible in the environment in which it is to be used. Positive attitudes from family, carers, teachers and healthcare professionals are crucial in motivating the child to use the equipment.

Safety

The equipment has to be stable. There must not be any sharp areas or places where fingers can be caught or trapped. Adjustment areas have to be secure. All equipment should comply with the relevant safety standard (CE Mark).

Other issues

- Durability and quality: equipment should be strong, well constructed and able to withstand rough handling and heavy use.

- Cleaning: it should be possible to clean and dry the fabric of the equipment thoroughly. Items with inaccessible corners or gullies should be avoided.

- Transportation and storage: if the equipment has to be moved, if should not be heavy or bulky. Heavy items should have wheels. Consider how much storage space is available for larger items.

- Repairs and spares: repairs should be readily available, with the costs of replacement components being kept at a reasonable level.

- Price: make a careful check with suppliers about the final price of any specialised equipment, especially where 'customised' alterations have been made. The guarantee and servicing agreement also needs meticulous consideration, as part of the whole assessment process.

What equipment is available?

Examples of equipment available to promote or support toileting programmes include:

- Support rails (there are many different styles available – wall mounted, drop down, different lengths, colours, shapes, etc.);

- Special toilet seats or adaptations (e.g. with smaller apertures, support harnesses, soft seats for skin problems, easy riser seats);

- Toilet training aids (e.g. musical potties, musical toilet trainers);

- Urinals (available for boys and girls);

- Commodes and potty chairs (there is a huge range available – height adjustable, bed attached, wheeled, static, etc.);

- Special toilets (with in-built washer-drier facility, automatic flushing, etc.). An example is shown in Figure 13.1.

- Toilet splash guards (designed for older boys who urinate in a sitting position);

- 'Shower chairs' which can be wheeled over the toilet or taken into the shower (see Figure 13.2 for an example).

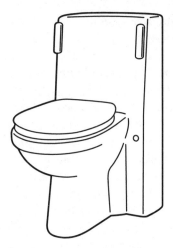

Figure 13.1 'Clos-o-Mat' type toilet with elbow pads
for activating flush/washing and drying facility and space
for an extended douche arm

Continence products for children

Products are not a cure for incontinence, however appropriate selection can make the problem more manageable. Thought should be given not only to the performance of a product, but also to its appearance and the ability products have to enhance quality of life.

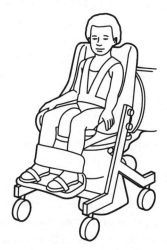

Figure 13.2 'Shower chair', which can be used over a toilet
or taken into the shower

Good Practice in Paediatric Continence Services: Benchmarking in Action (NHSMA 2003) suggests that indicators of best practice would ensure that healthcare personnel are proactive in anticipating the needs and preferences of children, their family and or carers and that choice is not restricted to number or type of product. Budgetary restraints may make it impossible to supply certain products free of charge, however providing information about the range of products that are available and where they can be purchased does not incur a cost.

Bladder and bowel problems are a burden not only to the child who is incontinent, but also to their siblings and other family members. Parents and carers have a constant need to arrange shopping trips or days out around clean accessible toilets. There will be problems in having friends to sleep over, and children with continence problems are rarely able to sleep at other people's houses. This issue alone may restrict the parents from going out for the evening and having 'adult' time, which is very often taken for granted by the majority of parents.

Using appropriate, discreet products can boost a child's self-confidence, enabling them to participate fully in activities with their peers without them finding out about their embarrassing 'problem'. 'The key is to ensure the product is suitable for the purpose for which it is needed' (White 2001).

Bedding protection

A study by Williams and colleagues (1996) interviewed 2962 children from primary schools in Sheffield, and found a strong association between bed-wetting and bullying. It is therefore essential that when bedding protection is suggested its appearance is not that associated with traditional waterproof covers.

Mattress protection

- Wide variety of mattress protection available from retail outlets and via mail order. It is essential to choose a protector that is breathable and does not rustle.

- Mattress protectors are available in a variety of sizes – bunk bed, single, double, king-size and some companies will make to order. Mattress protection is available to fit profiling beds.

- Protectors are available that fully encapsulate the mattress – these are ideal for children who insist on stripping the bed, as they are more difficult to remove. They are also available like a fitted sheet, to enable easy laundering.

■ Mattress protectors are available in pastel shades, which resemble a mattress and not a cover.

Waterproof mattresses

Waterproof mattresses are available, these can be purchased usually via mail order, from companies which supply products to residential or nursing homes. They are not expensive – similar in price to a good quality standard divan mattress. The mattresses can be purchased with the top only with waterproof covering, the top and sides, or fully waterproof. These products are particularly suitable for children with challenging behaviour.

Duvet protection

Duvet protectors are available, however they tend not to be as widely available in high street stores as they are from specialised mail order companies.

No-launder duvets and pillows

■ The cost varies from supplier to supplier, as it does with conventional duvets.

■ These products do not require laundering, they can be wiped over with a mild solution of soapy water and disinfectant. They are available in breathable fabrics.

■ Available mainly from mail order companies who would supply products to nursing and residential homes.

■ Pillows are available with feather and polyester insides.

■ If a conventional duvet were to get wet, it would be unlikely to fit into a domestic washer or dryer, therefore the cost of laundering and the time element to the parent or carer should be taken into account.

Pillow protection

Pillow protection is available from all the companies selling mattress protection.

Sleeping bag protectors

Several companies produce sleeping bag liners, which fit inside the bag and stop the bag from getting wet; however, they do not stop the child who is using them from getting wet. Ideally the sleeping bag liner should be used in conjunction with a body-worn disposable product.

Absorbent washable bed pads

Absorbent washable bed pads may be suggested as a means of managing incontinence at night. It is important that healthcare professionals advise parents or carers that the child wears nothing below the waist, to allow the urine to be absorbed by the bed pad. Very often this information is not relayed and the parents continue to put pyjamas on a child, which get wet and the bed pad is not effective.

- Bed pads are available with colourful cartoon prints, which may be suitable for young children.

- The majority of bed pads are available in pastel shades of blue or pink, and white is also available. For children of school age, it may be more appropriate to choose a bed pad the same colour as the sheet on the bed, as this would be more discreet.

- Bed pads which are sewn into a fitted sheet are also available; these may be more suitable for a child with learning difficulties who does not like change to his or her normal routine or surroundings.

- A top sheet is available with an integral lightweight absorbent pad. This would go over the child and is especially useful for boys who sleep on their back.

- A bed pad may also be useful if a child is using a handheld urinal in bed, as it would absorb any spillage.

Chair and wheelchair pads

Chair and wheelchair protectors are available from several companies. These are particularly useful when travelling in the car, going on holiday or visiting relatives. These products will ensure that, if the child has an accident, furniture would not get wet.

If the child is not incontinent but uses a urinal, these pads can be used to assist positioning, at the same time as absorbing any spillage that might occur.

Disposable pads

It is acknowledged that there is a gap in current product availability for a range of all-in-ones and shaped pads, specifically designed for children, however it is anticipated that an all-in-one product will be commercially available towards the end of 2005. Children do not need large toddler products, or extra, extra small adult products, they require a range of products specifically designed for them, which is in proportion to their body size.

- Current toddler and extra small adult products vary a great deal in size, fit around the waist and legs and as a result one product may absorb better than another. So it would be useful to contact companies for samples of equivalent products.

- Many parents prefer to use pull-ups as an alternative to the traditional nappy type product, however, due to cost implications many continence services do not provide these products. This should not stop healthcare professionals making parents and carers aware that they are available in larger sizes, as they may prefer to use this method of management – mixing different types of products in different situations.

- The 'rustle factor' should also be taken into account. Many companies are now manufacturing pads with a 'cotton feel' backing, which does not rustle like the traditional plastic-backed products.

Booster pads

Several companies provide pads with a non-waterproof backing, which can be placed inside all-in-one pads to increase the absorbency.

Booster pads or traditional sanitary pads may be useful for children who have severe diarrhoea, such as children with Hirschsprung's disease. The insert pad can be changed frequently, prolonging the life of the more expensive all-in-one pad.

Underwear with a built in pad; drop front underwear; reusable insert pads

Manufacturers working in this product area have greatly improved the design of products for this patient group. Until recently companies offered little choice in style and colour of products – white Y-fronts for boys and full briefs with a motif for girls. Currently there are several companies that sell trendy boxer shorts with wide elastic around the waist, in dark colours with discreet pads. The appearance of these garments is important; the style must be equivalent to those worn by their peers.

Knickers and underpants without an absorbent pad, but with a drop front are now available; these are particularly suitable for children who use intermittent self-catheterisation to manage their bladder problems or for children who use hand-held urinals.

Reusable insert pads are available in a variety of sizes; the small sizes can be a very cost-effective option and may be sewn into 'off the peg' underwear to provide added protection. This would enable the child to wear the same underwear as his or her peers.

Trainer pants

Reusable trainer pants have always been available, however these tended to be bulky with a waterproof outer layer and motifs that were unacceptable for children over toddler age. Recent product developments have introduced two discreet designs: a cost effective pant in white with a towelling inner layer, and a pant that resembles conventional underwear but with the added protection of an integral waterproof liner.

Sheaths, body-worn urinals and leg bags

Penile sheaths are available for boys; the smallest sheath is 18 mm in diameter, increasing in size by 2 mm to 40 mm. Male body-worn urinals are also available in paediatric sizes, they consists of a cone, which fits over the penis (it is similar to a sheath, but does not adhere to the penis), a flange, drainage bag and belt system which secures the urinal

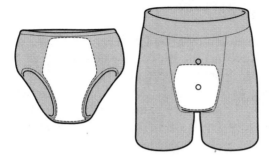

Figure 13.3 Examples of trainer pants and pads

to the body. Often healthcare professionals are not aware that sheaths and body-worn urinals are available in paediatric sizes, so they are not considered an effective method of managing urinary incontinence.

A range of discreet leg drainage bags are available which can be worn on the thigh. This may allow the child or teenager to be able to wear a greater variety in the style of clothes they can wear, such as shorts for the boys and shorter skirts for the girls.

Catheter valves

For young people who manage their bladder problems with an indwelling catheter, thought may be given to the use of a catheter valve, which would be a more discreet option than a leg drainage bag.

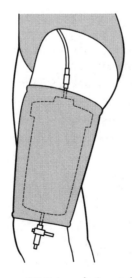

Figure 13.4 Leg drainage bag

Intermittent catheters

There is a wide range of intermittent catheters available: some are pre-lubricated, and others require water to be added in order to lubricate them. The child and their parents should be made aware of the various options available as one product may be more convenient than another. Several of the larger companies have introduced Catheter Kits to their product range. These can be particularly suitable when there is no access to toilets, and it can be helpful to take them on holidays.

Enuresis alarms – body-worn

There are many different models of enuresis alarms available, including ones which buzz or vibrate. More recent developments have enabled the parent or carer to record a message or music onto the alarm, which then alerts the child to go to the toilet. Bed alarms are also available.

Toilet-training alarms

For the younger child, potties are available which have a sensor. When the child urinates, this sensor is triggered and the child is rewarded with music. For the older child there is an equivalent reward alarm that fits inside a standard toilet bowl.

Urinals

There are very few urinals specifically designed for children, however some of those designed for adults will work perfectly well. For example, a mini funnel has been designed specifically for boys. It involves a funnel attached to a leg drainage bag, thus allowing the child to urinate when it is difficult to get to a toilet.

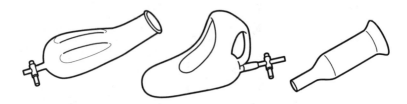

Figure 13.5 Different types of urinals

Miscellaneous

Sleepsuits
For children who smear faeces or interfere with their incontinence pads, a sleepsuit is available in a variety of fabric and designs. It fastens up the back, making it difficult for the child to open it.

Changing mats
Large changing mats are available from specialist rehabilitation companies, however these are very expensive. A more cost-effective solution may be to use an aerobics mat, which folds up concertina style. They are discreet and easily cleaned.

Swimwear
A variety of garments have been designed for children who are incontinent to wear under conventional swimwear, however these are not a very discreet option. A range of swimwear with integral pants is now commercially available; the swimsuits are very fashionable and discreet.

Watch alarm
A child's watch is available which incorporates an alarm that can be programmed to activate several times during the day to alert the child. This may be useful to indicate to a child when to go to the toilet or to self-catheterise.

It is very important that the item or appliance does not cause any harm, even slight harm, to the child using it. For example, is it likely that use, if prolonged, could cause soreness?

Clothing

Choice of clothing is extremely important for all people who have difficulty using the toilet (White and Holland 2001). Children and teenagers, in particular, want to wear clothes that are suitable for their age and look the same as those that their peers are wearing, and are fashionable. However, clothes for a child who has a disability, or problems with toileting, need to be hard-wearing, easy to put on and take off, and easy to launder. Children should be allowed sufficient time to dress and undress (Chester *et al.* 2001).

If the child's clothes are to promote continence and independent toileting, the following factors need to be considered:

- Material should be flexible. This will allow for any pulling or tugging while the child is transferring onto the toilet, for example.

- Choose items of clothing that are easy to remove or pull up and down.

- Fastenings should be kept to an absolute minimum. Alternative types of fastenings could be considered instead of fiddly zips and buttons. Opening the side seams of trousers and skirts and replacing them with strips of Velcro can make removing clothing much easier. This can be done to make either front-drop or back-drop trousers.

- If trouser zips are longer than standard ones, this will make it easier for a boy or a girl to use a urinal, or for an older boy to stand at the toilet.

- Drop-front or side-opening underwear can also be adapted from shop-bought items.

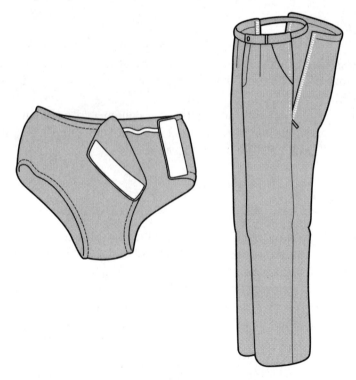

Figure 13.6 Clothing can be adapted using Velcro

Disability or special need should not necessarily dictate the style of clothing a child wears. Although specialist clothing is commercially available, it tends to be expensive. Many items of 'ordinary' clothing can be adapted with very little expert help but just a little 'know how'. Fashion does not have to be compromised just because a child has difficulty using the toilet or maintaining their continence (White and Holland 2001). Many Disabled Living Centres can give advice about clothing adaptations and how to access local alteration services.

Conclusion

It is essential to include all members of the multi-professional team in the assessment of the child and his or her family. It is crucial that this assessment does not just consider their current presenting difficulties but takes into account the many factors that will influence their emerging and future needs in the home, education and work situations. This cohesive and integrated approach serves to enhance the quality service given to children and their families.

References

Carvet J (1998) *People Don't Understand.* London: National Children's Bureau

Chester HJ, Freebody JS, Starkey SJ (2001) *Children with Disabilities.* Oxford: Disability Information Trust

Mandelstam M (1997) *Equipment for Older or Disabled People and the Law.* London: Jessica Kingsley

NHS Modernisation Agency (2003) Good Practice in Paediatric Continence Services – Benchmarking in Action. London: Department of Health. Website: www.modern.nhs.uk

Norton C (1996) *Nursing for Continence,* 2e. Beaconsfield: Beaconsfield Publishers

Vickerman J (2002) Thorough assessment of functional incontinence. *Nursing Times Plus,* 98 (28): 58–9

White H (2001) Continence Products in the Community: towards a more client-centered service. *Professional Care of Mother and Child,* 11 (5): 120–3

White H, Holland D (2001) Looking good and feeing good. *Nursing Times Plus.* 97 (20)

Williams K, Chambers M, Logan S, Robinson D (1996) Association of common health symptoms with bullying in primary school children. *British Medical Journal,* 313 (7048): 17–19

14 | Managing clean intermittent catheterisation

Rosie Kelly

Key points

- Thorough and sensitive preparation of patients and parents is essential if CIC is to be managed effectively.

- The child's dignity, right to choice and privacy should be respected at all times, by health professionals, teachers and family members.

- It is important to ensure that the child is using the correct techniques for self-catheterisation to prevent risk of infection.

Health promotion points

- Ensure cleanliness is rigorous and hands are thoroughly cleaned with either water or non-alcohol based wipes at every stage of the procedure.

Clean intermittent catheterisation (CIC) has been used as a means of emptying the bladder as far back as the ancient Greeks and Chinese. However, in modern times, it was the work of Lapides *et al* (1972) which led to the introduction of CIC as the preferred method of managing patients with incomplete bladder emptying. Since then, the variety of catheters which may be used for this procedure has increased significantly, allowing patients greater choice. Written literature is also available in abundance, as well as training tools for more thorough education.

CIC is most commonly used for patients with neuropathic bladder dysfunction, but may also be used to treat intractable incontinence in non-neuropathic cases where other treatment modalities have been unsuccessful.

Reasons for use

These can be listed as follows:

- Neuropathic bladder dysfunction (Aslan and Kogan 2002) secondary to:
  - spina bifida;
  - sacral agenesis;
  - transverse myelitis;
  - spinal cord tumours;
  - accidents and spinal trauma.
- Dysfunctional voiding syndromes (Homsy 1994):
  - daytime urgency/frequency syndrome;
  - lazy bladder syndrome;
  - Hinman syndrome – sometimes referred to as *non-neurogenic bladder syndrome* – dysfunctional voiding with associated renal impairment as a result of underlying psychological problems;
  - Ochoa syndrome – severe voiding dysfunction with associated inversion of facial expression.
- Post-operatively (Thomas 1997):
  - urinary retention;
  - bladder augmentation;
  - artificial urinary sphincter;
  - Mitrofanoff.

Catheter types

Nelaton catheters are the most commonly used for CIC, and may be either the pre-lubricated hydrophilic or non-hydrophilic variety (Winn and Thompson 1998; Pachler and Frimodt-Moller 1999; Smith 2003).

Pre-lubricated catheters must be immersed in water for at least 30 seconds prior to use to activate the lubricant. Some manufacturers have overcome the need for patients to have access to water in order to use their catheters by providing a pre-packed sachet of water/saline with the catheter, or providing pre-soaked catheters. This makes catheterisation easier for patients outside the home. Some non-lubricated catheters are provided with a small gel dispenser for simplicity, while others will require lubricating with an aqueous gel. Some of this latter type of catheter can be re-used for up to seven days, although this practice is becoming less common with the increasing number of once-only use catheters available (see Table 14.1). All of these catheters are available on the Drug Tariff, and may be obtained through community pharmacies.

Patients should be informed about the range of catheters available. Expert information about the most appropriate catheter for an individual should be provided by the nurse carrying out the training. Compliance with catheterisation depends largely on the patient's lifestyle and confidence when using a catheter. Careful selection jointly by the patient and nurse will reinforce this.

Psychological preparation

Children often respond with fear to the proposal to introduce CIC. Parents will also be filled with trepidation, concern and sometimes anger at the suggestion of such an invasive procedure. The first step in helping children and their parents to understand the need for CIC is to help them identify and understand the underlying bladder problem. This is part of the assessment process (Doherty 2001, p.66). Children who understand and – more importantly – accept that they have a bladder problem, are more willing to comply with the treatment modalities being suggested, including catheterisation.

Children need to feel part of the decision-making process, just as adults do. Allowing them to choose the type of catheter they will use, where they will catheterise and how often, helps children to feel in control, and empowers them to manage their own health (Borzyskowski *et al.* 2004). The same applies to parents who are being asked to catheterise children who are unable to catheterise themselves.

Many children prefer to learn to catheterise at home. This is a more familiar and relaxed environment, and there are likely to be fewer interruptions during the training process. It is also psychologically important for the child to realise how easy catheterisation can be at

Table 14.1 Catheter types

Hydrophilic coated (activate in water):	Prelubricated with gel:
Polyvinyl Chloride/Polyvinylpyrrolidone	*Polyvinyl Chloride*
Produced with a salt or urea base	Produced with or without silicone

home (see Case study below). Potential problems such as limited space and storage facilities can be addressed. Toilet and hand washing facilities may not be in the same room, so the child needs to explore how cleaning will be done prior to catheterising. The time taken to catheterise needs to be assessed as this may have an impact on other members of the family. The child may feel the need to rush using the catheter if other people are waiting in line! Advice can be given about the best times to catheterise to avoid having to queue for the bathroom, especially first thing in the morning.

CASE STUDY

Holly

Holly is a seven-year-old girl, who presented with day and night-time incontinence and recurrent urinary tract infections (UTI). Investigations revealed a bladder with high detrusor (bladder muscle) pressures, incomplete bladder emptying, and a poorly functioning right kidney.

Holly had taken prophylactic trimethoprim for a number of years. She had also been given anticholinergic medication to reduce her bladder pressures, and had undergone bladder retraining to facilitate complete bladder emptying. However she continued to have symptomatic UTIs. A Magnetic Resonance scan of her spinal cord was normal.

Holly lives with her parents and older sister and attends mainstream primary school. Both her parents are in full-time employment and there are several family members living close by. In order to prevent any further deterioration in renal function, and to reduce the number of symptomatic UTIs, it was recommended that Holly begin clean intermittent catheterisation (CIC).

A nurse specialist visited Holly at home, explained the reasons for catheterisation and helped Holly decide how and where she would catheterise. Holly also decided which catheter she preferred to use from a selection shown to her by the nurse specialist.

Holly was shown how to apply local anaesthetic gel to her urethra, and how to adopt a comfortable sitting position on the toilet for catheterising. She learned how to insert the catheter by feeling the top of her urethral opening and sliding the catheter in underneath. Holly's mother was present during every session to offer support, and to learn the procedure herself, to enable her to help Holly between the nurse's visits.

The nurse specialist also visited Holly's school and spoke to the staff, with Holly's permission. The school had recently installed a toilet for disabled children, as part of a refurbishment programme. This toilet was made available for Holly to use at lunchtime.

After several weeks, Holly was self-catheterising three times a day, including once at school. She has had no further UTIs, her renal function has stabilised, and she is continent during the day and at night.

Children are often unfamiliar with their genital area, and have no idea where the catheter needs to be inserted. Familiarising them with their own body, and the use of catheterisation models to practise on (Cobussen-Borkhorst *et al.* 2000) can help relieve anxiety and promote self-confidence in the child. Commercially available dolls can be prohibitively expensive. Many play specialists are adept at making play dolls that can be used for a number of procedures, including catheterisation. They can also help children discuss their fears and attain acceptance and understanding of the procedure. Some catheter manufacturers produce storybooks about catheterisation, which may be used to help prepare children for learning to self-catheterise.

The process of teaching children to catheterise is time-consuming for the professional. It usually requires weeks or even months of preparation and teaching. Failure to provide this time will usually lead to failure of catheterisation. Children must give their consent to catheterise or be catheterised if they are of an appropriate age (Pocock 2003). They can only do this if they understand the reasons for it and are given enough time to prepare for it.

Teaching methods

Preparation

Time and patience are the key elements required for teaching children to catheterise (Hunt *et al.* 1996; Seymour 1996). Parents who are going to catheterise young children may learn the technique relatively quickly, but also need education and reassurance to ensure compliance.

A number of issues need to be addressed prior to teaching CIC, as covered below.

Education

Ensure the child and parent are familiar with normal anatomy, and that they understand where the bladder is in relation to the kidneys and where the urethral opening is. Girls may find it helpful to use a mirror to familiarise themselves with the urethral opening and how best to visualise it prior to catheterisation. Boys who are not used to retracting the foreskin may wish to practise prior to learning to catheterise and they should be shown how to do this safely.

It is important to explain clearly to the family why CIC needs to be introduced, and the potential benefits it will bring. Many parents are concerned that catheterisation may increase the risk of UTIs, so this needs to be explored with them prior to starting CIC (see the 'Talking Point' box below).

TALKING POINT

The use of indwelling urethral catheterisation for more than six weeks often results in a UTI, due to colonisation of the catheter by organisms (Bray and Sanders 2006). However, studies of the presence of organisms in the bladders of patients using intermittent catheterisation (Lin-Dyken *et al.* 1992, Ottolini *et al.* 1995, Schlager *et al.* 1995) have found that, while bacteriuria ($>10 \times 5$ organisms per ml) is present in many urine samples, patients remain symptom-free, with no deterioration in previously normal renal function.

The conclusion therefore, is that CIC is a safe and effective form of treatment for incomplete bladder emptying (Aslan and Kogan 2002). Patients should only be treated for symptomatic UTIs, or when vesicoureteric reflux is present (Muller *et al.* 2002).

Multi-resistant organisms
Extended-spectrum B-lactamases (ESBLs) have become widespread in the United Kingdom since 2003. These new strains are capable of breaking down a wider range of antibiotics. *Escherichia Coli*, the common organism in most UTIs, is becoming resistant to multiple antibiotics, including penicillins and cephalosporins (Health Protection Agency 2006). This progression of multi resistant organisms makes the diagnosis of symptomatic UTIs and careful use of antibiotics even more important in patients using CIC.

Catheter size and selection
The age of the child will determine the catheter size (see Table 14.2). The catheter type should be selected based on patient choice and manual dexterity.

Table 14.2 Catheter size for urethral catheterisation

Age	Size
Neonates	5 or 6 Charrière (preferable) or 4fg feeding tube
Birth – 5 years	6–8 Charrière
6–10 years	8 Charrière
11–13 years	8–10 Charrière
14–16years	10–12 Charrière

Use of local anaesthetic
Local anaesthetic should always be used in boys who have normal sensation in the urethra (Doherty 2001). Girls may be offered the option of using local anaesthetic, although many decide against it because of the time it takes to work. Lidocaine takes at least five minutes to work effectively. It should be applied directly into the urethra for maximum benefit. Applying it to the tip of the catheter is ineffective. Warn the child that there may be some sensation as it is not always possible to achieve an anaesthetic effect as far as the bladder neck. Always check with parents that there is no history of allergy to previous lidocaine-based products prior to use (see Table 14.3).

Table 14.3 Precautions when using Lidocaine

Lidocaine should not be applied to a traumatised or inflamed urethra,
as it may be absorbed into the bloodstream causing systemic side effects
such as central nervous system disturbances, hypertension and bradycardia.

When used topically, Lidocaine is less likely to interact with other drugs,
but should be used with caution in patients taking:

Propanolol

Cimetidine

Diuretics

Anti-arrythmics

Anti-psychotics

Source: British National Formulary (2006)

Where CIC will take place

Children should be encouraged to catheterise on the toilet in the bathroom (or separate WC) wherever possible. This is where normal urination takes place and is therefore most appropriate. If the child is very young or has to be catheterised lying down, then a bedroom or the place where nappy changing takes place may be more appropriate. Encourage parents to think about the child's privacy (even in infants), and to avoid catheterising in front of other people, including members of the family.

Fears

The introduction of CIC is a daunting prospect for most families, so it is essential to spend time dealing with their fears and anxieties. Children tend to fear the pain that may occur or that they may hurt themselves during the procedure. They also fear 'being found out' by their peers. Parents may be concerned about causing their child pain or damage, and they also express concern about the long-term effects of CIC and the child's ability to cope outside the home.

Procedure

1 Begin by answering any questions the family may have about CIC.

2 Ensure the room is warm and private. There should be no observers for initial training sessions.

3 Ask the child to identify all the equipment needed: catheters, wipes, local anaesthetic. Then ask him or her to set everything out in an easily reachable place.

4 Identify a comfortable position for the child to adopt on the toilet. Girls can sit with legs straddling the toilet seat or with one leg raised on the seat to aid ease of insertion. Young boys may wish to sit on the toilet, older boys usually prefer to stand.

5 Ask the child to wash his or her genital area after removing underclothes. Girls should be instructed to wash from front to back and pay particular attention to the labia minora. Boys should be observed retracting the foreskin and shown how to clean the meatus.

6 Show the child (or parents) how to clean the hands effectively. Observe handwashing technique or, if preferable, wipes may be used.

7 Demonstrate the instillation of local anaesthetic gel – it must be left on for at least 5 minutes prior to catheterisation.

8 Allow the child to insert the catheter, offering reassurance and encouragement. Some girls have difficulty locating the urethral orifice, so offer gentle guiding by holding the child's hand to insert the catheter. Some practitioners advocate the use of a mirror to help visualise the urethral opening. This may be helpful, but remember that a mirror shows a reverse image, so girls may find this confusing. Boys should be advised to hold the penis at a slightly upward angle to visualise the urethral opening. Catheterising should be discontinued if the child experiences severe pain, frank bleeding or difficulty in inserting the catheter.

9 When urine begins to flow, advise the child to hold the catheter in place until the flow stops. The catheter should then be inserted a further centimetre to ensure complete emptying.

10 When the flow ceases, instruct the child to withdraw the catheter slowly. If urine begins to flow again, the child should stop withdrawal until the flow ceases. Continue this manoeuvre until the catheter has been completely withdrawn.

11 Show the child how to dispose of the catheter by reinserting it in the wrapper and putting it in the bin.

12 The child can then wash off any residual anaesthetic gel, replace underwear and wash hands thoroughly.

Troubleshooting

Trauma/bleeding

A small amount of blood may be visible on the catheter after removal. This is usually caused by irritation of the urethral lining and resolves as the child's technique improves. Frank blood in the catheter requires investigation and catheterisation should be discontinued (Bennett 2002).

Urinary Tract Infection (UTI)

Many children will have experienced recurrent UTIs prior to catheterisation. When the bladder is being emptied completely, the incidence should be reduced (Bakke *et al.* 1997).

Some children develop a symptomatic infection on introduction of CIC (Schlager *et al.* 1998). This is usually due to lack of experience with the technique, and, although most children will experience asymptomatic bacteriuria (Hunt *et al.* 1996), no treatment is required unless vesicoureteric reflux (VUR) is also present. Children with persistent VUR should remain on prophylactic antibiotic therapy until they are infection-free for one year (Thomas 2002, p.52).

Inability to retract foreskin

Some boys may experience difficulty retracting the foreskin. Encouraging them to practise while sitting in a bath of warm water may be effective. If the foreskin is visibly tight, the use of Daktacort (1% Hydrocortisone) cream, applied daily for six weeks may be of help. If these methods are unsuccessful, circumcision should be considered.

Sphincter spasm

Boys may have difficulty inserting the catheter through the sphincter and into the bladder. Gentle rotation of the catheter or relaxation techniques such as deep breathing or coughing may help open the sphincter. Gentle pressure may be applied to push the catheter through the sphincter, but force must never be used.

No drainage from catheter

If the child voids prior to catheterisation, the bladder may be empty. If this is unlikely, the child should withdraw the catheter slightly then reinsert it. In girls, the catheter may have been inserted into the vagina. The catheter should be withdrawn and inserted slightly higher, into the urethra. Most girls with normal sensation are able to identify the difference in sensation between the urethra and vagina, but if the problem continues, or the child does not have a sensate urethra, the catheterisation technique must be reviewed.

Catheterising during menstruation

Girls should be encouraged to continue catheterising during menstruation. The urethra may be more sensitive at this time, and some girls may wish to use anaesthetic gel for the procedure. Emphasise the importance of genital cleansing prior to CIC. Older girls may find it easier to catheterise if they are using a vaginal tampon as there is less bleeding.

Urinary incontinence may increase at this time due to fluid retention, and some girls may be advised to catheterise more frequently to overcome this.

Continuing urinary incontinence

If urinary incontinence remains a problem, the following possibilities should be considered:

- Unresolved constipation;
- The child is not catheterising frequently enough;
- UTI.

Anticholinergic therapy may be necessary.

Catheterising in school

Self-catheterisation or CIC by another person in school creates enormous anxiety for children. It also presents education and health professionals with many challenges which must be overcome if it is to be accomplished successfully.

Whenever possible, the child must be involved in the decision-making process, particularly in relation to who will perform or supervise the procedure.

Many school staff are concerned about learning to catheterise a child because of the intimacy of the procedure and the inherent child protection issues surrounding such care. All staff, the parents and, most importantly, the child, must feel fully supported, particularly during the initial introduction of the procedure at school (Fishwick and Gormley 2004).

An initial meeting between parents, school staff (including the school nurse) and the Continence Adviser/Nurse Specialist is essential, to explore all the issues involved in catheterisation, and to discuss concerns. The main aims of such a meeting are (Foulkes *et al.* 2004):

- To explain the child's condition and the need for CIC;

- To identify which school staff prepared to catheterise or supervise catheterisation;

- To identify a suitable private toilet with storage facilities;

- To start a training programme;

- To provide written educational material.

School staff may have to identify funding for refurbishment of toilet facilities and the employment of an additional member of staff to facilitate catheterisation in school, so the local education authority will also have to be involved.

Occupational therapy or physiotherapy input may also be required if special adaptations are required to enable the child to catheterise safely.

Some school staff are reticent about becoming involved in catheterising a child, so meetings must be held well in advance of a young child starting school to address this. Older children who can self-catheterise may not need any supervision, but will need reassurance about unobtrusive access to the toilet and information about obtaining a key if the toilet is usually locked.

Some education authorities insist on mandatory updating and training reviews for their staff, to be carried out by an experienced health professional. Other authorities will accept attendance at annual reviews of children with a Statement of Educational Needs. Clarification of the authority's rules should be obtained before a child starts CIC in school, so that these can be included in the child's School Health Care Plan.

It is advisable to restrict the number of people trained to catheterise to two members of school staff. This allows for sick leave etc. The child's parent should be designated as a further back-up if required. Allowing several members of staff to be trained breaks patient confidentiality and intrudes on the child's right to privacy. It is also unlikely that all members of staff, even if trained, would be catheterising regularly, and could not, therefore, be deemed competent with the technique.

A co-ordinated approach to planning leads to successful implementation, and allows the child to achieve independence while benefiting from full-time, mainstream education.

Mitrofanoff

The Mitrofanoff stoma was developed in the 1980s to provide an alternative to urethral catheterisation. It is particularly useful for children with a sensate urethra or for those in wheelchairs. It permits ease of access for CIC and promotes independence, as it allows children to self-catheterise easily and without discomfort. (See also Chapter 10 by Boddy, Affleck and Snell.)

The appendix, if available, is the tissue of choice (Kniest and McGovern 2002), and is inserted into the bladder with an anastamosis to the abdominal wall at the other end, to provide a channel for CIC. A valve is created within the channel to prevent reflux and leakage of urine. If the appendix is not available, other tissue such as the ureter or small bowel may be used instead (Malone 1997).

The siting of the stoma is extremely important as it must be visible to ensure ease of catheter insertion. The site should be identified prior to surgery with the help of the child, taking into account the most desirable position for CIC and the child's hand–eye co-ordination. If the child normally wears a spinal brace, arrangements may have to be made for a flap or hole to be made in the brace to allow insertion of the catheter without removing the brace. The most common stoma sites are the right iliac fossa or umbilicus.

Following construction of the stoma, a catheter is left in situ for two to three weeks. This may or may not be on free drainage, depending on local policy and if any other procedures were carried out at the same time. An experienced nurse must carry out the first catheterisation of the stoma to identify the route of the channel into the bladder. Most children catheterising by this method prefer to drain the urine into a jug or standing over a toilet.

The most common problem associated with a Mitrofanoff stoma is stomal stenosis (Rickwood and Malone 2002, p.146), usually at skin level. Most stomas are constructed to take a size 12 charrière catheter to provide complete bladder emptying. The stoma may stenose slightly following removal of the post-operative catheter, but should accommodate a 10 charrière or 12 charrière catheter. Anything less than this constitutes problematical stenosis requiring treatment. In some cases, dilation with graduated sizes beginning with size 8 charrière and working up to 12 charrière may be successful. The large catheter can be left in situ for a few days before recommencing intermittent CIC. If this is unsuccessful or stenosis becomes a persistent problem, a skin level revision may be required to prevent further problems.

The process of catheterising via a Mitrofanoff stoma is the same as for urethral catheterisation, paying particular attention to cleanliness and complete bladder emptying.

Latex allergy

True latex allergy is a reaction to the protein contained in natural rubber latex (ACA 2004). Not all products identified as latex contain this protein, so some may be used in patients previously identified as having a latex allergy.

In relation to urinary catheters, many catheters for intermittent use contain very little latex and most are now hydrogel-coated. Indwelling urinary catheters may be made of latex and coated with PTFE, silicone or hydrogel.

Patients who have been identified as having a latex allergy must undergo stringent precautions to ensure the use of all-silicone catheters and latex-free gloves. In patients exposed to prolonged use of latex-based products such as long-term indwelling catheters or major surgical procedures, the use of latex-free products is advisable.

Conclusion

Clean intermittent catheterisation is a safe, simple procedure designed to promote complete bladder emptying. It complements the use of anti-cholinergic therapy and reduces the incidence of symptomatic urinary tract infections.

Careful consideration must be given to the teaching methods employed with children, with particular emphasis on psychological support. Those teaching children to catheterise must be experienced in the technique, and be able to offer ongoing support to the child and family, as well as to any professionals involved in the child's care.

The primary aim of catheterisation must always be to enhance normal renal function. The secondary aim is to promote urinary continence and assist the child in leading a normal, independent life.

References

Association for Continence Advice (2004) *Urethral Catheterisation: notes on good practice*. Glasgow: ACA

Aslan AR, Kogan BA (2002) Conservative management in neuropathic bladder dysfunction. *Current Opinion in Urology*, 12: 473–7

Bakke A, Digranes A, Hoisaeter PA (1997) Physical predictors of infection in patients treated with clean intermittent catheterization: a prospective 7-year study. *British Journal of Urology*, 79: 85–90

Bennett E (2002) Intermittent self-catheterisation and the female patient. *Nursing Standard*, 17 (7): 37–42

Borzyskowski M, Cox A, Edwards M, Owen A (2004) Neuropathic bladder and intermittent catheterisation: social and psychological impact on families. *Developmental Medicine and Child Neurology*, 46: 160–7

Bray L, Sanders C (2006) Nursing management of paediatric urethral catheterisation. *Nursing Standard*, 20 (24): 52–60

British National Formulary 51e (2006) Section 14.2. London: British Medical Association and Royal Pharmaceutical Society of Great Britain.

Corbussen-Borkhorst JGL, Van der Weide M, Feitz WJF, DeGier RPE (2000) Using an instructional model to teach clean intermittent catheterisation to children. *British Journal of Urology International*, 85: 551–3

Doherty W (2001) Indications for and principles of intermittent self-catheterisation. In: Pope Cruickshank J, Woodward S (eds) *Management of Continence and Urology Catheter Care (BJN Monograph)*. Salisbury: Mark Allen Publishing

Fishwick J, Gormley A (2004) Intermittent catheterisation in school: a collaborative agreement. *Professional Nurse*, 19 (9): 519–22

Foulkes S, Oliver H, White M (2004) *Guide to Intermittent Catheterisation in Schools*. Gloucestershire: Astra Tech Ltd

Health Protection Agency report (2006) Investigations into multi-drug resistant ESBL-producing Escherichia Coli. Available online at: www.hpa.org.uk/publications/esbl_report

Homsy YL (1994) Dysfunctional voiding syndromes and vesicoureteral reflux. *Pediatric Nephrology*, 8: 116–21

Hunt GM, Oakeshott P, Whitaker RH (1996) Intermittent catheterisation: simple, safe and effective but underused. *British Medical Journal*, 312: 103–7

Kniest KR, McGovern P (2002) Using the umbilicus for catheterization. *Registered Nurse* 65 (8): 26–31

Lapides J, Diunko AC, Silber SJ, Lowe BS (1972) Clean intermittent catheterisation in the treatment of urine tract disease. *Journal of Urology*, 107: 458–61

Lin-Dyken DC, Wolraich ML, Hawtrey CE, Doja MS (1992) Follow-up of clean intermittent catheterization for children with neurogenic bladders. *Urology*, 40 (6): 525–9

Malone P (1997) The management of urinary incontinence. *Archives of Disease in Childhood*, 77 (2): 175–8

Muller T, Arbeiter K, Anfricht C (2002) Renal function in meningomylocele: risk factors, chronic renal failure, renal replacement therapy and transplantation. *Current Opinion in Urology*, 12: 479–84

Ottolini MC, Shaer CM, Rushton HG, Majd M, Gonzales EC, Patel KM (1995) Relationship of asymptomatic bacteriuria and renal scarring in children with neuropathic bladders who are practicing clean intermittent catheterisation. *Journal of Pediatrics*, 127 (3): 368–72

Pachler J, Frimodt-Moller C (1999) A comparison of prelubricated hydrophilic and non-hydrophilic polyvinyl chloride catheters for urethral catheterisation. *British Journal of Urology International*, 83: 767–9

Pocock M (2003) A critical analysis of legal and ethical issues regarding consent in childhood. *Nurse Prescribing*, 1 (4): 180–85

Rickwood AMK, Malone PS (2002) Neuropathic bladder. In: Thomas DFM, AMK Rickwood AMK, Duffy PG (eds.) *Essentials of Paediatric Urology*. London: Martin Dunitz

Schlager TA, Anderson S, Trudell J, Hendley JO (1998) Nitrofurantoin prophylaxis for bacteriuria and urinary tract infection in children with neurogenic bladder on intermittent catheterization. *Journal of Pediatrics*, 132 (4): 704–8

Schlager TA, Dilks S, Trudell J, Whitton TS, Hendley JO (1995) Bacteriuria in children with neurogenic bladder treated with clean intermittent catheterisation: natural history. *Journal of Pediatrics*, 126 (30): 490–6

Seymour J (1996) Self-catheterisation: a guide to this underused technique. *Nursing Times*, 92 (5): 46–8

Smith L (2003) Which catheter? Criteria for selection of urinary catheters for children. *Paediatric Nursing*, 15 (3): 14–18

Thomas DFM (1997) Surgical treatment of urinary incontinence. *Archives of Disease in Childhood*, 76: 377–80

Thomas DFM (2002) Vesicoureteric reflux. In: Thomas DFM, AMK Rickwood AMK, Duffy PG (eds) *Essentials of Paediatric Urology*. London: Martin Dunitz

Winn C, Thompson J (1998) Urinary catheters for intermittent use. *Professional Nurse*, 13 (8): 541–3

15 Transition through childhood and into adult life

Mary White

> ## Key points
>
> - Children have to undergo a series of transitions, of which the transition from paediatric to adult services is only one.
>
> - Transition is a topic that has been largely ignored by professionals, yet its importance cannot be overstated.
>
> - Since most of a child's life is spent in school, transition frameworks must be built around school life.
>
> - A multi-disciplinary approach to management is needed.

Child development is measured in milestones, the achievement of which mark the successful transition from one phase to the next. Routine examinations by health professionals at child health clinics record these milestones and identify any impairments which may affect or delay transition (White and Dobson 1999). Any developmental difficulties or special needs which may impact upon social, health and educational aspects of the child's life (or that of the family) should be addressed as soon as possible. Where appropriate, a multi-disciplinary approach to management should be sought.

Transition involves the process of changing from one state or style to another, and can be a period of some difficulty. Some familiar aspects must be left behind; other new and unfamiliar aspects accepted and assimilated. For a child in need of healthcare, 'transition' can also describe the process of being conveyed from one set of professionals to another and, perhaps back again. Ideally the child with identified special needs should be seen as a package, marked 'fragile', which requires safe passage throughout childhood.

Continence problems

Incontinence, whether it is short or long term, is one of the most isolating of childhood conditions. Problems may vary from occasional day and/or night-time wetting or constipation, to chronic bladder and/or bowel conditions requiring long-term interventions. In many cases, continence problems will be part of a wider problem which may be psychological or social. Or they may be related to mobility and other physical difficulties and, perhaps, learning impairment (White and Dobson 1999).

The impact of incontinence on a child's life can be underestimated as it is unlikely to be seen as causing risk to health or having a negative impact on personal safety. Neither can it be classified as either a developmental impairment, or a social impairment.

It does need to be appreciated, however, that incontinence *is*:

- Unhealthy – it can cause skin lesions as well as indicating the presence of urinary tract infection or even renal damage;

- Antisocial – being perceived as 'smelly', 'wet' or 'dirty' is likely to impede normal socialisation, lead to dependence, compromise education and distort relationships;

- Expensive – investigations and medication all have a cost; then there is the cost of supply and disposal of pads, which have both financial and environmental implications.

Transitions within the school system

The majority of children achieve control over their bladder and bowels before they start nursery school, but there are some who do not manage this, especially if they have a physical and/or a learning disability. If the disability is severe, continence care may be required for the whole of their childhood, and beyond. It is for these groups of children that *transition planning* is particularly important.

In some areas of the country, children are excluded from nursery school because they are not toilet trained. It is important, therefore, for professionals to be aware of local protocols and appeal procedures regarding the exclusion from nursery and primary schools of children who have bowel and bladder problems.

When continence problems have been identified, every effort should be made to ensure the admission of children with bowel and bladder problems to nursery and primary school without recourse to the law. Adequate time should be allowed for multi-professional assessment (MPA), statement of special educational need (SEN) and forward planning when a change of department or school is anticipated (for example, infant to junior, primary to secondary) in order to make sure the necessary facilities are in place. Local Authority education departments usually require at least one full academic year in order to process the requirement, and a further year to implement it. This means that, ideally, transition plans should commence two years before the change takes place.

Current situation

Good local services are required to deal with the long-term continence problems associated with physical and/or learning disability. However, the quality and quantity of children's services in this field does vary widely throughout the UK.

As curing the problem is not always a possibility, a good continence specialist will be keen to explore all available options for continence management. The most appropriate approach for any individual child may change from one year to the next, so regular multi-professional assessment is essential throughout the childhood years, with interventions scheduled to take place at the most appropriate time. Social and educational disruption should be kept to a minimum. Successful management requires professionals to work together, share information, and listen both to the child and to the family. Acute urology services should liaise with community continence and children's services. They, in turn, must work closely with schools and social services.

Even though there are, as yet, few integrated continence services for children in most areas of the country, local services should still be able to work together successfully in providing multi-disciplinary packages of care. For example, in some areas, consultant paediatricians with a special interest in bladder and bowel problems, are closely involved in drawing up Individual Education Plans (IEPs) which are designed to make use of multi-disciplinary services. Children do not have to have had a Statement of Educational Need (SEN) to have an IEP.

The National Service Framework (NSF) for Children and Young People (DH 2004) recognises that services are 'fragmented' and that there are 'big gaps in service provision'. The document recommends 'integrated community-based continence services' as discussed in *Good Practice in Paediatric Continence Services* (NHSMA 2003). Effective implementation of the NSF would enable children and young people with special needs and/or disabilities to have equal access to investigation and treatment programmes.

The Special Educational Needs and Disability Act (HMSO 2001) is only loosely interpreted by some education departments, so it may prove difficult for community health services to persuade schools that continence problems do constitute a special educational need impacting upon the child's ability to learn. While this point may be debatable, it is clear that children and families suffer while statutory services argue about responsibility. Multi-disciplinary co-operation can override local and national politics, and protect the child and family from the negative effects of continence problems in school.

Educational and social law

Transition planning involves thinking ahead and it is, frequently, in forward planning that gaps in services are identified. It is these gaps which prevent children from reaching their full potential and which cause them to be lost to follow up. If extreme difficulty is experienced in identifying and obtaining appropriate services and support, there is legislation (as described below) which can be used as a lever when other initiatives have failed.

In some areas, Children's Services will only carry out a Multi-Professional Assessment (MPA) if there is a learning disability, with physical disability seen as a health rather than an educational problem. This approach may fail to take into account those children with physical impairment, who may or may not have associated learning disability, requiring complex continence care in schools and perhaps adapted facilities and ancillary care support. It is unlikely that appropriate support will be made available without both MPA and a Statement of Special Educational Need (SEN), drawn up in accordance with the code of practice set out in the Special Educational Needs and Disability Act (2001). This Act strengthens the child's right to attend a tribunal hearing if required.

If a child is excluded from the full range of academic and social activities because of incontinence, every effort should be made at a multi-disciplinary level (and across services) to resolve the problem without resorting to the law. But if it is impossible to persuade the authorities to take appropriate action without legal help, the Disability

Figure 15.1 The Disability Discrimination Act

- Originally passed in 1995, this has now been extended to cover discrimination against disabled pupils and students.

- Since September 2002, children with a disability have the right not to be discriminated against in admissions, exclusions and in the provision of education at school.

- Children will have a right to require schools to remove such barriers as changing policies, practices and procedures but not adjustments to premises (Schools Access Initiative) or provision of auxiliary aids or services (covered by assessment and statement procedure).

- Children's Services (Education) and schools will be required to develop accessibility strategies to show how they will progressively increase the extent to which disabled pupils can participate in a school's curriculum, improve physical environment and improve delivery of education.

Discrimination Act (1995; 2001) is specifically designed to counter any discrimination.

Child protection

In the wake of the Laming Report on the Victoria Climbié case (Laming 2003) and its identification of incontinence as a trigger for abuse, child protection has moved up the agenda. Sexuality and body ownership must be protected and care plans, particularly during times of transition, should address physical and emotional needs. Continence management is necessarily invasive, so particular care must be taken to ensure that it is safe, respectful and not abusive in any way. Care must be taken to protect both the child and the professional.

While issues relating to child protection are explored in more detail in Chapter 1 by Maddie Blackburn, it must be borne in mind that particular care is needed during times of transition as so many more professionals are likely to be involved and links of communication or understanding can be lost. If we are to offer the children in our care safe transit from childhood to adult life, responsibility for continuing care should be passed from one reliable pair of hands to another, with identified professionals working together to maintain progress and avoid breakdown in service provision. When paediatric service responsibility ceases, a carefully planned transition to adult services should be executed. Problems often arise once a young person ceases to be the responsibility of paediatric services and becomes another 'adult service user', with no discernible 'handover' to ensure that previously identified needs will continue to be met (Miller 1995; Baldessano *et al.* 2002; Fleming 2002; Watson 2005; Shribman 2007). If the young person is discharged from paediatric care without referral on to appropriate services for young adults, their future needs are unlikely to be met (White 2000).

If long-term continence problems are seen as a disability, however, they will attract the same protection in law for the child as any other disability.

Assessment

Pre-school

There are a number of congenital and acquired conditions which will, almost certainly, affect bowel and bladder function. Once identified, children with these conditions should have access to specialist units which should take the lead in planning care and in providing advice and training for those professionals from health, education and social services who may be involved. These conditions include:

- Spina bifida (open and closed) (Hunt and Oakshott 2003);
- Other neural tube defects;
- Spinal cord tumour;
- Spinal cord injury;
- Sacral agenesis;
- Cerebral palsy.

A full assessment may be necessary, covering the following aspects:

- Mobility;
- Behaviour;

- Co-ordination;

- Sensation (or lack of it) in the lower limbs;

- Manual dexterity;

- Sexuality and sexual function (which will certainly become important when the child becomes a teenager and young adult);

- Spatial awareness;

- Vision;

- Hearing;

- Developmental stage;

- Independence and life skills;

- Motivation.

It is unusual, however, for specialist units to instigate a multi-disciplinary assessment (MPA) which precedes the statement of special educational need (SEN). This decision is usually taken by community paediatric services.

A diagnosis and treatment plan should included in an individu-alised daily care plan, designed for use in the home, which can be adapted later for use in school.

Educational assessment

As well as the variations in quality and quantity of paediatric conti-nence care, there are also regional variations in the level of educa-tional assessment and ancillary support available for children throughout their education.

CASE STUDY

Gemma during infancy and early childhood

Gemma was born in 1985 with SB (myelomeningocele) and hydrocephalus.

The lesion was closed immediately and an intra-ventricular shunt inserted at 4 weeks to control her hydrocephalus.

Paediatric Urology Centre
The baby was referred to specialist paediatric urology services
(30 miles away) for full assessment and the decision was taken to
instigate intermittent catheterisation with immediate effect.
Her mother was instructed in the procedure using a nasogastric tube
size 4FG.

Follow-up appointments were given at 6-monthly intervals with
periodic scans and urodynamic studies.

Local Child Development Centre
As a small child, Gemma was closely monitored by local paediatric
services but suffered from only occasional urinary tract infections
over the next few years. A tendency to constipation was managed by
a series of measures.

Particular issues at different stages

Continence issues at 3–5 years

Incontinence is not, in itself, a reason for assessing and statementing a
child but, if the acquisition of toileting skills is elusive, action may need
to be taken. Many nursery schools insist that children are clean and
dry on entry, which means that they may not have any provision for
toilet training. These entry criteria put parents in the position of either
being unable to place their child or having to conceal the problem by
using continence products to cover the period that the child is at
school. As a result, the child is at risk of failing to be toilet trained by
the time full-time education starts.

If continence needs are simple and short term, there is usually no
requirement for the assessment procedure. Local continence services
should be able to assess and deal with the problem and follow up at
least six monthly until it is resolved. If the child is not fully continent by
the time they enter primary school, school health will have to be
involved and a decision taken whether or not to proceed on to a MPA.

If needs are complex, an MPA is usually initiated by a community-
based healthcare professional, ideally two full years before the child is
due to start school. This should allow the Children's Services sufficient
time to identify funding for adaptations and ancillary support as

appropriate. The SEN should describe the child's identified needs and the steps which will have to be taken in order to meet them. An annual review date will be selected, and all the professionals involved should have the opportunity to contribute to these reviews so that any necessary changes can be made to the level of support being provided.

Whether or not the child is placed in mainstream or special education will depend upon the level of need, the availability of appropriate multi-disciplinary support and parental choice. Although inclusive education is considered by many to be the ideal, in practice the child with complex special needs may be disadvantaged by the expectations within the mainstream. Special schools do provide education which is in line with the national core curriculum, and the additional services offered may be beneficial to both child and family. Other benefits include access to all areas of the building and to the curriculum, the availability of appropriate equipment and on site expertise.

Mild to moderate learning disability will not necessarily be a barrier to the acquisition of continence, but extra support may be necessary to enable the child to be toilet trained in time for school.

If the assessment (MPA) reveals the child's needs to be complex, a care assistant may be appointed to deal with toileting and changing in school. Training is usually provided by the local continence or specialist urology services, especially if toileting procedures include intermittent catheterisation (White and Oliver 1997; Clarke *et al.* 2005). Further information can be found in the *Guide to Intermittent Catheterisation in Schools* (Foulkes *et al.* 2003; see also Chapter 14 by Rosie Kelly).

The role of care staff

While it is important to ensure the availability of care staff to supervise toileting as necessary, to deal with the effects of incontinence at school or nursery and to carry out agreed programmes of independence training, there are pitfalls which can and should be avoided. One way of ensuring the best possible outcomes is for care staff to:

- Receive training relevant to the child's assessed need;

- Be employed in one-to-one support capacity in exceptional cases only;

- Have terms of employment that are clear and concise;

- Not have terms of employment linked to the child's potential level of dependence;

- Be included in the annual review.

Some children will be so disabled that care staff will be a permanent fixture in their lives but, no matter how severe the disability, every effort should be made to ensure the acquisition of maximum independence. To achieve this, care staff should be trained by appropriately qualified health professionals to meet the child's physical needs while encouraging as much independent self-care as possible.

Where a pupil is severely disabled, care staff should be trained to supervise the programme daily until the child becomes proficient and eventually able to meet his or her own toileting needs reliably and independently. Progress should be evaluated at each annual review and the level of care increased or reduced as necessary. It is important to remember that strange environments may cause confusion and a failure to adhere to routines, so the transition plan should allow for increased support when major changes occur throughout the child's life.

Care assistants responsible for attending to the toileting and changing needs of children risk becoming redundant if they are really good at what they do. If success results in loss of employment, it may prove difficult to motivate a care assistant to work in a way that promotes the young person's independence.

A particularly rewarding relationship between child and carer at school may be threatened by a change of school. It is unusual for carers to move with a child. Usually, a new carer is appointed and this can compromise the progress previously made.

Continence issues at 5–7 years

Once the child is settled in school, independence training routines should be established which place as much responsibility as possible upon the child. If there is a learning disability, programmes should be made as simple as possible, broken down into easy steps and progress monitored and recorded. While this is usually carried out by health professionals and/or care staff, there are some excellent educational programmes designed and implemented by teachers.

Whenever possible, care assistants should be appointed to *supervise* a programme of independence training, rather than simply to carry out care.

Annual reviews should include an update on the management plan from the specialist unit. If reconstructive bowel and/or bladder surgery is planned, ideally timing should be discussed with the school so that the child's education is not disrupted any more than absolutely necessary.

Continence issues affecting ages 7–11 years

For many children, there is a marked transition from infants to juniors. There may even be a change of school. If considerable changes are to be made in environment and personnel, plans should be drawn up well in advance. If mild learning disability or lack of short-term concentration are a feature, it may be difficult to transfer the skills previously attained to the new setting. Extra support may be required at least for the first term.

Ideally, planning should be started two full years before a child makes the transition from junior to senior school. Adaptations will need to be made to the environment. Staffing changes may be necessary and appropriate training should be completed before the child arrives.

Where a child has complex physical needs, it may be necessary to consider counselling and age-appropriate sex education (Blackburn 2002). Consideration should also be given to progress with independence training in toileting, self-care and life skills (Blackie 1998). Continence nurse specialists are able to design daily toileting programmes, which are appropriate for use at home as well as in school. It is very important to avoid deterioration in independence during school holidays.

Continence problems in school should be seen as a multi-disciplinary concern and it is important that different professionals feel able to communicate and collaborate. Staff should be given appropriate support and in-service training to help them fulfil their role.

CASE STUDY

Gemma's school years

Gemma's development was delayed, her health visitor noted her failure to meet her developmental milestones. By the age of 3 years, she had few words, was only able to drag herself around and showed a minimal interest in colourful toys. The decision was taken to undertake a Multi Professional Assessment (MPA) in preparation for entry into primary school in just under 2 years' time.

Double incontinence was identified as well as mild to moderate associated learning disability and a full-time care assistant was employed to assist with toileting, catheterisation (trained by a nurse specialist) and learning support. Gemma was admitted to her local primary school.

Annual reviews took place each year until Gemma's ninth birthday when transition plans were high on the agenda. A comprehensive school was selected which was 8 miles from Gemma's home. Her care assistant was invited to apply for the post at the new school.

Independence skills remained relatively poor with Gemma showing very little inclination to take responsibility for her own toileting needs.

The new school built a toilet specifically for Gemma's use but sited it on a main corridor with the door opening outward. Not only was this a danger to children on the move from one class to another, it also gave opportunity for disruptive pupils to deliberately obstruct the doorway so that Gemma could not get out. Episodes of bullying were frequent and few meaningful friendships were formed.

Transition from primary to secondary school

All parents of school-age children are aware of the enormity of the move from primary to secondary education. How much greater then is the change for a disabled child? The size of the school, noise level, poor standard of toilets and the increased risk of bullying should be considered (Vernon *et al.* 2003). If the secondary school has a split site, how many accessible toilets will be required to meet the young person's needs? If transition plans are not undertaken early enough, it is unlikely that the change of school will be anything less than traumatic for the child with special needs. The need to use urinary catheters and to change pads and the effects of occasional 'accidents' if management routines break down can conspire to make life exceedingly difficult for the child, parents and school staff alike (White and Oliver 1997).

Incontinence in any school, but particularly in secondary schools, may lead to a number of problems for the child, as listed below:

- Behavioural problems;

- Bullying;

- Damaged self-image;

- Staffing problems;

- Interruption of lessons;

- Inability to keep up with the rest of the class;

- Loss of socialising time;

- Exclusion from field trips;

- Difficulties with disposal of continence equipment;

- Discrepancy in level of actual need as opposed to that described in SEN and areas of service responsibility.

Challenges for the school may include:

- The quality of the annual review;

- The need for revised personal and social education and counselling;

- The need for peripatetic support;

- Organising appropriate in-service training for staff;

- The necessity for multi-disciplinary working;

- The challenge of enabling the child to participate fully, across the curriculum and in extra-curricular activities.

If a new carer is to be in place in time for the new academic year, training must be completed in advance.

Adolescence

Teenage years are difficult for most young people. Physical impairment and other obstacles to independence may add to the frustrations experienced. Incontinence may affect self-image, self-awareness and sexuality; counselling may be required. If sexual function is likely to be an issue, individual sex education and counselling may be necessary (Blackburn 2002). This should be considered when transition plans are drawn up for the change from primary to secondary school.

Obstacles to independence

There are a number of stumbling blocks commonly found throughout mainstream education nationwide, which can hinder progress to independence. These include:

- No suitable programme of toileting available;

- Insufficient number of toilets;

- Poorly sited, inadequate or badly designed toilets;

- Toilet key held in school office;

- Lack of care staff;

- Staff terms of employment (which make it difficult or impossible to involve them in helping with toileting problems). In addition, if a care assistant is employed to work on a one-to-one basis with a particular child, there may be insufficient motivation to succeed. Success, after all, will lead to redundancy.

- Insufficient effort made to involve the child in planning or to gain the child's consent for care procedures (DH 2001).

There are examples of excellent multi-disciplinary working within schools which enable the most disabled children to strive for, and achieve, independence in toileting. One of these is at Uffculme School in Birmingham which offers an impressive service, designed and implemented by teachers, for autistic children (see Chapter 16, by Lynne Conboy, Lizi Snushall and Charlotte Kerslake). This was described at the Trent Region Children's Continence Special Interest Group in March 2004. Success in this area tends, however, to be more marked at junior school level, with mounting difficulties at secondary school.

Continence issues affecting ages 14–16 years

Most secondary schools have a transition from lower to upper school. For some, this may mean a change of site as well as department, teaching staff and streaming for academic subjects. It is important to use the annual reviews to think and plan ahead so that incontinence does not get in the way of field trips and extra-curricular activities. If there are mobility and other problems, attention must also be given to the health and safety of staff when lifting disabled pupils.

At the annual review nearest to the child's 14th birthday, there should be appropriate representation from health, current and further education (FE) and social services. This is the stage at which obstacles to independence should be discussed.

For some young disabled people, a period of further education in a residential setting may be required to enable social and life skills to be sufficiently well developed for the young person to live independently in adulthood. The selection of the type of higher education required should be considered by the multi-disciplinary team in conjunction with the child and family. For many children, this will be the first time away from home and every effort should be made to provide the college of FE with as much information as possible. Funding will need to be secured if applications are being made to suitable establishments.

Since young people cease to be the responsibility of Children's Services on reaching their 16th birthday, transition plans should be drawn up for continuing urological healthcare as well as education. Transition to adult services is an area that has been identified as one that is badly served at present (Shribman 2007).

CASE STUDY

Gemma's school years

There were many problems which needed addressing at Gemma's 14+ review. A full multi-disciplinary presence was achieved to discuss:

- Poor academic progress;

- Social isolation;

- Bullying;

- Obesity;

- Independence training;

- Sibling behavioural problems;

- Marital stress on the part of her parents.

Both of Gemma's parents attended and were very open about their difficulties. Gemma was invited in to part of the meeting but looked to her classroom assistant to explain her situation.

A three-year placement at a college of FE was agreed though funding was expected to be an issue. Gemma's parents were given a quantity of literature and possible appropriate placements.

Work began immediately to identify a suitable placement.

With good multi-disciplinary liaison and much encouragement for Gemma, a suitable college was found and information provided. The spotlight was also shone onto the transition of healthcare from paediatric to adult services. Because of geographical and other difficulties, the responsibility for care remained with the paediatric unit throughout Gemma's placement and liaison was fairly good between college and unit.

Now in her final year at college, Gemma has lost weight, is much more independent, has revealed a strong and likeable personality and is considering whether or not to return to the family home or live independently. Her parents remain fully supportive. Her urology care is to be transferred to an appropriate adult service when this decision is made.

At the end of the current academic year a report will be prepared and sent to wherever Gemma chooses to live.

Continence issues affecting children of 16 and over

On arrival in a residential college of further education, records of previous education, paediatric healthcare and social care should be available. This is particularly necessary for those with complex needs because much valuable educational time may be lost in trying to obtain the relevant information required for successful integration and smooth transition of care. In some cases, this may lead to a loss of skills previously attained. If the young person has communication difficulties and, perhaps, some degree of learning impairment, there is little chance of resolving problems which could, and should, have been avoided.

Currently, it appears that few FE colleges receive full medical and educational documentation in time for the new academic year even though it is clear that insufficient information will extend the settling in period and impair progress. But there are examples of good practice. The Transition Service at NHS Lothian (Lothian PCT 2000) offers a full assessment and care plan, which covers all aspects of care including continence. This document accompanies the child into higher special education.

The Adults with Incapacity (Scotland) Act 2000 clearly states the legal requirement for the health service to provide care for young people on reaching adulthood. A similar legal requirement would be beneficial across the United Kingdom.

Most residential courses in special needs colleges of FE are for a period of three years. Changes of staff and key workers may compromise progress, so particular care should be taken to document progress and produce a final report of independence and toileting needs which can be used as the basis for provision of appropriate health and social care wherever the young adult chooses to live on leaving college.

A questionnaire was given to all students/families at a College of FE for students with special needs in Lancaster in 2000 (Denny 2003). The students are drawn from all over the country and so the study is representative. Apart from many disappointing remarks about the absence or poor quality of continence services during childhood, there was also the perception that 'transition had been smooth because nobody had told them otherwise' when the reality was that although the young person had been discharged from paediatric care, they had not been referred on to an appropriate adult service.

Among the few examples of good practice is a combined effort between paediatric urology and nephrology services and their adult counterparts at Nottingham City Hospital (NHSME 2003). This service, which is available to young adults living in Nottingham, has resulted in an impressive transition clinic for 16 to 25-year-olds.

Conclusion

Continence problems may be short term and resolve with maturity but, equally, continence care may be a central issue in the management of complex conditions throughout life. Particularly when the latter situation is involved, it is impossible to overstate the importance of transition when managing continence care.

Paediatric continence/urology nurse specialists in the acute and community care sectors have a vital role to play. However, transition and rehabilitation services for young people are in short supply, and limited respite services mean that the burden of care continues to rest with parents.

It is essential therefore that effective transition planning is built in to paediatric care, and this can only be achieved by close co-operation between health, education and social services. It is the final transition from paediatric to adult care that will set the standard and provide the last opportunity to influence the quality of care and support which is to be made available to young adults. Their quality of life from now on may depend upon it.

References

Baldassano R, Ferry G, Griffiths A, Mack D *et al.* (2002) Transition of the patient with inflammatory bowel disease from paediatric to adult care: Recommendations of the North American Society for Pediatric Gastroenterology, Hepatology and Nutrition. *Journal of Pediatric Gastroenterology and Nutrition*, 34 (3): 245–8

Blackie C (1998) Promoting health in young people. *Nursing Standard*, 12 (36) May 27: 39–46

Blackburn MC (2002) *Sexuality and Disability*. Oxford: Butterworth Heinemann (now Elsevier)

Clarke SA, Samuel M, Boddy SA (2005) Are prophylactic antibiotics necessary with clean catheterisation? A randomised controlled trial. *Journal of Paediatric Surgery*, 40(3): 568–71

Denny A (2003) Beaumont College Study. Paper presented at the RCN CCF Conference, 23 October 2003, International Centre, Telford

Department of Health (2001) *Consent - What You Have a Right to Expect. A guide for children and young people*. Norwich: The Stationery Office

Department of Health (2004) *National Service Framework for Children, Young People and Maternity Services*. Norwich: The Stationery Office

Fleming E (2002) The transition of adolescents with diabetes from the Children's Healthcare Service into the Adult Healthcare Service: a review of the literature. *Journal of Clinical Nursing*, 5 (Sept 11): 560–67

Foulkes S, Oliver H, White MC (2003) *Guide to Intermittent Catheterisation in Schools*. Stonehouse, Glos: Astra Tech Ltd

Hunt G, Oakshott P (2003) Outcome in people with open spina bifida at age 35: a prospective community based cohort study. *British Medical Journal*, 326 (June 21): 1365–6

Laming WH (Chair) (2003) *The Victoria Climbié Inquiry*. Norwich: Crown Copyright. Website: www.victoria-climbié-inquiry.org.uk

Lothian PCT Community Rehabilitation Service (2000) *The Transition Service Health Needs Assessment + Care Plan Transition Service*. Lothian Primary Care NHS Trust

Lothian PCT (2001) *A Guide to The Adults with Incapacity (Scotland) Act 2000*. Lothian Primary Care NHS Trust

Miller S (1995) Adolescents' view of outpatient services. *Nursing Standard*, 9 (17) Jan 18: 30–2

NHS Modernisation Agency (2003) *Good Practice in Paediatric Continence Services –
Benchmarking in Action*. London: Department of Health.
Website: www.modern.nhs.uk
Shribman S (2007) *Making it Better for Children and Young People: Clinical case for
change*. London: Department of Health
Vernon S, Lundblad B, Hellstrom AL (2003) Children's experiences of school
toilets present a risk to their physical and psychological wellbeing. *Child: Care,
Health and Development*, 29(1): 47–53
Watson AR (2005) Problems and pitfalls of transition from paediatric to adult
renal care. *Paediatric Nephrology*, 20 (Feb): 113–17
White MC (2000) A Contract For Care. Unpublished MA Dissertation, University
of Keele
White MC, Dobson P (1999) *Bladder and Bowel Management in Children with
Special Physical Needs*. Bristol: ERICWhite MC, Oliver H (1997) Developing
Guidelines on Catheterisation in Schools. *Professional Nurse*, 12 (12): 855–8

Legislation
Disability Discrimination Act 1995 (as amended by the Special Educational Needs
and Disability Act 2001). Part 4: Code of practice for Schools
The Special Educational Needs and Disability Act 2001

Continence issues in schools

16

Lynne Conboy, Lizi Snushall and Charlotte Kerslake

Key points

- Continence issues are common in children with special educational needs.

- Comprehensive assessments – looking at a whole range of issues – are essential.

- Individualised programmes need to build on children's strengths and interests, and take account of individual family situations. Lateral thinking and creativity are important.

- A multi-disciplinary approach is needed – involving teaching staff, teaching assistants, parents, speech and language therapists and other relevant agencies.

- Toilet training should be linked to other areas of learning such as communication, for a holistic approach.

Continence issues present problems in special schools, but they can also challenge teachers and support staff in mainstream education. This chapter, written by two teachers from a special school and a Paediatric Continence Adviser working with schoolchildren generally, looks at pioneering work being carried out at one special school in Birmingham, and considers the strategies that might be useful in the wider field.

The Uffculme approach

Uffculme School is a primary school in Birmingham LEA for children with autistic spectrum disorder (ASD). The school population represents the spectrum of autism, from children with severe learning difficulties and severe autism through to the children with Asperger's Syndrome. The school is funded for 120 children. Many pupils experience difficulties in achieving full continence. Their difficulties are not related to medical problems, but are encompassed within the all-pervading nature of the specific difficulty of autism. Some of the principles used may be applied to children with other cognitive impairments.

At Uffculme School, the approach to toilet training takes account of the difficulties and strengths of children with ASD. In our experience, traditional toilet training methods often lead to limited success. Not taking account of the specific nature of autism can lead to frustration and failure by all involved. The Uffculme toilet training approach is a continuation of the teaching methods used in all other curriculum areas. Our approach is one that is continually evolving as each individual child and family situation presents new and specific needs and difficulties. We believe that the teacher should be instrumental in developing toilet training programmes as the skills needed are inseparable from all other functional areas of learning.

Health promotion

Most of the health issues promoted in Uffculme school are basic health principles, which many children with autism find difficult. The school is involved in the Healthy Schools Initiative, with groups of staff and children working on projects to promote healthy choices for eating and for physical activities. The school has water dispensers in the corridors and children are encouraged to drink water wherever appropriate. Where pupils are not toilet trained, drinks are offered within a timetabled routine. Scheduling the drink times rather than providing drinks continuously throughout the school day seems to help children to empty their bladder in a large amount rather than trickling into their nappy continuously. The school also takes part in the free fruit scheme, where children are encouraged to eat fruit regularly at snack times. Many children have self-imposed diets which can impact greatly on regular bowel movements or any toilet training programme.

Definitions

Toilet training success can be achieved at different levels:

- *Habit trained* or *toilet regulated* is when the child learns to empty the bladder or bowels at a set time, but they are unable to indicate a need to go to the toilet at other times.

- *Toilet trained* is when the child is able to:
    - recognise the need to go to the toilet;

☐ communicate this need to others or find the toilet independently;

☐ complete the toilet sequence independently.

Habit training may be the ultimate achievement for some of our children; it may be an initial achievement for others. Any level of toilet training means greater social acceptability and dignity.

Prevalence

Over the past ten years, the school's pupil population has gradually changed from children with moderate learning difficulties (not necessarily autistic) to a predominance of children at the more severe end of the autistic spectrum, with increasingly complex needs – all with a diagnosis of autistic spectrum disorder (ASD).

In September 2001, out of 20 children within the nursery and reception classes, only one child was fully toilet trained (see Figure 16.1). The majority of these children had complex difficulties – our familiar toilet training methods were not going to work. It was at this stage that the Reception class teacher sought help, which arrived in the form of one of ERIC's private consultants and a nurse from the continence team in Birmingham. With their knowledge and expertise in the field of toilet training, and ours in the field of autism, we changed the philosophy of our toilet training radically and devised an approach that has given us much greater success and is still continuing to evolve. Each year the new intake of children present with ever more complex behaviour and needs, which require us to develop ever more complex individual toilet training programmes.

The issue of toilet training and continence is not confined to the younger children within the school. Small numbers of children were remaining incontinent through their primary years (see Figure 16.1). The toilet training programmes have been implemented with pupils throughout the school.

Pathways and care

Why do children with autism need a specific approach to toilet training?

We have many children who have joined us at the age of 3 or 4 already trained successfully at home. Other children arrive with parents readily

Figure 16.1 Number of pupils toilet trained in September 2001

Class (age)	Already toilet trained	NOT toilet trained
Nursery (3–4yrs)	1	9
Reception (4–5 yrs)	0	10
Year 1 (5–6 yrs)	4	8 (2 partially)
Year 2 (6–7 yrs)	11	(1 partially)
Year 3 (7–8yrs)	14	1
Year 4 (8–9yrs)	12	2
Year 5 (9–10 yrs)	22	3
Year 6 (10–11 yrs)	12	4

admitting that they have never tried – or have tried but given up. For many, the exhausting daily challenges involved in bringing up a child with autism mean that toilet training is not high on their priorities.

The problems that the majority of pupils with ASD encounter in achieving continence are directly related to their autism as opposed to being related to their level of maturity or physiological or neurological development. Figure 16.2 shows how some continence issues relate specifically to the specific difficulties of autism as identified by the 'Triad of Impairment'.

Accompanying medical and sensory issues frequently compound the difficulties. Some children may be hyper- or hypo-sensitive to smell and sounds. This can cause potential behaviour difficulties associated with the toilet. Some children find the noises, smells and the close environment difficult, and so don't want to go into the toilet area. Other children may crave these sensations, which can lead to behaviour difficulties as the child seeks sensory input involved with the toilet training process (smearing, obsessive toilet flushing, licking or smelling surfaces, etc.).

Many children with ASD have a self-imposed diet which means that increasing fluids and fibre intake as a means to facilitate toilet training and continence can be nigh on impossible to implement successfully. Other children may have motor difficulties that make it difficult for them to organise and sequence the motor actions needed to use the toilet successfully. Anxiety may be related to any of these factors, or

Impairment of communication and language leads to:
Difficulty in recognising and communicating needs appropriately;
Literal understanding of instructions such as 'go to the toilet'
(the child may go into the toilet – but not use it)

Impairment of flexibility of thought leads to:
Resistance to changing well-established behaviours/behaviour sequences (e.g. using a nappy as the toilet), and changing toilet routines and sequences;
Fear of the toilet area (hand driers blowing unexpectedly, echoing small areas, fear of water, fear of the toilet flush).

Impairment of social interaction leads to:
Lack of empathy with the feelings of others;
No awareness of the social inappropriateness of wearing a nappy, or of age-appropriateness issues;
Poor understanding of the social conventions associated with the toilet.

Figure 16.2 The 'Triad of Impairment'

may also be related to difficulty accepting changes to familiar routines and practices. Challenging behaviour may be sufficient for parents and staff to feel that the possible creation of more difficulties is reason enough for not attempting to toilet train. In view of these difficulties, toilet training suddenly appears as an insurmountable challenge rather than an achievable milestone.

The key to our toilet training programme is the setting up of appropriate routines. In Nursery and Reception classes, the children are routinely taken to the toilet area and their nappy changed. The whole sequence is seen as being critical to the success of the programme. From the day a child enters the school, he or she is encouraged to tolerate as much of the normal toilet routine as possible: entering the toilet area; pulling down their clothes; sitting on the toilet; pulling up their clothes; flushing the toilet; washing and drying hands. Some children may only be able to accept part of this, and this will become part of the information gathering process leading to the development of individualised objectives. Certain elements within the sequence may become specific objectives as a means of working towards toilet training, for example, the dressing sequence can be actively worked on when dressing/undressing for PE – this then supports the clothing element of the toilet routine.

Assessments and information gathering

Careful and thorough assessments are essential to the development of individualised programmes. Maria Wheeler's *Readiness Assessments* (Wheeler 1998) ensures collection of basic information: the child's level of awareness; physiological factors and medical conditions. Wheeler also suggests collection of information about specific characteristics that will inform the individualised programme. This information should be gathered from all involved with the child, and should include strengths and weaknesses in, for example:

- Communication status and needs;
- Rigidity of behaviours and reliance on routine;
- Levels of anxiety;
- Rewards and motivators;
- Sensory difficulties.

We use these assessment criteria for guiding our observations, and gathering information from teachers, teaching assistants, speech and language therapists and parents to ensure that we obtained a full picture of the child. These assessments enable us to prioritise which child should begin working on a toilet training programme and how their individual programme should be devised (see Figure 16.3). It is an extremely time-consuming process and thus we cannot work with all pupils to the same degree, some pupils continuing to work on other parts of the toileting process. The assessments are also a tool in explaining to parents why it is we are or are not working with their child at the present time. It helps them to see their child within the context of their own development rather than in the context of usual time scales in toilet training children without these difficulties. Parents are invited in for parent workshops in order to discuss their child and their role. These workshops are invaluable. They mean we are working on common agreed goals; we have a shared understanding of the problems and tasks ahead, and also, importantly, a shared commitment and mutual support.

The initial assessments lead us to further investigations and recording.

Recording of the amount and time of fluid intake and when the child

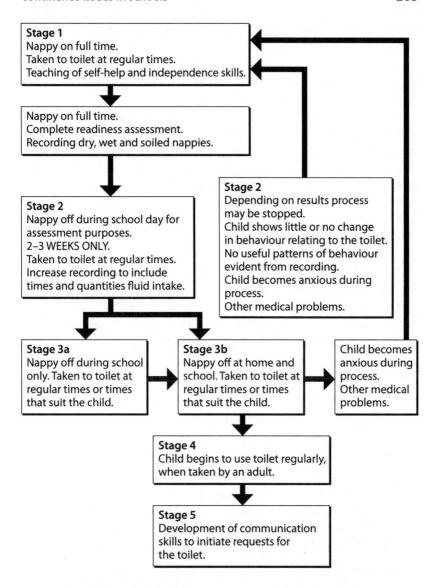

Figure 16.3 The process of introducing and implementing
a toilet training programme

actually urinates or soils, rather than recording when the wet nappy is
changed, allows staff to pinpoint the child's individual pattern of elimination, and hopefully their bladder capacity. Our success in using electronic alarms for gathering this data has been limited; our preference is
to gather this information by removing the child's nappy for a period of

approximately 2–3 weeks. An additional factor at this time is that many children exhibit quite dramatic changes in behaviour (both positive and negative), once their nappy is removed. The nappy has always been there, a safe warm environment, where they never feel wet or uncomfortable. We are breaking into a habit that was established at birth.

When the nappy has been removed for this assessment period, the toilet routine is not changed. Toilet training is not being sent to sit on the toilet every half an hour. Being truly toilet trained is being able to empty the bladder when it is full. The child still goes to the toilet at the same routine times, wet accidents and fluids drunk are recorded and then the subsequent toilet times may be altered. Making the connection between passing urine and using the toilet is a tricky one. Some children watch others, or we magically catch them at the right time. But, whenever it happens, it is an amazing moment.

With some children, it may be apparent that they are not ready for toilet training as such. However, these children can still be working towards toilet training in a variety of ways: learning to use and respond to photographs of activities; increasing the time they will sit on the toilet; independent dressing and undressing.

CASE STUDY

Catherine

Catherine has been diagnosed with ASD. She uses 2–3 word utterances, and can comprehend instructions using two or three key words. She can make her needs known using pictures and the spoken word. Catherine was one of the first group of children involved in our new toilet training philosophy; her parents attended the first parent group.

Catherine's difficulties are such that she is an extremely rigid in her thinking and is a non-compliant little girl. She is very self-directed and has an extreme dislike of adult direction – which often resulted in her being verbally and physically abusive to adults. Toilet training had been a very negative experience with her often refusing to go into the toilet area, not sitting appropriately and staying on the toilet for only one or two seconds. It was a meaningless activity for her. She had no understanding of what was expected or the purpose of it. It had become a battleground. However assessments showed some positive aspects, particularly that she showed awareness of being wet and didn't like it, and she didn't like nappies. She had some imitation skills and liked playing with dolls, and she could tolerate changes in her routine when supported with the photographic timetable pictures.

The objectives we worked on were:

- Sitting on the toilet for longer – the aim was for about 10–15 seconds;

- Accepting wearing pants;

- Communicating the need for the toilet;

- Connecting the process of having a wee with the toilet – giving it some meaning.

The 'toilet bag' was introduced to encourage her to sit on the toilet – she was only allowed the bag once sitting on the toilet. The bag was chosen specifically for Catherine – and so was filled with items that would interest her with toys and books of things she liked – mainly Disney items. This increased her time sitting from 2–35 seconds, which was quite a breakthrough. Alongside this, the staff made detailed recording of what she drank and the times she was wet. We planned to remove the nappy completely both at home and at school.

A photographic timetable sequence was used to show her what she was doing and to enable adults to direct her non-verbally if necessary. Catherine enjoyed playing with dolls, and had shown us that she was able to imitate actions from an adult. She accepted playing with a doll that wet as a model, but it wasn't very realistic as the water went through straight after dolly drinking. Catherine was pleased to have her nappy off – and was very proud of her 'Disney' pants. Parents were making changes at home to support Catherine's toilet training – they made the toilet a place where Catherine would enjoy being. A date was arranged for the nappy to be discarded at school and at home. On the first day, after a few wet accidents in the morning, Catherine did her first wee on the toilet. She was rewarded with praise and chocolate. Success at home followed quickly, and Catherine soon progressed to being fully toilet trained – indicating her need to go to the toilet, rather than being taken there as a timetabled activity.

CASE STUDY

Zak

Zak came to us having never used the toilet and following extremely negative experiences at his pre-school nursery. On entry to Uffculme he was anxious about the whole toilet process, but he responded positively to the photographic timetable sequence for the daily routine activities, and he soon became familiar with the nappy changing process and was even sitting on the toilet for a short time. However he was very resistant to changes and very attached to his nappy. He would become tearful if the nappy was removed.

Zak is diagnosed as having ASD and is quite a verbal child. He can make his needs known effectively to choose snacks and activities, using a combination of speech and picture token exchange. One of his strengths is that he can read, and is extremely interested in books. He has the level of symbolic understanding to be able to understand symbols and line drawings both of people and of objects.

The main aim for Zak was to reduce his anxiety. An individualised book was prepared for Zak detailing the toileting process and he was encouraged to read this with an adult before and during toilet time. His tolerance was also increased by putting pants on under his nappy, which enabled him to experience 'being wet' while still having the security of his nappy. Finally the nappy was removed and the photo book changed to correspond to the alterations in routine. An individualised toilet bag was also used to encourage him to sit for longer.

Within two days of the nappy being removed, Zak had used the toilet and was happy about it. He hasn't looked back since. For a long time afterwards he would use the book in school, reciting the words on each page as he did the action.

Investigations and developments

The Uffculme toilet training programme is continually evolving, taking account of individual needs and experiences both in school and from the home situations. After our initial successes we moved on to working with other children, but didn't do parental workshops as we had at the

CASE STUDY

Neil

Neil was 10 years old, and not toilet trained. He was one of our pupils with severe autism and severe learning difficulties. Staff involved agreed that they should work towards achieving habit training for Neil. Assessments informed us that Neil had awareness of being wet and didn't like wet clothes. He accepted sitting on the toilet as part of the routine in the toilet area, but had never used it. Neil had been with the same staff for several years. They knew him well and were sure that he urinated as soon as a clean nappy went on. Neil had only a very basic receptive understanding of a few familiar photographs. He had no means of making his needs known other than behaviour. He was a child with very set routines, and exhibited very rigid behaviours.

The main objective of the programme implemented was for all staff consistently to use an individual toilet photo when taking Neil to the toilet. The class staff also worked on breaking into his toilet routine by encouraging Neil to tolerate sitting back onto the toilet once his nappy was on – staff identified a special chocolate as a motivator. Once accepting of this change, the staff began to cut small slits into the nappy, so that when he sat back onto the toilet and started to wee, urine came out of the nappy. Neil tolerated this, and did begin to show an interest.

The size of the hole was gradually increased.

Unfortunately other factors led to an increase in challenging violent behaviour. All agreed that the programme had to be halted – temporarily we hoped.

Within weeks, Neil's Mum phoned to tell us that he had woken her up in the night clutching his toilet photo, and sure enough his nappy was wet and warm. Neil moved on rapidly to finding his toilet photo to indicate that he needed to go to the toilet before being wet.

beginning. The process was explained and discussed over the phone. We continued to achieve success with children but also encountered difficulties arising from our lack of direct parental involvement. In one case, the parent was quite keen for us to work on toilet training. We removed the nappy and used absorbent pants. We carried on with our recording, but after two months it became quite obvious to us that we were getting nowhere and we talked to the parent about stopping the programme. She was quite adamant that she didn't mind the washing and desperately didn't want to go back to nappies. Another child and parents were keen for us to toilet train their child but once we removed the nappy and started sending home bagfuls of wet clothes they were horrified at the amount of washing they were faced with. In both cases we had assumed they had understood the implications of the programme and were working from the same baseline as us. This has had a profound effect on how we present our toilet training programme to parents. We now always do a workshop and invite parents of a specified group of children who are showing toilet training readiness.

Information for parents and carers

As with the direct work with the children, our work with parents in parental workshops and meetings has ensured that our procedures have evolved to meet individual needs – and to take account of parental feedback and experiences. At the workshops the parents are given an information pack containing the school's policy on toilet training, a flow chart of the process, definitions of toilet training and examples of the assessments. We discuss each part and listen to their thoughts, comments and experiences on toilet training. We have also been privileged to have some parents, whose child has successfully been toilet trained at school, attend these meetings. They were keen to tell other parents that it can be done, even when (as they thought) the task looked impossible.

An invaluable development has been the implementation of a parental questionnaire. A questionnaire is sent home for parents to fill in before the workshop. This provides school staff with information on how parents approach nappy changing, and the toilet procedure. It also enables staff to determine any differences in expectation and experiences between home and school, enabling staff to give very individual advice and support to each parent to help them to introduce the routines that work so well in school.

The parents are then able to enter the process with realistic expectations and aware of what may or may not happen next. A 'Home–School Agreement' is agreed by parents and staff. This indicates what objectives are to be worked on at home and at school, giving time scales and review dates. Often the parents are working on different objectives to school, but it is important for all to work on something and for the parents to be proactive in toilet training their child. The feedback on these workshops has been very positive.

When the staff at Uffculme first embarked on this project, we had no idea that toilet training was such a complex issue. The more we learn and do, the more we find we need to learn and do! Our work on toilet training has brought us into contact with many different professionals from the health services – a new experience for us working in the field of education. Our knowledge and understanding of continence issues has been greatly enhanced by our involvement in health service conferences, and through meeting many different professionals. Through these contacts we also realise what a privileged position we are in. We are able to apply a holistic approach to toilet training, with our knowledge of the child's skills and abilities of one area of learning being used to support and guide developments in other areas. Each new child and his or her specific needs and experiences is a new challenge; our toilet training programmes are therefore continually evolving and developing.

A nursing view of continence problems in schools

As a Special School, Uffculme has particular challenges and particular resources. In the wider sphere however, the emphasis being placed on education departments to educate children with special needs in mainstream schools has affected teaching staff and school nurses (DeBell and Jackson 2000). Some schools have access to a Continence Adviser, but unfortunately this resource is not available to all. While the policy agenda promotes provision of a multi-disciplinary, integrated continence service, the reality falls short (NHSME 2003).

Some of the facilites at Uffculme are simply in line with recommendations for good practice, such as the provision of water dispensers in all corridors. The provision of accessible drinking water in state schools has been shown to be woefully inadequate according to a survey carried out on behalf of the CPHVA (Madge and Franklin 2003). Indeed the only place where drinking water could be accessed in one third of the schools surveyed in another study was in the toilet area itself (Croghan 2002). The Bog Standard campaign, aimed primarily at teachers, works to raise awareness of the links between provision of acceptable toilet facilities and drinking water, and children's health. This has been fuelled by the additional access problems experienced by children with special needs in mainstream education, but all pupils stand to benefit.

Depending on national discrepancies and regional differences, many children with special needs who are in mainstream education do not have funded individual support. This is causing increasing anxiety and pressure on parents, teaching staff and children where a child is unable to manage his or her own continence needs. Concerns from teaching staff often centre around 'child protection' issues (DfES 2003), and the necessity of balancing the needs of the child against risk factors for teaching staff. Parental worries are not only concerned with the ways in which continence issues might affect their child's education but also how they will affect relationships with their peer group.

Where Paediatric Continence Advisers are available, they usually work within a multi-disciplinary team alongside teachers, special education needs co-ordinators (SENCos), teaching assistants and nursery nurses within the school and nursery setting. There is also an extended role of liaison with occupational therapists, physiotherapists, school nurses and social service departments, and in some cases with medical or surgical specialists – as in the Portsmouth area for example (NHSME 2003).

Currently, many services have an open referral system (as recommended in *Every Child Matters*, DfES 2003). Following referral, the child is added to the waiting list and a detailed assessment undertaken as soon as possible by the Paediatric Continence Adviser, with emphasis on the very specific individual needs of each child.

Figure 16.4 shows the information sheet used after assessment by one Trust's Continence Service; other authorities will have similar tools. The child's social, birth and medical/surgical history must all be taken into account when planning care and treatment pathways.

Uffculme School is unusual in that the pupils all have variants of the same disorder – ASD. In mainstream education, a wider variety of physical and learning problems will be found and these will impact on continence in different ways. The majority of a Paediatric Continence Adviser's work is with children with special educational needs and this frequently involves working with parents or families who also have learning difficulties and possible communication problems. These families require individualised care and support, and may require very frequent input, sometimes needing weekly visits or telephone calls to help them attempt or support appropriate toilet training programmes. In some cases, nursery nurses can also be invaluable in working with this client group on a follow-up basis.

Bedfordshire Continence Service
[Contact phone numbers]

Date:

Re: Name and DOB and Address

Points Discussed at Meeting on   at   School

(1) Toileting after *all* meals.

(2) To encourage sitting on the toilet using a footstool if possible.

(3) Distraction techniques whilst 'sitting' on the toilet, e.g. picture symbols.
(Child's name) likes *Toy Story*.
Possible use of visual distraction, e.g. egg timer if appropriate or suitable for (Child's name).

(4) (Child's name) to wear *underpants under* the nappy to help increase awareness of being wet or soiled.

(5) Use of *'gamgee'* padding in *back* of underpants if (Child's name) experiencing increased soiling.

(6) Continued use of communication symbols e.g. toilet sign and the sitting on the toilet sign.

(7) Continued encouragement with drinks throughout the day.

Signed: _____ [Name]
                                         Paediatric Continence Adviser

Copied to: Parent/Guardian of .... Address
                  School Staff .... School Address
                  Community Nurse .... Address

Figure 16.4 Information sheet used by Bedfordshire Continence Service for Paediatric Assessment

Further assessment involves taking detailed information about fluid intake, noting how the child is fed, asking about their dietary intake and whether the diet may play a part in some of the problems being experienced (e.g. constipation with or without overflow). The child's current developmental stage of toileting and bowel habits are noted, and questions should be asked about whether advice or input from GP has been sought with regard to medication as appropriate, or whether the child has had a physical examination to exclude any underlying abnormality.

Information regarding diagnosis, medication, mobility/dexterity and general overall development, or any delay, all play a relevant part in the assessment process and the further individualised care plans are drawn up in consultation with parents and carers and other professionals.

Continence is a very emotive subject and problems with continence may cause various behavioural problems in any child whatever other problems they may or may not have. The possibility of abuse, although hopefully rare, should not be forgotten and relevant referrals and correct action taken as necessary according to local policy and guidelines (DfES 2003).

THE PAEDIATRIC CONTINENCE ADVISER

"Approximately 5% of children on my caseload are in mainstream education, have no obvious learning difficulty but have complex bowel or bladder conditions. These clients are usually seen in specialist centres and my involvement is follow-up, support and possible training of staff involved in the child's care (e.g. clients with spina bifida requiring intermittent catheterisation) and general follow-up/support of family and child. Today greater emphasis is placed on helping young people with complex needs develop self-help and independence as much as they are realistically able, and this often requires the support of a multi-disciplinary team."

Communication is probably the most relevant aspect of the role of the Paediatric Continence Adviser in schools (see also Chapter 2 by Ruth Emery). Individual care plans may be drawn up on the basis of a full assessment, and include a communication element depending on need and appropriateness. This can vary from written advice or tips to help the family, the gradual introduction of one or two communication symbols, or detailed 24-hour care plans using communication symbols (e.g. Picture Exchange Communication Symbols (PECS), or other communication systems such as Widgett). Figure 16.5 gives an example of a 24-hour care plan.

Child's Name _____

Date _____

To try – Regular toileting with underpants under nappy to increase awareness of being wet.

Time	Routine	Picture	Comments	Star/sticker
6.30am	Washed and dressed. Toilet			
7.30–7.55am	Drinks. Toilet			
9.20–9.30am	Arrival at school – try the toilet – sit for 5 minutes			
	Breaktime			
11.10am	Drink			
11.20am–11.30am	Toilet (encouraged to sit for 5 minutes)			
12.30pm	Lunch (note food/drink)			
1.15–1.30pm	Toilet (to be encouraged to sit for 5 minutes)			
2.15pm	Breaktime drink			
2.30–3pm	Toilet – flexible time depending on timetable			
4pm	Drink and toilet			
5.30pm	Tea and drink			
6pm	Toilet sit for 5 minutes			
7.30–8pm	Bath/shower. Toilet before and after			
9pm	Toilet then bed			

Bedfordshire Continence Service

Figure 16.5 24-hour care plan

Depending on the child's individual level of understanding, a more simple 'step chart' may be used for the child and other family members to follow (see Figure 16.6). This can be adapted at a pace suitable for the individual child, in order to help him or her move forward at a comfortable pace to the next stage of toileting.

All this can be very time-consuming, and progress can be slow. It can even go backwards if the child is upset or unwell, or if a change in routine takes place. At assessment, we explain to parents, carers and staff that acquiring toileting skills can take children with special needs (especially those with ASD) a long period of time – months or

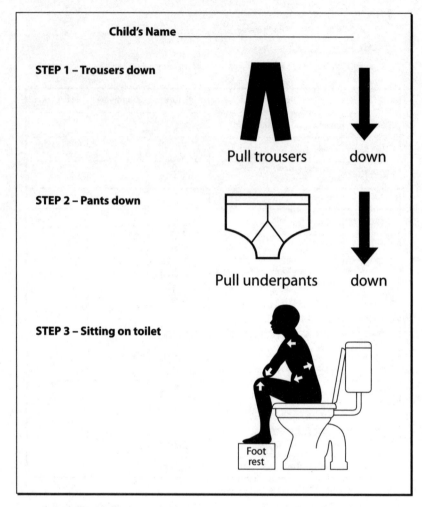

Figure 16.6 Step chart for tracking toilet training progress

even years – with slow individual steps of progress. The intention of these explanations is not to put parents off, but to give them a realistic overview of what to expect. Consistency and perseverance are probably the most important aspects of toilet training alongside praise/reward systems as appropriate to the individual.

Professionals (and parents) also need to be aware that a number of children will continue to have continence issues and require assessment for continence products. This may be because the child is unsuitable for toileting programmes due to functional problems or lack of cognitive awareness. Alternatively, it may be because the child is unable to acquire the relevant skills despite routines or programmes.

Paediatric Continence Advisers attempt to offer ongoing advice and support for all families, schools and children with continence issues. This includes practical advice, implementation of training programmes, support or simply being a listening ear at the end of the telephone. Advisers may also be asked to give advice and teaching to parents, school nurses and health visitors. In many parts of the UK, they assist medical colleagues, such as the Community Consultant Paediatrician, with monthly bowel clinics and are involved with referrals to specific enuresis clinics (NHSME 2003).

Conclusion

Addressing toileting and continence problems for children with ASD or other special educational needs will always require a multi-disciplinary approach.

The main elements of establishing a successful toilet training programme, such as the one at Uffculme School, are:

- Establishing a routine;
- Effective assessments that lead on to the development of individualised programmes;
- Working in close contact with parents.

Toilet training programmes are at their most productive when all involved are working on common agreed goals, but progress can equally be made when working on agreed individual goals towards a common end.

The same principles can also be applied to working in mainstream education, though there may be additional challenges when working with children with special needs in an environment that is not specifically designed to help address their difficulties. There is no age or time limit for attempting toilet training with special needs clients, although reviewing an individual's care should take place on a regular basis in consultation with parents and teachers. These are the people who are most likely to be aware of recent developments or signs that a child may have acquired skills that indicate readiness for further assessment.

References

Croghan EC (2002) A survey of drinking and toilet facilities in local state schools. *British Journal of Community Nursing*, 7: 76–9

DeBell D, Jackson P (2000) *School Nursing within the Public Health Agenda: A strategy for practice*. London: CPHVA

Department for Education and Skills (2003) *Every Child Matters*. Norwich: The Stationery Office. Website: www.dfes.gov.uk/everychildmatters

Madge N, Franklin A (2003) *Change, Challenge and School Nursing*. London: CPHVA

NHS Modernisation Agency (2003) *Good Practice in Paediatric Continence Services – Benchmarking in Action*. London: Department of Health
Website: www.modern.nhs.uk

The Bog Standard Campaign Website: www.bog-standard.org

Wheeler M (1998) *Toilet Training for Individuals with Autism*. Arlington TX: Future Horizons

17

Strategy for developing integrated paediatric continence services

Liz Bonner

Key points

- Continence problems prevent children from reaching their full potential.

- A large number of different professionals need to be involved if continence problems are to be managed effectively.

- Multi-disciplinary teams need a motivating leader and clearly defined terms of reference.

- Everyone benefits if paediatric continence services can be integrated.

Health promotion points

- A large number of different professionals from health and social care, and education, may be involved in a child's care. It is important to prepare parents for this.

- Parents are the experts on their own children, and should be encouraged to regard themselves as essential members of the caring team.

'The importance of politics in nursing can not be over estimated' (Antrobus and Kitson 1999). Professionals have lobbied for many years for integrated paediatric continence services. They have seen, all too closely, the protracted efforts many families have to make if they are to access the most appropriate health professionals to help with the management of long-term bladder and bowel dysfunction. They are all too well aware of the extent to which continence problems can damage self-esteem and prevent children from reaching their full potential.

Social and educational opportunities are likely to be limited if help is needed for toileting, catheterisation or changing continence products.

Bladder and bowel problems can cause distress, frustration and strain relationships and may lead to bullying at school, as well as causing emotional and behavioural problems, so it is important to provide responsive accessible services (Cavat 1998). Emerging findings from the report following the inquiry on the Victoria Climbié case (Laming 2003) suggest that effective early intervention optimises the child's health, social, emotional and cognitive functioning and educational achievement, leading to better outcomes for the whole family.

The limits of practice

According to the NHS Modernisation Agency (2003), there are examples of good practice in paediatric continence services across the UK, but many of these address part of the problem only. For example, they may focus on particular specialisms (such as enuresis or encoporesis), or they may be particularly concerned with the provision of continence products. The Department of Health paper *Good Practice in Continence Services* (2000) makes the case for an Integrated Paediatric Continence Service to be commissioned by each Primary Care Trust (PCT). Such a service should provide accessible, evidence-based assessment, treatment, management and containment programmes for any child with a bladder and/or bowel problem. In a multi-centre study carried out on behalf of the Continence Foundation, Thomas (2004) found that PCTs had limited access to paediatric continence advisers. Only 10% of the Primary Care Organisations she interviewed could state that children with difficulty maintaining continence were *not* being excluded from school. The study identified only a small number of PCOs that have established ways of working in collaboration, using agreed paediatric continence assessment and referral pathways between primary and secondary care (Thomas 2004).

The *National Service Framework for Children, Young People and Maternity Services* (DH 2004:30) recognises that current paediatric continence services are 'fragmented', as shown in the paragraphs quoted in Figure 17.1. The section focusing on 'The Ill Child' has identified the major issues for PCTs to focus on when developing multidisciplinary integrated paediatric continence services.

The document *Good Practice in Paediatric Continence Services* (NHSMA 2003) argues for an integrated, community-based paediatric

Figure 17.1 From *The NSF for Children, Young People and Maternity Services*, Module: 'The Ill Child' (DH 2004:30)

10.17 There are at least 500,000 children who suffer from nocturnal enuresis and a significant number with daytime wetting and faecal incontinence, yet services are currently fragmented and often made up of a collection of professionals providing different levels of intervention in both the community and hospital. This currently results in gaps in service provision, inappropriate hospital/specialist referrals, and a waste of money in providing products instead of expertise.

10.17 Incontinence is distressing for children and young people and can be indicative of both physical and emotional problems; it can lead to bullying at school and cause emotional and behavioural problems.

continence service. This needs to begin by taking into account the large number of different professionals who might need to be involved in the care and management of one individual child with continence problems (see Figure 17.2).

A child under the care of different professionals may be individually assessed by each service, with the same information being collected repeatedly. This can be both time-consuming and frustrating for children themselves and those who care for them. Poor communication between services can delay treatment, increase the number of appointments (with a knock-on effect on school attendance). Such needless repetition is neither reassuring for the patient and family, nor an efficient use of scarce resources. Many services have long waiting times, and follow-up appointments may be considerably wide of the two week standard (Morgan 1993; Bonner 2001).

Combined assessment processes

As a result of the Children Act 2004 and *Every Child Matters* (DfES 2003), the Common Assessment Framework (CAF) has been developed to address these issues by developing the children's workforce and the integration of front-line delivery.

The Common Assessment Framework (CAF) is a key part of delivering front-line services that are integrated and focused around the needs of children and young people. The CAF is a standardised

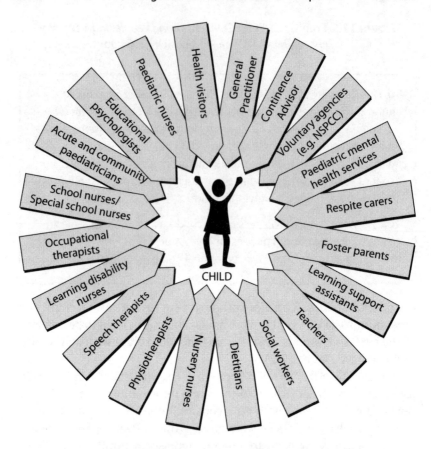

Figure 17.2 Which professionals are involved in caring for the child with continence problems?

approach to conducting an assessment of a child's additional needs and deciding how those needs should be met. It can be used by practitioners across children's services in England.

The CAF will promote more effective, earlier identification of additional needs, particularly in universal services. It is intended to provide a simple process for a holistic assessment of a child's needs and strengths, taking account of the role of parents, carers and environmental factors on their development. Practitioners will then be better placed to agree, with the child and family, about what support is appropriate. The CAF will also help to improve integrated working by promoting co-ordinated service provision. All local authority areas are expected to implement the CAF between April 2006 and the end of 2008 (DfES 2003).

Services could be further streamlined by the development of an evidence-based, basic paediatric continence assessment tool, preferably in electronic format, that can be used across different services and professional groups. Minimising duplication during the initial assessment process allows all relevant professionals time to focus on treatment and management. An appropriate, shared referral process can put the child in touch with the most appropriate services without wasting time. The resulting efficient and tailored approach is likely to make children (and their families) feel they are valued and taken seriously. This is particularly important when the condition itself undermines self-esteem and consequently motivation.

Good Practice in Paediatric Continence Services (NHSMA 2003) lists 11 indicators for best practice which can be used to benchmark service provision. More information about these is given in Chapter 18 by June Rogers and Liz Bonner.

The *NSF for Children, Young People and Maternity Services* (DH 2004) puts forward a ten-year plan to ensure that services offer the best possible solutions for children and their families. If inequalities in services are to be reduced, and standards met, health, social services and educational services are going to have to work together to develop and provide integrated paediatric continence services. Other guidelines and policy documents (see Figure 17.4) support the implementation of an integrated paediatric continence service.

Historically, a form of 'professional apartheid' has restricted practitioners to a traditional range of activities (Glen and Leiba 2002). *The NHS Plan* (DH 2000b) introduced a strategic framework for improving healthcare by setting national standards with clear accountability

---

- ■ An integrated community-based paediatric continence service informed by *Good Practice in Paediatric Continence Services – Benchmarking in Action* (NHSME 2003) ensures that accessible, high quality assessment and treatment is provided to children and their parents/carers in any setting, including for example looked-after children and children at boarding schools.

- ■ Children and young people with special needs and or disabilities have equal access to investigation and treatment programmes.

Figure 17.3 Markers of Good Practice, as defined by the National Service Framework for Children, Young People and Maternity Services (DH 2004a)

- Morgan R (1993) *Guidelines on Minimum Standards of Practice in the Treatment of Enuresis*. Bristol: ERIC

- Continence Foundation (2000) *Making the case for investment in an integrated continence service*. London: The Continence Foundation

- Department of Health (2000a) *Good practice in continence services*. Norwich: The Stationery Office

- Department of Health (2000b) *The NHS Plan*. Norwich: The Stationery Office

- Bonner L (2001) *Childhood Soiling. Minimum Standards of Practice for Treatment and Service Delivery: Benchmarking Guidelines*. Bristol: ERIC

- Department of Health (2001) *Essence of Care: Patient Focused Benchmarking for Healthcare Practitioners*. Norwich: The Stationery Office

- Department of Health (2002) *Liberating the Talents*. London: The Stationery Office

- Pollock D. (2002) *Making the Case for an Integrated Continence Service*. London: The Continence Foundation

- Department for Education and Skills (2003) *Every Child Matters*. Norwich: The Stationery Office

- NHS Modernisation Agency (2003) *Good Practice in Paediatric Continence Services: Benchmarking in Action*. London: Department of Health

- Department of Health (2004) *National Service Framework for Children, Young People and Maternity Services*. Norwich: The Stationery Office

- Department of Health (2004) *Standards for Better Health*. Norwich: The Stationery Office

- The Children Act 2004. Norwich: The Stationery Office

- NHS Modernisation Agency (2004) *Ten High Impact Changes for Service Improvements and Delivery*. London: Department of Health

- Shribman S (2007) *Making it Better for Children and Young People: Clinical Case for Change*. London: Department of Health

Figure 17.4 Summary of guidelines and policy documents

- Give children, young people and their parents increased information, power and choice over the support and treatment they receive and involve them in planning their care and service.

- Focus on early intervention based on timely and comprehensive assessment of a child's and family's needs.

- Improve access to services for all children according to their needs particularly by co-ordinating services.

- Promote and safeguard the welfare of children and ensure staff are suitably trained and aware of action to take if they have concerns about a child's welfare.

Figure 17.5 NSF for Children, Young People and Maternity Services (DH 2004a) Core Standards

and increased flexibility to cut across boundaries. The NSF for Children (DH 2004a:38) draws attention to the fact that many health professionals with no paediatric training are currently providing 'care, advice and treatment without the necessary knowledge base, skills or competencies'. In the same document (page 4), Professor Aynsley Green acknowledges there needs to be pressure for change to provide co-ordinated services between and across sectors and agencies. The Core Standards (see Figure 17.5) should underpin all services for children.

A multi-disciplinary taskforce

As each area in the UK has different paediatric continence services, a local needs assessment will direct future service development and provision. Engaging key stakeholders from across all disciplines, and agreeing a common goal, will be a challenge. Change can be threatening; barriers tend to be erected in response to it. So it is important that all those affected by the changes feel involved in the process. They must know that their voices carry the same weight as those of others, that good practice will be acknowledged and built upon, that gaps in knowledge and service will be identified. Change must be seen to improve service provision and role satisfaction.

A multi-disciplinary taskforce of key stakeholders requires a Lead with a talent for moulding and motivating the group, so they can move projects forward to completion. At the first meeting, stakeholders will

Figure 17.6 Terms of Reference

REPORTING STRUCTURE

Accountable to (Name of the Board/organisation) as the lead organisation, reporting to partner organisations as listed:

PCT

PCT

Hospital NHS Trust

Hospital NHS Trust

Mental Health and Learning Disability Community NHS Trust

Local Authority Representatives

Education, Social Services

Parent/Carer

Voluntary Organisations

Postgraduate Training Institute

A chair and secretary is to be agreed by the group, this is to be reviewed annually.

Terms of reference are to be agreed and reviewed annually.

Meetings will be quarterly in an agreed venue.

Each member is responsible for seeking support and agreement from their organisation's governing board for service development, pilot projects and submitting funding proposals to the organisation's local development plan.

Each member is responsible for providing a baseline report of current paediatric continence services, budgets and equipment available.

Members unable to attend meetings will provide reports to the chair as requested and raise any issues for discussion in writing or agree tools for printing in writing prior to the agreed meeting dates.

Minutes of all meetings will be circulated to all members and any other person responsible for commissioning paediatric services for information.

Each member is responsible for identifying service gaps against National guidance for service provision.

Members will develop a strategy for developing an integrated paediatric continence service with common paediatric continence assessment and referral pathways from primary to secondary care.

Members will monitor and guide activity in relevant areas working towards implementation of *Good Practice in Continence Services* (DH 2000), *Essence of Care* (DH 2001), *Good Practice in Paediatric Continence Services: Benchmarking in Action* (NHSMA 2003) *National Service Framework for Children, Young People and Maternity Services* (DH 2004a).

Members will agree priorities for joint bids to fund service developments to meet identified gaps in services. Bids will be processed using the local financial framework for developing services.

Members will develop sub-groups to develop a common paediatric continence assessment tool and referral pathways for diurnal enuresis, nocturnal enuresis, neurological bladder and bowel problems, constipation, encoporesis, soiling, delayed toileting, toileting problems related to physical and or cognitive dysfunction, behavioural problems related to toileting.

To receive reports from relevant sub-groups in order to monitor progress and support development of evidenced-based paediatric continence assessment tool and referral pathways.

Agree final generic paediatric continence assessment tool and referral pathways and organise printing.

Agree implementation programme for introducing generic paediatric continence assessment tool and referral pathways to all organisations.

Influence post-graduate training institutions to provide competency-based multi-disciplinary modules to support the implementation of an integrated paediatric continence service.

Agree joint training programme.

Ensure the paediatric continence assessment tool and referral pathways are audited in line with each organisation's clinical governance framework after one year.

Influence the development of Information Technology systems to monitor paediatric bladder/bowel dysfunction across the area, ensuring common coding systems that are known to all professionals, including those in Hospitals, Social Services, Education and Community.

Agree priority areas for research and development.

Figure 17.6 Terms of Reference (*continued*)

CORE MEMBERSHIP

List all members, their contact details and their reporting structure.

(e.g. the Professional Lead for Health Visitors reports to the Director of Patient Services, Strategic Health Authority)

Dissemination of Information

List all professionals receiving minutes for information.

NHS Direct to be kept informed of service developments.

Quorum

A quorum will not be required. A recommendation can be made if a member from each organisation is present or provides agreement in writing.

All organisations will endeavour to send a representative to each meeting.

---

need to agree a chair secretary and terms of reference that detail the time span, purpose and scope of the project. Terms of reference (see Figure 17.6) are particularly important when more than one organisation is involved. Membership and reporting pathways need to be documented to ensure minutes are distributed to key leads in each organisation. The number required at a meeting before a decision can be made (quorum) must be decided. Dates and venues of future meetings will need to be agreed for the duration of the project, along with arrangements for reporting back to the group in writing and what processes need to be adhered to by those members unable to attend meetings. Some of those involved will also require secretarial support, particularly if they are involved with the taking and distribution of minutes, or the inputting of new data.

The Lead, in partnership with the taskforce, needs to agree a strategy for achieving an integrated paediatric continence service. Most importantly the agreed strategy must identify any cost pressures or new service developments that will require funding. The strategy will form the basis for a report (see Figure 17.7) that can be presented to the Board of each contributing organisation for ratification. Board

Figure 17.7 Template for Board Report

Board Report front page, dated, with title of report, name and job title of strategy lead, contact details (many Boards have a preferred pro forma)

Executive summary

Recommendations (e.g. partnership working, service developments)

Contents page

Introduction

Supporting policy documents

Local implementation plan of an integrated paediatric continence (service level agreement). Include the number of children to be served and total service costs. Do NOT use jargon

Patient-focused outcomes

Conclusion

Recommendations

References

approval is essential to ensure that the development of the initiative is incorporated into the organisation's business plan, enabling its progress and implementation to be monitored. Table 17.1 provides a framework to guide the development of a strategy that could be adapted to fit any organisation. A business plan will be essential if funding is required and must meet the specifications of practice-based commissioners.

A first step for the taskforce is to investigate the local prevalence of paediatric bladder/bowel problems found in their services, provide a report on existing services and identify service gaps.

The next step is to complete a paper exercise benchmarking the existing services against *Good Practice In Paediatric Continence Services* (NHSMA 2003) – (see Chapter 18 on 'Ensuring proficiency' by June Rogers and Liz Bonner). The baseline information will guide the development of the strategy document. The strategy document in turn needs to provide a summary of why the change is necessary, list the partnership organisations, and detail how the change is to be managed.

Table 17.1 Strategy development: developing a service

Rationale	Supporting documents
Prevalence	■ Number of children accessing local services (including admissions for 'clear out' to hospital, A&E admissions, 'abdominal pain', etc.)
Current service provision	■ Number and type of clinics, identify all staff (including clerical support) providing paediatric continence services ■ Identify service budgets for equipment, incontinence products, health promotion, patient information leaflets, information technology, training, clinic space and staff costs ■ Identify current referral pathways and assessment paperwork used by all organisations
Clinical governance (NHS organisations are accountable for quality and safety of care) Healthcare Commission Assessment for Improvement Contains 24 Core and 10 development Standards: Seven Domains: • Safety • Clinical and cost effectiveness • Governance • Patient focus • Accessible and responsive care • Amenities and environment • Public health	■ Audit – Collect any completed service audits which demonstrate a systematic review of care against explicit criteria ■ Risk assessment – early identification of conditions that may cause long-term health problems (e.g. vesico-ureteric reflux, parental intolerance) ■ Protocols – description of the steps taken to deliver care or treatment to a patient. This could also be covered by the service level agreement ■ Safeguarding children policy ■ Consent policy ■ Staff training and updating to provide evidenced-based services
Every Child Matters (DfES 2003) – Identify risks and benefits using key outcomes	■ Be healthy ■ Stay safe ■ Enjoy and achieve ■ Make a positive contribution ■ Achieve economic well-being

Table 17.1 (*continued*)

Scope of integrated services (It is important to involve doctors and surgeons providing secondary care from the outset)	■ Agree terms of reference that specify the remit and responsibility of members and time frame
	■ Identify key targets that could be achieved by all the key stakeholders, e.g. for:
	  □ Constipation
	  □ Soiling
	  □ Encoporesis
	  □ Urinary tract infections
	  □ Diurnal enuresis
	  □ Nocturnal enuresis
	  □ Vesico-ureteric reflux
	  □ Delayed toileting problems
	  □ Toileting problems related to disability
	  □ Toileting problems related to cognitive dysfunction
	  □ Children with behaviour problems related to continence
	  □ Children with neurological conditions that may cause bladder and bowel conditions
	■ Develop a generic baseline paediatric continence assessment form that could be used by all areas
	■ Develop multi-disciplinary care pathways and referral pathways – these are tools that include guidelines, protocols, locally agreed best practice and evidence-based practice

Service Level Agreement	■ Identify and cost service gaps ■ Identify all organisations and service provision ■ Include all costs of service provision ■ Seek support from a service commissioner to ensure the document provides the organisation with the relevant information
Partnership working 'It is important that children's and parents' views are sought and recorded and taken into account when assessments are undertaken and plans made' (DH 2003)	■ Children and young people will have a method of commenting on service provision by means of comment boxes, questionnaires or focus groups ■ Parents and carers will also have an opportunity to comment on service provision and places should be available on the Strategy Group.

Table 17.1 (*continued*)

Patient-focused outcomes	■ Work with service users to provide user-friendly information
	■ Improve waiting times
	■ Reduce replication of assessment
	■ Monitor effectiveness of treatment interventions
	■ Improve communication between professionals, children and their carers

Conclusion

This chapter has discussed a range of options for engaging the key stakeholders required to develop integrated paediatric continence services. Professionals need to share the challenges and successes of service development with groups such as Paediatric Continence Forum RCN, Paediatric Specialist Interest Group Association of Continence Advisers.

There is an opportunity to improve paediatric continence services over the next ten years by developing professional roles, multi-disciplinary working and listening to the service users. It is important that the opportunity to improve children's continence services is taken even though it may take time to identify the resources to provide integrated paediatric continence services.

References

Antrobus S, Kitson A (1999) Nursing Leadership influencing and shaping health policy and nursing practice. *Journal of Advanced Nursing*, 29: 746–53
Bonner L (2001) *Childhood Soiling. Minimum Standards of Practice for treatment and service delivery: benchmarking guidelines*. Bristol: ERIC
Cavet J (1998) *People Don't Understand*. London: National Children's Bureau
Continence Foundation (2000) *Making the Case for Investment in an Integrated Continence Service*. London: The Continence Foundation
Department for Education and Skills (2003) *Every Child Matters*. Norwich: The Stationery Office. Website: www.dfes.gov.uk/everychildmatters
Department of Health (2000a) *Good Practice in Continence Services*. Norwich: The Stationery Office. Website: www.doh.uk/continencesevices.htm
Department of Health (2000b) *The NHS Plan*. Norwich: The Stationery Office

Department of Health (2001) *Essence of Care: Patient Focused Benchmarking for Healthcare Practitioners.* Norwich: The Stationery Office

Department of Health (2002a) *Liberating the Talents.* London: The Stationery Office

Department of Health (2004a) *National Service Framework for Children, Young People and Maternity Services.* Norwich: The Stationery Office

Department of Health (2004b) *Standards for Better Health.* Norwich: The Stationery Office

Glen S. Leiba T. (2002) *Multiprofessional Learning for Nurses, Breaking through the Boundaries.* Basingstoke: Palgrave

Laming WH (Chair) (2003) *The Victoria Climbié Inquiry.* Norwich: Crown Copyright. Website: www.victoria-climbie-inquiry.org.uk

Morgan R (1993) *Guidelines on Minimum Standards of Practice in the Treatment of Enuresis.* Bristol: ERIC

NHS Modernisation Agency (2003) *Good Practice in Paediatric Continence Services: Benchmarking in Action.* London: Department of Health. Website: www.modern.nhs.uk

NHS Modernisation Agency (2004) *Ten High Impact Changes for Service Improvement and Delivery.* London: Department of Health. Website: www.modern.nhs.uk

Pollock D (2002) *Making the Case for an Integrated Continence Service.* London: The Continence Foundation

Shribman S (2007) *Making it Better for Children and Young People: Clinical Case for Change.* London: Department of Health

Thomas S (2004) *Is Policy Translated into Action?* London: The Continence Foundation and Royal College of Nursing

Legislation
The Children Act 2004

18

Ensuring proficiency

June Rogers and Liz Bonner

Key points

- Standards of care, and ways of measuring achievement against them, are fundamental to good practice.

- *Good Practice in Paediatric Continence Services: Benchmarking in Action* (NHSMA 2003) has provided a framework for benchmarking standards.

- Looking to the future, consolidation and creative approaches to achieving and maintaining standards are reliant on a competent workforce.

Standards of care

It has long been recognised that there must be well-defined standards for patient care, along with a means of measuring the reality against them. In her 1860 book *Notes on Nursing*, Florence Nightingale emphasised the importance of clean air, hygiene and nutrition (Skretkowicz 1996). The focus on measurable quality in basic nursing care informs today's writing too, particularly *Essence of Care* (DH 2001, 2003) and *Good Practice in Paediatric Continence Services: Benchmarking in Action* (NHSMA 2003). Both detail the standards of care necessary for the provision of the best possible services in paediatric continence. Central to achieving this aim is the effective translation of knowledge into practice, and ensuring all aspects of care are evidence-based and up to date.

In common with the Codes of all UK healthcare regulatory bodies, the Nursing and Midwifery Council (NMC)'s *Code of Professional Conduct, Performance and Ethics* states that practitioners must be personally accountable for maintaining professional knowledge and competence. Article 5(2) (a) of the code requires the NMC to:

> . . . establish the standards of proficiency necessary to be admitted to the different parts of the register being the standards it

considers necessary for safe and effective practice under that part of the register. (NMC 2004a)

Competence is defined as: 'possessing the skills and abilities required for lawful, safe and effective professional practice without direct supervision'. Lack of competence, meanwhile, is defined as: 'a lack of knowledge, skill or judgement of such a nature that the registrant is unfit to practise safely and effectively in any field in which the registrant claims to be qualified or seeks to practise' (NMC 2004b).

Competence and proficiency

The NMC is beginning to replace the term 'competence' with that of 'proficiency'. This includes specific targets for students at pre-registration level. These students should be able to demonstrate the following (NMC 2004c: 5):

- Sound clinical judgement across a range of differing professional and care delivery contexts;

- Knowledge of effective inter-professional working practices which respect and make full use of the contributions of members of the health and social care team;

- Effective mastery of key skills;

- A commitment to the need for continuing professional development and personal supervision activities in order to enhance knowledge, skills, values and attitudes needed for safe and effective nursing practice.

Continence care requires multi-disciplinary working, so all staff should be trained to agreed standards with recognition across disciplines of particular and shared skills. Standardisation of training using competency or proficiency frameworks (such as 'benchmarking' – see below) will optimise the efficiency and effectiveness of services. Patient experience will be improved, unnecessary duplication of assessment avoided, and care pathways streamlined.

'Skills for Health'

The Skills for Health Council is a new body which aims to support such initiatives. Established to become the sector skills council for health, it is one of more than 20 sector skills councils covering every aspect of the UK economy. Its remit covers identification of sector workforce needs, and promoting workforce development by investing in education to meet those needs. The Skills for Health Council will also be responsible for developing competency frameworks that link health and education, providing national sector skills agreements and regional skills partnerships. The agreed competencies will form the basis of National Occupational Standards that will be grouped together to form National Qualification Frameworks.

Measuring tools

Umiker (1999) found assessing practice-based competency required resources to fund competency assessment training. Another essential was adequate time for observing and discussing practice with the learner. This requires additional staff cover as the time health professionals have to carry out their professional tasks will inevitably be reduced.

Storey and colleagues (2002) developed a method of measuring proficiency levels in completing particular tasks, as outlined in Table 18.1.

Table 18.1 Proficiency levels (Storey *et al.* 2002)

Level 0	Does not form a part of the current or future role of the worker
Level 1	Foundation
Level 2	Intermediate
Level 3	Proficient
Level 4	Advanced
Level 5	Expert

How can frameworks be used?

Competency or proficiency frameworks can be useful in identifying the full range of skills required to provide a service, and in identifying gaps in service. They can also be used to help establish the skill mix required for service development, identify new ways of working and define or redesign job roles. If the spread of talent is right, not every team member will need to have the full set of defined competencies for an efficient service to be provided.

Skills for Health links in with the *Knowledge Skills Framework* (DH 2004) which is designed to identify the knowledge and skills that individuals need to apply in their post, help guide the development of individuals and provide a fair and objective framework on which to base review and development of staff. For the first time, this staff development programme also provides a framework for pay progression within the service.

One author (Payne 2004) has looked at practical applications of competency frameworks to clinical situations, and lists the following issues as specific areas to target:

- Identify all the activities to be carried out in order to provide a particular service;

- Ensure workforce planning takes these into account, and all competencies are covered by the staff skill mix;

- Design jobs, draw up person specifications, selection criteria and assessment processes for recruitment, around the frameworks;

- Review individual and team learning needs on a regular basis;

- Encourage self-assessment related to the competency framework headings;

- Appraisal and development planning should also be based around the frameworks;

- As should education and training programmes, qualifications and assessment strategies;

- Identify which key activities are not being carried out effectively;

- Ensure that individual team members maintain their role within the team.

The Knowledge and Skills Framework: The Development and Review Process (DH 2004b) aims to advance the development of a skilled National Health Service workforce that can deliver appropriate patient-focused care effectively. The Department of Health has established a number of care group workforce teams to support the National Workforce Development Board to deliver service development and identify competency frameworks. The care group workforce teams will identify the skills required to deliver services to defined standards using such guidelines as The *Essence of Care* (DH 2001, 2003) and *Good Practice in Paediatric Continence Services: Benchmarking in Action* (NHSMA 2003).

'Essence of Care'

'Essence of Care' is a national programme originally launched in 2001. It was developed from a commitment to explore the benefits of benchmarking in improving the quality of the most fundamental and essential aspects of care. The *Essence of Care* document lists nine key areas of care that have been identified by patients and carers as needing attention. These include self-care, personal and oral hygiene, food and nutrition, continence, pressure ulcers, safety of people with mental health needs, record keeping, privacy and dignity, and communication.

Each of the benchmarks focuses on a number of areas that need to be addressed and these areas are then rated from A to E, with A being the benchmark of 'best practice'. The benchmarks can be used, not only as tools for identifying best practice, but also to highlight areas that need addressing. They provide an excellent mechanism by which the profile of 'Cinderella' services such as continence can be raised.

In a further development, in collaboration with the then NHS Modernisation Agency, benchmarks have been adapted to relate specifically to paediatric continence promotion. The National Service Framework (NSF) for Children, Young People and Maternity Services (DH 2004a), has identified the need for Trusts to set up integrated paediatric continence services and has laid down recommendations for best practice in paediatric continence services. There is now an obligation on all Primary Care Trusts to ensure that services are developed in line with these recommendations.

By looking at service provision in line with the Essence of Care benchmarking 'best practice' tool, Trusts will be able to identify clearly deficits in service provision. By sharing 'best practice' with other areas and linking in to work together to improve services, paediatric continence promotion services should be much better placed to ensure the best possible treatment outcomes for children in their care.

The *Essence of Care for Paediatric Continence Promotion and Bladder and Bowel Care* (NHSMA 2003) includes 11 'Agreed patient-focused outcomes' to ensure patients' bladder and bowel needs are met. Benchmarking information relating to each of these factors is detailed below.

Factor 1: Information for children, families and carers

The continuum is as shown:

Patients and or carers have evidence-based information about bowel and bladder care	**Benchmark of best practice** Patients and or carers have free access to general evidence-based information about bowel and bladder care

E ————————————————→ A

To stimulate discussion about the quality of care delivered in your centre, you may find it helpful to consider the following indicators of best practice:

- A range of child-focused information is available for children, young people, parents and other carers. This should include national and local information, and information in a variety of formats to suit their individual needs. Some examples may be story books, dolls, pictures, videos or DVDs and CD-ROMs.

- All available opportunities are taken to promote ensure that children and young people, parents and carers know about this information and where to find it.

- User acceptability of information is audited, surveyed and analysed. Feedback from this exercise is used in practical ways.

- A databank of evidence-based information is available. It is regularly reviewed and evaluated to ensure it is up to date and consistent.

Factor 2: Access to professional advice about continence and bladder and bowel care

The continuum is as shown:

	Benchmark of best practice
Patients do not have access to professional advice re professionals who can meet their continence needs	Patients have direct access to professionals who can meet their continence needs and their services are actively promoted

E ⟶ A

To stimulate discussion about the quality of care delivered in your centre, you may find it helpful to consider the following indicators of best practice:

- Professional advice and services are available that meet the individual continence needs of children and young people.

- Children and young people, their families and carers are able to self-refer, and to access services.

- Policies, procedures and referral protocols to specialist paediatric services are all available.

- Response times for referrals or appointments are met, and within ERIC guidelines.

- All necessary provisions have been made to ensure that continence services are fully accessible, particularly to vulnerable groups such as children with special needs.

- Service providers are aware of any barriers that prevent needs being met locally (such as language problems, lack of interpreters, waiting lists, difficulty in obtaining products or equipment, lack of knowledge and interpersonal skills). It should also be clear what is being done to address these.

- Strategies incorporate education and training programmes for healthcare personnel, to enable them to provide advice.

- Children with special needs, for example learning disabilities, have full access to all services such as enuretic clinics.

Factor 3: Individual assessment of patients

The continuum is as shown:

Patients are not asked a trigger question related to bladder and bowel continence needs within their general health assessment

Benchmark of best practice Patients' positive response to the trigger question always leads to an offer of an initial bladder and bowel continence assessment which if accepted by the patient is completed

E ————————————————▶ A

The trigger question should be asked at all initial contacts (for example, standard health visitor assessment at 3 years, school health interviews). A trigger question could be 'Are you having any problems with potty training, wetting or soiling?'

All children presenting for help with continence problems have automatically given a positive response to the trigger question.

To stimulate discussion about the quality of care delivered in your centre, you may find it helpful to consider the following indicators of best practice:

- A trigger question determines assessment, and there is evidence of audit to ascertain whether trigger questions have been used.

- Trigger questions are asked as part of, for example, school health checks, routine assessments or admission, opportunistic screening.

- The use of trigger questions is promoted among colleagues and other team members.

- The child or young person's understanding or acceptance of the trigger question is assessed, and any adaptations made to the trigger question used are described.

- Assessment tools have been adapted for use within paediatric groups.

Factor 4: Planning, implementation and evaluation of care based on the bladder and bowel assessment

(This section is to be completed only if an assessment has been performed.)

The continuum is as shown:

There are no patients' plans of care to meet the bowel and bladder needs identified in the continence assessment

Benchmark of best practice The effectiveness of patients' care is continuously evaluated and leads either to the patients' needs being met or the modification of the care plan (e.g. referral on)

E ————————————▶ A

Care is expected to be evidence-based, and planned jointly with the patient, family and/or carers.

To stimulate discussion about the quality of care delivered in your centre, you may find it helpful to consider the following indicators of best practice:

- Care plans or care pathways are used, and outcomes are measured.
- Young people and their parents or carers are involved in developing their own care plan and in setting their own outcome measures, including action to remove barriers such as the use of interpreters, support for children with special needs.
- Protocols or evidence-based guidelines are used for care interventions.
- Details are used about referral rates, re-referral rates, complaints and patient survey results.
- Record keeping and evaluation is maintained and audited, including the extent of patient access to records (see the benchmark for record keeping, below).
- Clinical audit is undertaken; the results of this are disseminated and inform the development of practice.

Factor 5: Education for professional assessors and care planners

The continuum is as shown:

	Benchmark of best practice
Patients are not assessed or do not have care planned by a health professional	Patients are assessed and have care planned by professionals who have received specific continence care training and are continuously updated

E ——————————→ A

To stimulate discussion about the quality of care delivered in your centre, you may find it helpful to consider the following indicators of best practice:

- Roles and responsibilities are defined for those carrying out assessment and planning of care. It should be clear who performs the assessments and plans care.

- Children are assessed and have care planned by professionals with a paediatric background, who have received specific continence care training and keep up to date with continuous professional development.

- The following are all in regular use: initial and continuing education and training opportunities, programmes, policies and training analysis, peer group review, supervision and personal development plans. Peer group review and/or supervision arrangements are clearly stated.

- Training packages, information and communication channels are all used; training records are maintained.

- Children and young people's views and expectations are included in any training programme, as are links with self-help or user groups.

- The impact of any training is assessed and evaluated.

- The education content and outcomes include consideration of any individual needs, for example learning needs in children, language difficulties in children, parents or carers.

Factor 6: Promotion of continence and a healthy bladder and bowel

The continuum is as shown:

There is no attempt to promote patients' continence and a healthy bladder and bowel	**Benchmark of best practice** All opportunities are taken to promote continence and a healthy bladder and bowel among patients and the wider community

E ————————————————————▶ A

To stimulate discussion about the quality of care delivered in your centre, you may find it helpful to consider the following indicators of best practice:

- Any 'risk' groups are identified locally. These may include children with special needs, school-age children, children immediately following surgery or other procedures.

- Information is available as to what will be done to target these groups.

- Inter-professional or inter-agency working is assured, along with an understanding of how this promotes continence.

- The content (evidence-base) and format of promotion strategies (e.g. videos, pictures, story boards, written materials) is clear, as is the way they are used to promote knowledge and understanding within the wider community. The 'wider community' here includes subsections of the community that are hard to reach, such as children or parents with special needs, black and minority ethnic communities.

- A variety of measures are taken to promote continence services, including links with self-help, user groups and health promotion units, the displaying and use of posters and leaflets.

- Children and young people with special needs have the same access to all services as their mainstream peers.

- Audits are undertaken, educational links and ongoing research are maintained.

- Links with local user or self-help groups are used to raise awareness.

- Any local awareness initiatives are capitalised upon. This may include making use of national promotional opportunities such as 'Healthy School' campaigns, 'Water is cool in school' campaign, National Continence Week.

- Practitioners are actively involved in raising awareness and promoting healthy bladders and bowels among all children, their families, carers, schools and the wider community.

Factor 7: Access to continence supplies

The continuum is as shown:

Patients do not have access to supplies that assist in the management of their incontinence	**Benchmark of best practice** Patients have access to appropriate 'needs specific' supplies to assist in the management of their incontinence

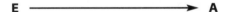

E ⟶ A

To stimulate discussion about the quality of care delivered in your centre, you may find it helpful to consider the following indicators of best practice:

- Healthcare personnel are proactive in anticipating the needs and preferences of children, other family members and carers, and that choice is not restricted to number and type of product.

- Sufficient time is given to enable children to communicate their needs and preferences. Explicit or expressed consent is obtained from patients prior to treatment or care.

- Patients and their parents or carers have access to specialist knowledge and skills and have access to supplies that assist in the promotion of continence.

- Technology is available and is used to meet patient needs, for example, electronic prescriptions.

- The use of services is monitored – for example, by regular audit.

- Arrangements are in place for cleanliness, maintenance and replacement of equipment.

- Children have access to appropriate 'needs specific' supplies to assist in the management/promotion of their continence and they are only supplied following a full documented assessment.

- Children with special needs have access to specialist equipment they may require such as musical potties, wetting alarms.

Factor 8: Education of the care deliverers

The continuum is as shown:

Patients are cared for by carers with no continence training	**Benchmark of best practice** Patients are cared for by carers who have undertaken continence care training which includes ongoing updating

E ⟶ A

NB: Education should involve regular practice and peer review.

To stimulate discussion about the quality of care delivered in your centre, you may find it helpful to consider the following indicators of best practice:

- Children are cared for by practitioners who have a paediatric background.

- The training needs of those who give care are assessed. The way in which care is carried out is monitored to ensure caregivers have undertaken continence care training which includes ongoing updating.

- Intended learning outcomes are clearly identified and the impact of training is assessed and evaluated.

- Peer group review, supervision and personal development plans are used.

- The views and expectations of children and young people are included in training programmes, including links with self-help or user groups.

- Appropriate training packages, information and communication channels are used.

- Training of children and young people, their parents, carers or support groups takes place. A range of teaching aids is available for children with special needs.

- There is a facility where staff can shadow 'local experts'.

Factor 9: A physical and social environment conducive to continence and a healthy bladder and bowel

The continuum is as shown:

The environment is not conducive to the patients' individual needs	**Benchmark of best practice** All bladder and bowel care is given in an environment conducive to the patients' individual needs

E ──────────────→ A

NB: Consideration of individual needs (e.g. children with 'special needs') is paramount, however this may need to be balanced with meeting the needs of other users of the same facility. Use with the Privacy and Dignity benchmark.

To stimulate discussion about the quality of care delivered in your centre, you may find it helpful to consider the following indicators of best practice:

- Attempts are made to make the environment child-friendly and adaptable for different age groups.

- The environment is conducive for the child's individual needs. Lighting, cleanliness and heating adaptations should all be adequate. Curtains should meet.

- Facilities should be age-appropriate and sensitive to religious and cultural expectations.

- The views on the environment are sought from children and young people, their families or carers. Feedback is acted upon, and action taken to remove any barriers.

- Consultation with specialist continence professionals will include informed assessment of the environment.

- The environment is adapted to meet the individual needs of patients – for example, children with disabilities or mobility problems.

- There is evidence of attempts to make the environment conducive to the individual, such as disability access.

Factor 10: Patient to patient support

The continuum is as shown:

	Benchmark of best practice
Patients and/or carers have no access to other patients and/or carers for support	Patients and/or carers have the opportunity to access other patients who can offer support and this is actively promoted

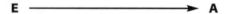

E ⟶ A

To stimulate discussion about the quality of care delivered in your centre, you may find it helpful to consider the following indicators of best practice:

- Children and their families and or carers have the opportunity to access patient/family support groups both locally and nationally.

- Information about support groups is given to children and families.

- Measures have been taken to set up or support a local self-help or user group. Investigations have been carried out as to whether there are any barriers to forming or maintaining such a group.

- There are good links between services and local groups.

- Strategies are in place to put families in touch with each other, and to make them aware they can contact other families in a similar situation.

Factor 11: User involvement in service delivery

The continuum is as shown:

No user feedback or involvement sought	**Benchmark of best practice** Users are always involved in planning and evaluating services, and their input is acted upon

E ————————————➤ A

The term 'user' is taken to mean 'patient', 'relative', 'family member' or 'carer'. Wherever possible, users should be involved in all aspects of care planning and delivery.

To stimulate discussion about the quality of care delivered in your centre, you may find it helpful to consider the following indicators of best practice:

- Methods are used to secure the involvement of children and young people. This can be achieved through focus groups, user forums, etc., and should include consideration of religious, cultural, language, age-related and special needs issues.

- The views of children, their family or carers are sought. They are informed about the ways in which satisfaction with continence services is assessed and how complaints are addressed.

- There is evidence of inter-agency involvement and networking between all interested parties.

- Strategies are used to involve users from isolated communities, or communities that are hard to reach, such as travellers or children in care.

- The views of children themselves, and of their parents and carers are sought when planning and evaluating services. Their input is acted upon.

The way forward

The Knowledge, Skills Framework (DH 2004a) and The Agenda for Change (NHMSA 2004) will influence the future of professional health education moving towards assessment inclusive of academic and competency and or proficiency factors. The Health Care Commission (HCC 2005b) has identified key targets and performance indicators which when assessed will provide healthcare organisations with a performance rating (star rating). One of the performance indicators will be the achievement of risk management standards that supports the assessment of competence to practise: 'an appropriate training programme is an important means of assessing competence and helps ensure compliance with safe working practices' (NHSLA 2005). The NHS Litigation Authority (HCC 2005a) rationalises that achieving risk management standards will ensure quality of healthcare is maintained and improved, which in turn will reduce the scope for negligence claims. However, a recent report (Shribman 2007) indicates there is still some way to go.

Bedfordshire Continence Service has initiated the development of a competency framework for specialist continence advisers to help develop induction programmes for new staff, and identify training needs during individual performance review. The intention is that this will become part of the assessment for moving through the payment bands fitting in with Agenda for Change (NHSMA 2004) and The Knowledge Skills Framework (DH 2004a). Bedfordshire Continence Service has eight continence advisers of various grades who have all participated in the development of locally agreed competencies for paediatric practice. These are shown in Table 18.2, below. The competency level assessment is based upon the practical guidance developed by Storey and colleagues (2002) for developing competency frameworks.

Table 18.2 Competencies required for a Paediatric Continence Adviser (PCA) (Bedfordshire Continence Service 2005)

Competency	Method of Achievement	Method of Assessment	Competency Level
To have knowledge and understanding of the anatomy and physiology of the normal urinary system and gastro-intestinal tract	Formal training Personal study Observation of Continence Advisers (CA) teaching	Qualification Questioning Observation of PCA teaching	
To demonstrate knowledge of normal childhood continence development	Formal training Personal study Observation of CA teaching	Qualification Questioning Observation of PCA teaching	
To demonstrate knowledge of normal cognitive development and to recognise developmental delay	Formal training Personal study Observation of CA completing a continence assessment	Qualification Questioning Observation of PCA assessing	
To understand how physical/cognitive disability affects continence development	Formal training Personal study Observation of CA teaching	Qualification Questioning Observation of PCA teaching	
To have an understanding of how diet and fluid intake affects bladder and/or bowel function	Formal training Personal study Observation of CA teaching	Qualification Questioning Observation of PCA teaching	
To understand the importance of urinalysis and be able to take appropriate action if abnormalities detected	Formal training Personal study Observation of CA teaching	Qualification Questioning Observation of PCA teaching	
To understand the importance of bowel diaries using Bristol Stool Chart, monitoring and taking appropriate action	Formal training Personal study Observation of CA completing a continence assessment	Qualification Questioning Observation of Observation of	

Table 18.2 Competencies required for a Paediatric Continence Adviser (PCA) (Bedfordshire Continence Service 2005) (*continued*)

Competency	Method of Achievement	Method of Assessment	Competency Level
To demonstrate knowledge of the effects of medication on the bladder and bowels	Formal training Personal study Observation of CA teaching	Qualification Questioning Observation of PCA teaching	
To demonstrate knowledge of various toilet training programmes and demonstrate ability to plan individual toileting training programme	Formal training Personal study Observation of CA teaching and assessing	Qualification Questioning Observation of PCA teaching and assessing	
To demonstrate knowledge of paediatric toileting aids and adaptations available and referral pathways	Formal training Personal study Observation of CA teaching and assessing	Qualification Questioning Observation of PCA teaching and assessing	
To demonstrate knowledge of paediatric containment products, criteria for supply, product assessment and fitting, home delivery system	Formal training Personal study Observation of CA teaching and assessing	Qualification Questioning Observation of PCA teaching and assessing	
Able to identify symptoms that require direct referral to a general practitioner or paediatrician	Formal training Personal study Observation of CA completing an assessment	Qualification Questioning Observation of PCA assessing	
To demonstrate knowledge of the Child Protection Policy and how to liaise with key stakeholders if a child protection issue is identified	Formal training Personal study Observation of CA teaching and assessing	Qualification Questioning Observation of PCA teaching and assessing	

Competency and Proficiency frameworks are in early stages of development in many areas around the United Kingdom. In the longer term, the Skills for Health Council may develop a nationally agreed skills framework for providing an integrated paediatric continence service. This will lead on to the development of national competencies which, in turn, would influence the provision of in-house training and University-run modules on continence. Standardisation of education programmes and agreed competencies, accompanied by a record of proficiency attainment, will improve the calibre of the workforce and reduce the need for retraining every time a health authority boundary is crossed.

References

Department of Health (2001) *Essence of Care.* Norwich: The Stationery Office
Department of Health (2003) *Essence of Care: Patient Focused Benchmarking for Healthcare Practitioners.* Norwich: The Stationery Office
Department of Health (2004a) *The National Service Framework (NSF) for Children and Young People.* Standard 6 Children and Young people who are Ill. Norwich: The Stationery Office
Department of Health (2004b) *The NHS Knowledge and Skills Framework and the Development Review Process.* Norwich: The Stationery Office
Health Care Commission (2005a) *NHS Litigation Authority.* Norwich: The Stationery Office. Website: www.healthcarecommision.org.uk
Health Care Commission (2005b) *NHS Performance Indicators.* Norwich: The Stationery Office. Website: www.healthcarecommision.org.uk
Laming WH (Chair) (2003) *The Victoria Climbié Inquiry.* Norwich: Crown Copyright. Website: www.victoria-climbie-inquiry.org.uk/
NHS Litigation Authority (2005) *Risk Management Standard for Primary Care Trusts.* Norwich: The Stationery Office. Website: www.nhsla.com/Publications
NHS Modernisation Agency (2003) *Good Practice in Paediatric Continence Services: Benchmarking in Action.* Norwich: The Stationery Office. Website: www.modern.nhs.uk/home/key/docs
NHS Modernisation Agency (2004) *Agenda for Change.* Norwich: The Stationery Office. Website: www.modern.nhs.uk/home/key/docs
Nursing and Midwifery Council (2004a) *Code of Professional Conduct, Performance and Ethics.* London: NMC. Website: www.nmc-uk.org
Nursing and Midwifery Council (2004b) *Reporting Lack of Competence: A Guide for Employers and Managers.* London: NMC
Nursing and Midwifery Council (2004c) *Standards of Proficiency for Pre-Registration Nursing Education.* London: NMC
Payne B (2004) Developing a Competence Framework for Renal Services. *British Journal of Renal Medicine,* 9 (1): 26–8

Shribman S (2007) *Making it Better for Children and Young People: Clinical case for change*. London: Department of Health

Skretkowicz V (1996) *Florence Nightingale's 'Notes on Nursing': Edited with an Introduction, Notes and Guide to Identification*, revised edn. Harrow: Scutari Press

Skills for Health. *The Sector Skills Council for Health*. Available online at: www.skillsforhealth.org.uk (last accessed March 2007)

Storey L, Howard J, Gillies A (2002) *Competency in Healthcare: A Practical Guide to Competence Frameworks*. Oxford: Radcliffe Medical Press

Umiker W (1999) The Challenge of Competency Assessment. *Health Care Supervisor*, 17(3): 11–17

19

Governance and standards for better health

Mandy Wells

Key points

- Clinical governance is an essential element of ensuring excellence in clinical care is delivered to children with bladder and bowel problems.

- Clinicians need to ensure they keep up-to-date with the research evidence that underpins their practice.

- Clinicians need to ensure their skills and knowledge are kept up-to-date.

- The voice of the child must always be listened to. Children need to be involved in deciding about provision of services.

- Clinical supervision and leadership are essential to delivering and monitoring care, and ensuring high standards.

This chapter aims to explain Standards for Better Health in relation to Children's bladder and bowel care, while relating the Standards to other NHS initiatives (NHSMA 2003). Standards for Better Health are linked to the NHS Priority Areas (see Figure 19.1, page 324) to which specific national targets have been set either as Core Standards or Developmental Standards. The Standards apply to people equally, and to all groups unless specified. This means that there is an intrinsic link to 'the Child'. A number of these Standards can have a specific impact on service provision for the child with bladder and/or bowel problems.

Essence of Care Standards (see Chapter 18 on 'Ensuring proficiency' by June Rogers and Liz Bonner) make up another important element of healthcare delivery that is fundamentally linked to all Standards for Better Health (DH 2001; NHSMA 2003). In addition, the National Primary and Care Trust Development Programme (natpact) published a competency framework for nurses, midwives and health visitors in January 2005. This is intrinsically linked to Standards for Better Health (see Table 19.1).

Table 19.1 PCT Competency Framework for nurses, midwives and health visitors

Competency statement	Examples of evidence
N1. Organisational maturity	
N.1.2 Ns, MWs and HVs have produced risk-management strategies in relation to statutory risk reduction requirements and where new roles need to be risk assessed	N.1.2.2 Health and safety N.1.2.3 Child protection N.1.2.4 Moving and handling N.1.2.5 Managed innovation N.1.2.6 Clinical supervision
N.1.3 All Ns, MWs and HVs understand and implement child protection policies and procedures, and are aware of the named child protection nurse	
N.1.4 The expertise of Ns, MWs and HVs is used to shape PCT decision-making	N.1.4.1 There is effective N, MW and HV leadership at all levels including the board and PEC N.1.4.2 N, MW and HVs are involved in drawing up and are signed up to the PCT's strategy for clinical developments within the context of national strategies
N.1.6 Ns, MWs and HVs are provided with protocols and policies whilst being supported to exercise professional judgement and independence when appropriate e.g. PMS pilots	N.1.6.1 A system is in place for the development, dissemination and implementation of clinical policies N.1.6.2 Where professional judgement and independence indicates a variation from protocols and policies the rationale is documented
N.2 Primary care	
N.2.1 The PCT has a documented strategy for inclusive primary care nursing	N.2.1.1 The strategy document contains an implementation plan with lead responsibilities at board level and identified timescales N.2.1.2 The strategy is developed through engagement of all key partners and is owned by all staff groups
N.2.3 There is a whole system approach to service development, which recognises that changes in nursing will require change across the organisation, other services and professional groups	N.2.3.1 The lead nurse works closely with senior nurses in local NHS Trusts, NHS Direct, other providers and the SHA to ensure whole system development and integration with hospital and other services

Table 19.1 (*continued*)

Competency statement	Examples of evidence
N.2.4 Effective management and leadership arrangements are in place	N.2.4.1 The model of management and leadership is clearly described, and has been developed with local engagement N.2.4.2 Nurses are undertaking leadership training, e.g. LEO, RCN, local programmes N.2.4.3 There are formal systems in place for PEC nurses, lead nurse and nurse managers to discuss nursing business/networks N.2.4.4 There is development of professional practice, new knowledge and innovation
N.2.5 Staff have the time and support needed to examine current practice, consult users, review evidence, try out new ways of working and have the freedom to be innovative	N.2.5.1 Nurses are working in new ways that deliver PCT priorities and the NHS Plan, e.g. nurses are providing intermediate care, advancing practice to encompass roles traditionally provided by clinicians, improving care for excluded groups, participating in nurse-led PMS pilots N.2.5.2 There are specialist nurses in primary care centres N.2.5.3 Local innovation is taking place; staff are developing new roles and a mix of skills ensures that patients' and communities' needs are met flexibly and safely N.2.5.4 Staff are taking advantage of opportunities offered by PMS, nurse prescribing, public health, CNOs' ten key roles, Nurse Consultants
N.2.6 The PCT encourages Ns, MWs and HVs to explore new ways of working together across organisational boundaries to deliver patient-focused services	N.2.6.1 Engagement with midwifery, the acute sector and nursing homes is evidenced by the use of integrated care pathways, joint working arrangements and other collaborative initiatives N.2.6.2 There are workshops, seminars and training sessions that engage staff in organisational developmental opportunities

Table 19.1 (*continued*)

Competency statement	Examples of evidence
N.2.6 (contin'd)	N.2.6.3 Team working and development initiatives (e.g. Sure Start) are in place N.2.6.4 There is a clear plan for implementing the NHS Plan's 'ten key roles'
N.2.7 The PCT works with GPs to ensure that practice-employed nurses can contribute to service development and are provided with professional and clinical support to develop their services	N.2.7.1 Cross practice and community joint working is encouraged by the PCT
N.2.8 There are systems in place to involve frontline staff in planning and delivering service improvements	N.2.8.1 The lead nurse has overall responsibility for establishing these systems and ensuring staff involvement N.2.8.2 Staff feel they have ownership of the changes and are involved in improving services for their local community N.2.8.3 Decision-making is devolved to frontline staff, e.g. community budgets, skill mix changes
N.2.9 Patients and communities are provided with flexible teams with fewer handovers, both within the practice team and across a neighbourhood	N.2.9.1 Individual staff have the confidence, skills and knowledge to be able to assess needs, plan care and provide treatments/ interventions involving a wider range of skills N.2.9.2 Patients are being presented with fewer titles and can understand the role and responsibilities of the nurses, midwives and health visitors providing their care
N.3 Service Provision **N.3.1** The potential of Ns, MWs and HVs is fully developed by the PCT and utilised to create new approaches to delivering care	N.3.1.1 There is a reduction in turnover rates and an ability to fill posts N.3.1.2 Clinical audit outcomes and patient satisfaction surveys demonstrate effective nursing care

Table 19.1 (*continued*)

Competency statement	Examples of evidence
N.3.2 The PCT provides fast and convenient access to care, tailored to the needs of individuals and the local community, and delivered to a consistently high standard	N.3.2.1 Nurses, midwives and health visitors have the equipment and tools they need to deliver effective care to their patients
N.3.3 The PCT supports general practice teams to make the most of their nursing resource	
N.3.7 Leadership and management are in place throughout the organisation that are facilitative, enabling, devolve authority to frontline staff and support change	N.3.7.1 A range of registered, specialist and advanced level nurses and AHPs is providing and leading programmes of care and public health programmes to meet PCT priorities, e.g. reducing admissions, enabling earlier discharge, providing ambulatory care, such as dermatology services, diabetes, providing first contact services
N.3.8 Ns, MWs and HVs are integrated with social care and secondary care services focusing on the patient pathway and the local community	N.3.8.1 Ns, MWs and HVs are contributing to the delivery of NSFs, meeting inequalities targets and improving the patient's experience of the NHS
N.3.9 Where there are benefits to the patient in terms of fast and convenient access to medicines, nurses are trained to prescribe	
N.4 Securing Service Delivery **N.4.3** The PCT works with providers to redesign services so that the contribution of Ns, MWs and HVs is maximised, traditional demarcations are broken down and the opportunities provided by *Making a Difference* (DH 2001) are fully used	N.4.3.1 The PCT commissions Ns-, MWs- and HVs-led services where appropriate, such as dermatology, continence, diabetes, first contact assessment N.4.3.2 A care pathway approach to commissioning is taken and Ns, MWs and HVs are involved across organisations reflecting the patient journey and experience

Table 19.1 (*continued*)

Competency statement	Examples of evidence
N.5 Partnership	
N.5.1 The PCT enables and empowers the nursing, midwifery and health visiting workforce to work across organisational and professional boundaries to plan and deliver effective care and public health programmes	N.5.1.1 Staff are participating in multi-agency and multi-disciplinary teams and initiatives to deliver NSFs (particularly Older People and Mental Health), family support and initiatives such as Sure Start, National Healthy Schools, Child Protection and Free Nursing Care N.5.1.2 The lead and PEC nurses participate in the Local Strategic Partnerships and other inter-agency planning teams N.5.1.3 Staff work at neighbourhood level with multi-agency partners to identify needs and plan services
N.5.2 Nursing, midwifery and health visiting services are integrated with social care and secondary care services focusing on the patient pathway and the local community	N.5.2.1 There are posts are in place that straddle organisational boundaries
N.5.3 Practical measures are in place that remove the barriers to partnership working for nurses, e.g. single assessment, shared information systems and pooled budgets	N.5.3.1 GP-employed and PCT-employed nurses undertake joint CPD and work together on planning, co-ordinating patient care, public health and service provision
N.5.4 All Ns, MWs and HVs who work in the PCT have the opportunity to acquire the skills and knowledge to enable them to work in partnership	N.5.4.1 Staff are participating in multi-professional and multi-agency education and training
N.6 Public Health	
N.6.1 The PCT involves, utilises and develops Ns, MWs and HVs across the health community to enable them to deliver health improvements and reduce inequalities in health	N.6.1.1 Ns, MWs and HVs have a range of knowledge and skills that reflect local health needs and priorities
N.6.5 The PCT has clear public health	N.6.5.1 Services are supported by a public health team, led by the DPH, which includes Ns, MWs and HVs N.6.6 The PCT supports evaluation strategies, and frontline staff are given reports about progress

Table 19.1 *(continued)*

Competency statement	Examples of evidence
N.7 Community engagement	
N.7.1 The PCT ensures that Ns, MWs and HVs facilitate and promote community engagement and involvement	N.7.1.1 Staff are involved in community engagement processes and structures, e.g. in identifying and responding to health needs and developing patient information N.7.1.2 Staff's knowledge of community and patient needs and their local networks is utilised by the PCT
N.7.2 The PCT ensures that N, MW and HVs facilitate and promote patient involvement and self-care	N.7.2.1 Staff are involved in programmes to develop expert patients and promote self-care and patient education N.7.2.2 Patients' involvement in their care is demonstrated by family health plans and patient-held records
N.7.3 The PCT promotes effective methods of community engagement that are accessible to all segments of the community	
N.7.4 N, MW and HVs receive training and advice on public and patient participation	N.7.4.1 Patients are involved in evaluating and shaping nursing services and report that they are given information, choice and feel involved in their own care N.7.4.2 There are formal processes in place that allow practitioners, within a framework of clinical supervision, to reflect on the role of the patient in self-care and how this could be improved
N.8 Clinical Quality	
N.8.1 The PCT provides the nursing, midwifery and health visiting workforce (both PCT and GP employed) with a clinical and professional working environment that supports the continuous development of high standards of clinical and professional practice and ensures public safety	N.8.1.1 The public is assured that systems are in place to protect the public and ensure N, MW and HVs deliver high standards of care N.8.1.2 Patient satisfaction with N, MW and HV services is known from GP and PCT surveys N.8.1.3 Systems are in place for whistle blowing, complaints, child protection, measuring quality of nursing care and using evidence-based practice

Table 19.1 (*continued*)

Competency statement	Examples of evidence
N.8.1 (cont'd)	N.8.1.4 A PCT statement indicates how the organisation will learn from staff feedback
N.8.2 All Ns, MWs and HVs, regardless of employer are able to review their clinical practice, participate in CPD, clinical governance activities and professional networks	N.8.2.1 Ns, MWs and HVs are aware of and working within the NMC Code of Professional Conduct and The Midwives Rules and Code of Practice, and are provided with a practice environment that supports the continuous development of high standards of clinical and professional practice N.8.2.2 All Ns, MWs and HVs receive clinical supervision and mentorship and clear accountability arrangements are in place
N.8.3 Service level agreements and contracts with providers include quality specifications and measures such as *Essence of Care* (DH 2001)	N.8.3.1 A senior lead nurse is in place to provide clinical and professional nursing leadership across the PCT. Team working with Midwives will need to recognise the LSA function and midwifery supervision N.8.3.2 The PCT uses tools and systems to measure and review standards of care and poor performance is identified and addressed
N.8.4 Frontline nurses are involved in PCT and local clinical governance activities	N.8.4.1 Critical and adverse incidents involving Ns, MWs and HVs are tracked and common themes identified and acted upon N.8.4.2 Ns, MWs and HVs are accessing and using evidence when planning and delivering care N.8.4.3 Ns, MWs and HVs messages from CHI and NICE reviews are distilled and acted upon
N.9 Workforce **N.9.3** The PCT is delivering on specific nursing, midwifery and health visiting policies derived from the NHS Plan and *Making a Difference*	N.9.3.1 These include recruitment and retention of nursing staff N.9.3.2 The 10 key roles (new roles and Chief Nursing Officer

Table 19.1 (*continued*)

Competency statement	Examples of evidence
N.9.3 (cont'd)	N.9.3.3 The PCT demonstrates that it is actively considering and starting to implement new roles for nurses, including the following: Nurse Consultants, Nurse leadership, Modern Matrons, Agenda for Change
N.9.4 The PCT works with the WDC and in partnership with Teaching PCTs (tPCTs) to ensure training commissions for Ns, MWs and HVs are in place to meet future service needs	N.9.4.1 Programmes are in place for recruiting, retaining and encouraging returners. These are linked to local regeneration by creating access to nursing careers for local people reflecting local diversity and ethnicity e.g. cadet schemes, peer educators, expert patients
N.9.5 The PCT workforce has sufficient nurse mentors and practice educators in place and undertakes regular skills audits	N.9.5.1 A programme is in place to increase skill mix and encourage N, MW and HVs to acquire new and advanced clinical skills and that ensures patient safety N.9.5.2 Nurses in training benefit from high quality practice-based learning (pre- and post-registration) across a range of settings

Relating the standards to children's needs

Standards for Better Health that relate to bladder and bowel services or care for children are listed below. 'C' indicates a Core Standard; 'D' indicates a Developmental Standard.

Safety

C2 Healthcare organisations protect children by following national child protection guidance within their own activities and in their dealings with other organisations.

With bladder and bowel problems it is important to remember that not only can voiding or incontinence lead to abuse but abuse can also lead to bladder and bowel problems. Vicious circles can and do arise. All healthcare professionals working with children need to undertake

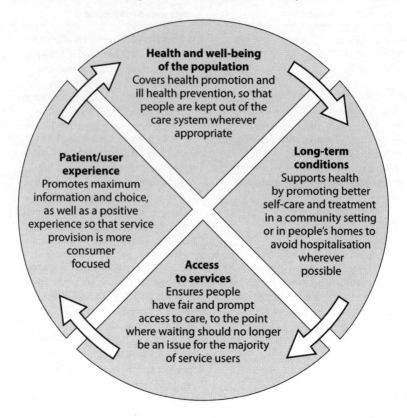

Figure 19.1 NHS priority areas

training in Child Protection and be properly Police-checked. It is imperative that local protocols are identified for reporting any concerns that staff may have about any forms of abuse.

It must be remembered that urinary and faecal incontinence was one of the root causes of the abuse of Victoria Climbié (Laming 2003). It resulted directly in her being made to sleep in the bath, and even being wrapped in a black plastic rubbish sack. While it is not known whether Victoria suffered from primary or secondary incontinence, it is clear that her symptoms worsened as the abuse increased.

Staff need to be aware that, when they are assessing bladder or bowel problems, children may become very upset or 'clam up'. These are not necessarily indications of abuse but cannot be ignored. Conversely, many healthcare professionals find ways of developing a unique rapport with individual children. This rapport enables the children to feel trust, and gives them 'permission' to speak openly.

Clinical and cost-effectiveness

C5 Clinical care and treatment are carried out under supervision and leadership.

Clinical supervision is a core component of monitoring patient care to ensure that it meets the highest and safest standards possible. All professional groups should be actively enabled and allowed to have clinical supervision, and it is the responsibility of health service managers to ensure that this happens.

A new concept that is starting to become regular is *practical supervision*. This involves a member of a healthcare team sitting in with another member to ensure that their interaction with the patient, as well as their clinical competence, is appropriate and once again of a high standard.

Both clinical and practical supervision are essential elements of ensuring clinical practice is delivered to meet the needs of the patient, and this is especially important when the patient is a child. It is also a critical component of any clinical governance activities.

Leadership is essential to any service delivery. Leadership in itself is different to management and is being established as the direction for healthcare delivery. There are a number of reasons for the high profile of Leadership. Although numerous styles of leadership have been described (Daft 2002), ranging from autocratic, democratic, trait and dyadic, authoritarian and participative. In the early 1980s, there was a shift in the models of leadership from 'transactional' to 'transformational' (Gaughan 2001).

The old paradigms of task-orientated or relations-orientated leadership, directive or participative leadership, and autocratic leadership, ignored effect on leader–follower relations of sharing a vision, symbolism, imaging and sacrifice.

In addition the newer paradigm of transformational leadership extols influencing skills and the empowerment of staff in decision-making. It is inclusive and developmental, so as to allow clinical staff to feel actively involved in all healthcare delivery processes.

One problem with this core standard, however, is the paradigm to which a healthcare organisation is working, as there are still a large number that make use of a more transactional, objective-based style. The standard does not state what type of style is encouraged. This allows for a less empowering style to be interpreted as leadership, whereas it is actually more of a management style.

Healthcare professionals need to be aware of the difference in these paradigms and ensure that effective leadership models are implemented. This is particularly important in the care of children – an area that requires a great deal of vision especially with the advent of Children's Trusts. A facilitative approach is necessary to engage all practitioners who might have their own vested interests.

C5 Clinicians continuously update skills and techniques relevant to their clinical work.

Although not stated as being linked to the Knowledge and Skills Framework that is an integral part of *Agenda for Change*, the Framework is key to allow clinicians to update skills and techniques.

In particular this relates to the Core Dimension 2 in the Knowledge and Skills Framework of Personal and People Development (Table 19.2). This dimension is important because it puts the onus on healthcare professionals to develop themselves in order for services to 'continue to meet the needs of patients, clients and the public'. It makes it clear that they must take individual responsibility for this.

This continual professional development links seamlessly to other dimensions which although not core are still imperative for the clinician to meet. The main domains related to clinicians' knowledge and skills relate to Dimension HWB2: Assessment and care planning to meet health and well-being needs (Table 19.3). This being an area where child protection issues might easily be picked up.

HWB6: Assessment and Treatment Planning (Table 19.4) and HWB 7: Interventions and Treatment (Table 19.5) also relate to the skills that are needed in order to deliver evidence based and effective care to all children. These dimensions ensure that healthcare professionals work towards becoming advanced and expert practitioners who deliver high quality care to all patients.

C5 Clinicians participate in regular clinical audit and reviews of clinical services.

Clinical audit should be a part of every healthcare professional's routine practice and should be embedded in the culture of all services. However, there have been very few published audits of children's bladder and bowel care or services.

Audit and research is needed to evaluate the effects, particularly of primary care-led bladder and bowel care services for children, in the light of shifting the balance of care from secondary to primary care services. The majority of such primary care children's services are

Table 19.2 Core Dimension 2: Personal and people development

OVERVIEW	
Status	Core – this is a key aspect of all jobs as everyone needs to develop themselves in order for services to continue to meet the needs of patients, clients and the public.
Levels	1 Contribute to own personal development 2 Develop own skills and knowledge and provide information to others to help their development 3 Develop oneself and contribute to the development of others 4 Develop oneself and others in areas of practice.
Description	This dimension is about developing oneself using a variety of means and contributing to the development of others during ongoing work activities. This might be through structured approaches (e.g. the NHS KSF development review process, appraisal, mentoring, professional/clinical supervision) and/or informal and ad hoc methods (such as enabling people to solve arising problems). Progression through the levels in this dimension is characterised by: ■ taking greater responsibility for your own personal development ■ this includes more reflectiveness and self-evaluation, and addressing own development needs ■ increasing involvement in supporting others and their development including a wider range of people with different backgrounds ■ having a greater understanding of own and other's learning needs and preferences, styles of learning and how to facilitate learning and development.
Examples of Application	Personal development includes taking part in: ■ the development review process (reviewing what you are doing well now and areas for development) ■ identifying own learning needs and interests and how to address these ■ on-job learning and development including: learning through doing, reflective practice, participating in specific areas of work, learning from others on the job, learning from developing others, professional supervision, undertaking qualifications in the workplace, networking ■ off-job learning and development on one's own including: e-learning, private study, distance learning ■ off-job learning and development with others including: induction, formal courses, scenario-based learning, role play, learning sets, undertaking qualifications in education settings ■ evaluating the effectiveness of learning and its effect on own work.

Table 19.2 (*continued*)

Examples of Application	Others, who might support an individual's development or who the individual might help to develop, will include: ■ patients and clients ■ carers ■ the wider public ■ colleagues in immediate work team ■ other colleagues ■ workers from other agencies.
Links to other KSF dimensions	This dimension is supported by: ■ *Core 1 Communication:* This dimension is different from dimensions: ■ *G1 Learning and development* which focuses on more formal approaches to learning and development ■ *G7 Capacity and capability* which focuses on developing collective capacity and capability rather than the development of individuals.

nurse-led. There is a need for robust measurement to determine which model of service is preferred, both by children and by parents, as well as for auditing clinical outcomes.

D2 Treatment and care take into account a patient's individual requirements and meet their physical, cultural, spiritual and psychological needs and preferences.

It is essential to take into account children's individual requirements in the care-giving situation, even though these may sometimes conflict with parents' requirements. For example, parents might require a child with enuresis to be dry by the age of 3, but this could be impossible for the child. There can also be differences in what a child actually wants, and what the parent – or even the healthcare professional – wants. The importance of listening to the voice of the child cannot be overstated (see below).

Cultural and spiritual issues also must be considered in our multi-cultural society. For example, some Muslim families expect their children to be dry by the time they are walking. Leininger (1994) has studied toilet training practices within an Iranian village and reported on this culture's perception of bodily wastes being considered unclean and defiling. Babies are trained before they are one year old and expected to defecate outside of the home by the time they are walking.

Table 19.3 Dimension HWB2: Assessment and care planning
to meet health and well-being needs

OVERVIEW	
Status	Specific – it will relate to some jobs but not all.
Levels	**1** Assist in the assessment of people's health and well-being needs **2** Contribute to assessing health and well-being needs and planning how to meet those needs **3** Assess health and well-being needs and develop, monitor and review care plans to meet specific needs **4** Assess complex health and well-being needs and develop, monitor and review care plans to meet those needs.
Description	This dimension relates to assessing the health and well-being needs of people – individuals and groups (including families). This assessment focuses on the whole person in the context of their community, family, lifestyle and environment. It may take place in any setting. In undertaking this work staff will need to be aware of their legal obligations and responsibilities, the rights of the different people involved, and the diversity of the people they are working with. Progression through the levels in this dimension is characterised by: ■ increasing complexity of health and well-being needs and an understanding of how these can be addressed ■ increasing demands for inter-agency and inter-professional working ■ increasing involvement in the planning, monitoring and review of programmes of care (as contrasted with making a contribution to the assessment).
Examples of application *These may be relevant to all levels in this dimension*	Health and well-being needs may be: ■ emotional ■ mental ■ physical ■ social ■ spiritual. Legislation, policies and procedures may be international, national or local and may relate to: ■ carers ■ children ■ criminal justice ■ disability ■ domestic violence ■ duty of care ■ education ■ human rights ■ mental health ■ mental incapacity ■ medicines ■ vulnerable adults.

Table 19.3 *(continued)*

Links to other KSF dimensions	This dimension is supported by: *Core 1 Communication* which focuses on effective communication with people during assessment of their health and well-being needs ■ *Core 6 Equality and diversity* which focuses on promoting equality and valuing diversity and supporting people's rights ■ *G2 Development and innovation* which focuses on testing and developing new and innovative forms of assessment. This dimension is different from dimensions: ■ *HWB4 Enablement to address health and well-being* – which focuses on the enablement that might take place as part of the programmes developed in this dimension ■ *HWB5 Provision of care to meet health and well-being needs* – which focuses on the various care interventions that might take place as part of the programmes developed in this dimension ■ *HWB6 Assessment and treatment planning* – which focuses on assessing and diagnosing physiological and psychological functioning.
Terminology	*Health:* a state of complete physical, social and mental well-being, and not merely the absence of disease or infirmity. Health is a resource for everyday life, not the object of living. It is a positive concept emphasising social and personal resources as well as physical capabilities. A comprehensive understanding of health implies that all systems and structures which govern social and economic conditions and the physical environment should take account of the implications of their activities in relation to their impact on individual and collective health and well-being. (World Health Organization) *Care plans:* overall plans for the protection, enablement and care that people require to meet their health and well-being needs.

Table 19.4 Dimension HWB6: assessment and treatment planning

OVERVIEW	
Status	Specific – it will relate to some jobs but not all.
Levels	1 Undertake tasks related to the assessment of physiological and/or psychological functioning 2 Contribute to the assessment of physiological and/or psychological functioning 3 Assess physiological and/or psychological functioning and develop, monitor and review related treatment plans 4 Assess physiological and/or psychological functioning when there are complex and/or undifferentiated abnormalities, diseases and disorders and develop, monitor and review related treatment plans.

Table 19.4 (*continued*)

Description	This dimension is about assessing physiological (e.g. autonomic nervous system, cardio-vascular, gastrointestinal, musculo-skeletal, respiratory) and/or psychological functioning and any treatment planning associated with this, within the context of that person as an individual. It includes clinical history taking and examination, and a range of tests and investigations, including various forms of imaging and measurement of body structures, and tests of physiological and psychological functioning. It also includes diagnosis and treatment planning.
	It involves interactions using a variety of communication methods with individuals and carers (either face to face or at a distance, e.g. by telephone) and may require the use of equipment and technology, including computer-assisted tools.
	Progression through the levels in this dimension is characterised by:
	■ the move from tasks or specific activities to more complex procedures with higher levels of associated risk
	■ the move from undertaking delegated tasks to planning assessment, informing diagnoses and the planning of treatment, making diagnoses, planning treatment
	■ increasing levels of clinical, technical and interpretive skills and knowledge
	■ greater complexity in presenting cases and/or the ability to make diagnoses of undifferentiated abnormalities, diseases and disorders.
Examples of application *These may be relevant to all levels in this dimension*	Legislation, policies and procedures may be international, national or local and may relate to: ■ carers ■ children ■ consent ■ criminal justice ■ disability ■ equality and diversity ■ health and safety ■ information ■ ionising radiation ■ medicines ■ mental health ■ mental incapacity ■ technology and equipment ■ the practice and regulation of particular professions ■ vulnerable adults.

They are punished if they soil, and the punishment is seen as part of the training.

Another study (Kelleher and Hillier 1996) of Bangladeshi people living in the East End of London reported on how urinary incontinence was seen as an illness what was outside of the scope of medicine but was caused by the '. . . influence of extra forces . . .'. Many Bangladeshi mothers reported they used the help of the Mullah or spiritual healer to help their children with wetting, and they did not like to speak to the GP about it.

This misconception is important for healthcare professionals to address by educating mothers. A good place for this to happen is in the local Bangladeshi Women's Centres (where children can also be seen). An unpublished needs analysis of Bangladeshi women in the Central London Trust showed that this group of women prefer to have service delivery and education for this taboo subject within their own community (Wells *et al.* 2003). In addition, Bangladeshi women felt that they had little information of what services were available and that there was a need for health promotion in local centres so that community members became more aware of their own and their families health needs so they would feel more confident about taking up services.

D2 Treatment and care are well co-ordinated to provide a seamless service across all organisations that need to be involved, especially social care organisations.

Seamless cross-boundary/interface services have already been discussed and examples of structures and processes described in Chapter 18 by June Rogers and Liz Bonner.

This is an important area for future and continuing development of services to children and all healthcare professionals can use this domain as a catalyst for initiative in service delivery.

D2 Treatment is delivered by healthcare professionals who make clinical decisions based on evidence-based practice.

Although medical care is generally considered to be based on evidence, there are areas where care is delivered because it has historically been done that way. Nursing care is in an even worse situation, as until recently little research has been carried out in this profession. Although this is changing gradually there is still the culture of 'this is how we do it and how we have always done it'.

There have been a number of studies on the care of the child with

Table 19.5 Dimension HWB7: Interventions and treatments

OVERVIEW	
Status	Specific – it will relate to some jobs but not all.
Levels	**1** Assist in providing interventions and/or treatments **2** Contribute to planning, delivering and monitoring interventions and/or treatments **3** Plan, deliver and evaluate interventions and/or treatments **4** Plan, deliver and evaluate interventions and/or treatments when there are complex issues and/or serious illness.
Description	This dimension is about intervening and treating individuals' physiological and/or psychological needs in the context of the whole person. The interventions and treatments that are undertaken are within an overall treatment plan – the development and monitoring of the overall treatment plan is covered in dimension HWB6. Interventions and treatments may take a variety of forms including ongoing monitoring of the individual's condition to identify a need for possible intervention at a later date. Progression through the levels in this dimension is characterised by: ■ the move from routine tasks or specific activities to more complex procedures with higher levels of associated risk ■ increasing levels of clinical and technical skills and knowledge ■ greater complexity in or seriousness of the conditions being treated.
Examples of application *These may be relevant to all levels in this dimension*	Interventions and treatments may relate to physiological and/or psychological functioning and might include: ■ advice, explanation and reassurance ■ application of energy (e.g. radiation) ■ application of materials and substances ■ exercise ■ extraction/removal ■ manual treatments ■ medicines ■ modification ■ ongoing monitoring ■ palliation ■ psychotherapeutic approaches ■ rehabilitative approaches ■ replacement ■ restoration ■ supporting and supplementing body functioning ■ surgery ■ therapeutics (not included above)

Table 19.5 (*continued*)

Examples of application	Legislation, policies and procedures may be international, national or local and may relate to: ■ carers ■ children ■ consent ■ counselling and therapeutic regulation ■ criminal justice ■ disability ■ equality and diversity ■ health and safety ■ information ■ ionising radiation ■ medicines ■ mental health ■ mental incapacity ■ the practice and regulation of particular professions ■ vulnerable adults.

enuresis, a few on the child with encoporesis; and a limited number for other groups of children with bladder or bowel problems. Unfortunately, however, a large number of these studies have been badly designed. Although they purport to give sound clinical evidence, the opposite could in fact be the case.

The Cochrane Database of Systemic Reviews has published a number of reviews related to children. A review of simple behavioural and physical interventions for nocturnal enuresis in children (Glazener and Evans 2005), has concluded that simple behavioural methods are commonly used. These may be better than doing nothing, but from the studies reviewed there is insufficient evidence to show that they are better than other means of treating nocturnal enuresis (such as desmopressin). While the studies reviewed are generally poor in quality and have small sample numbers, Glazener and Evans do feel that simple behavioural and physical interventions such as lifting, waking and star charts should be considered as first line treatment. They go on to conclude, however, that such methods require a high level of parental involvement that can sometimes be stressful. They advise that the main benefit would be to encourage a positive family culture in response to dry nights rather than a negative atmosphere of blame and punishment for wetting.

Two other Cochrane reviews have also looked at bladder and bowel problems in children. Brazzelli and Griffiths (2005) reviewed the behavioural and cognitive interventions with or without other treatment disorders in children and Glazener *et al.* (2005) reviewed the complex behavioural and educational interventions for nocturnal enuresis in children.

Glazener *et al.* (2005) again found that trials were mostly small and some had methodological problems. They reviewed complex interventions such as dry bed training or full spectrum home training on their own or with an alarm and the use of an alarm on its own. These authors concluded that although dry bed training and full spectrum home training were better than no treatment when used in combination with an alarm, there was insufficient evidence to support their use without an alarm. An alarm on its own was better than dry bed training on its own, but there was some evidence that combining an alarm with dry bed training was better than an alarm on its own, suggesting that dry bed training may augment the effect of an alarm. They found some evidence that contact with a therapist might enhance the effects of an intervention (see also Chapter 7 on 'Nocturnal enuresis' by Jonathan Evans).

The paucity of good research-based evidence has been described by Butler *et al.* (2004) who believe that one of the reasons is due to the debate as to what constitutes successful treatment and on how to document improvement. They argue that a lack of an agreed definition of outcome reduces confidence in comparing studies, with of course serious clinical and research implications. They have suggested a banding system referred to as a 'dryness scale', which focuses on the percentage of dry nights accomplished at a point in time, thus eliminating the need to compare current levels of dryness with a baseline. Whether researchers will agree on this 'dryness scale' is of course another debateable question and only time will show the outcomes of their suggestion.

Brazzelli and Griffiths (2005) concluded that there is no evidence that biofeedback training adds any benefit to conventional treatment in the management of encopresis and constipation in children. They found that there is some evidence that behavioural interventions plus laxative therapy, rather than behavioural intervention or laxative therapy alone, improves continence in children with primary and secondary encopresis.

In addition to these Cochrane Reviews, Sureshkumar *et al.* (2006) have developed a protocol for a review of the treatment of daytime urinary incontinence in children.

Patient focus

C13 Healthcare organisations have systems in place to ensure that staff treat patients, their relatives and carers with dignity and respect.

The importance of privacy and dignity has been highlighted as an area of care that tends to get forgotten as is highlighted by it being one of the ten *Essence of Care* Standards (DH 2001) and the fact that it has been included as a Core Domain in *Standards for Better Health*.

Children and adolescents can need more privacy and dignity in their care delivery due to the embarrassment of being examined (if this is a necessary procedure) as well as the embarrassment of discussing a problem that might have led to them being bullied at school.

C13 Appropriate consent is obtained when required for all contacts with patients and for the use of any patient confidential information.

This is a controversial area where children are concerned. Kuther (2003) highlights the way in which the healthcare practitioner–patient relationship is a partnership in which patients and physicians work together to make healthcare decisions. She continues to argue that, although adults receive considerable encouragement to become active participants in medical decision-making, children and adolescents often have little voice in such decisions and are granted limited access to confidential medical care.

Where consent is concerned, the healthcare professional must include minors and respect their autonomy. They must walk a fine line between respect for minors' autonomy, respect for parental rights, and the law.

C14 Have systems in place to ensure that patients, their relatives and carers have suitable and accessible information about, and clear access to, procedures to register formal complaints and feedback on the quality of services.

All healthcare Trusts have complaints arrangements. Clinicians should be aware of how complaints can be made and should have information in clinical areas of how this can be done.

It is always important to ensure that there are leaflets around and also preferably posters in a number of languages) so that patients, relatives and carers can write down a number in case they feel too annoyed or embarrassed to ask.

Patients' liaison

C16 Healthcare organisations make information available to patients and the public on their services, provide patients with suitable and accessible information on the care and treatment they receive and, where appropriate, inform patients on what to expect during treatment, care and after-care.

ERIC (the Enuresis Resource and Information Centre based in Bristol, see Appendix 1) has a large array of specialist literature that should be given out to all. Any service or clinical area that sees children with bladder or bowel problems is recommended to keep a selection of this literature. It must be assured when giving out literature that it is in a style that children find appropriate, readable and non-derogatory or condescending. The literature written and supplied by ERIC fulfils all these essentials.

There is minimal information for children who have bladder or bowel incontinence due to special needs either learning or physical.

Erickson and Ray (2004) have described a 'Parenting and Childhood Chronicity Model' which describes the work of raising a child with myelomeningocele with continence problems. This includes medical care, adapted parenting, dealing with systems, caring for siblings, maintaining relationships and personal coping (keeping yourself going). Erickson and Ray discuss the importance of setting appropriate expectations, providing parents with accurate information, ensuring that the focus on continence is not at the expense of other important aspects of the child's functioning, and supporting parents in their interaction with the school system. They do not detail any written information, however.

Try looking at the websites of some of the main consumer organisations for children with disabilities. The chances are you will find it extremely difficult to find any information about bladder or bowel problems. If the task is difficult for you as a healthcare professional, think how difficult it must be for the parent and child.

D9 Patients, service users and, where appropriate, carers receive timely and suitable information, when they need and want it, on treatment, care, services, prevention and health promotion and are encouraged to express their preferences; and supported to make choices and shared decisions about their own healthcare.

This is a particularly sensitive area for the child in that the voice of the children is often forgotten. There have been a number of research studies into how the voice of the child is heard by healthcare professionals as well as strategies that can be employed to improve the way in which they can respond to the child's voice.

It is no understatement to say that the child's voice frequently goes unheard. Curtis *et al.* (2004) found young people aged between 4 and 19 years from community and clinical settings including those 'hard to reach' such as asylum seekers and those with learning difficulties are able to comment helpfully on their experience of service provision (even those as young as 4–5) if a range of flexible and age-appropriate techniques are used. Alongside planning and environment issues, young people particularly emphasised the impact of communication and relationships with staff on their experience of services.

D10 Patients and service users, particularly those with long-term conditions, are helped to contribute to planning of their care and are provided with opportunities and resources to develop competence in self-care.

This is a particularly contentious area of care where children are concerned. A number of studies have described the 'voice' of children and how, despite the best of intentions by healthcare professionals, the parents' voice tends to be dominant. This happens in all clinical areas whether in primary care, in GP surgeries or in hospital settings.

Some interesting research has detailed the problems the child has in having a 'voice' no matter how old they are. Sartain and colleagues (2000) describe a qualitative study aimed at exploring children's, parents' and health professionals' experience of childhood chronic illness. Seven families and their professional carers participated in semi-structured interviews. The children's interviews were augmented with a 'drawing' technique. These authors found that research and data collection with children can be effective in giving them a voice. They found that many children are able to put their feelings into the drawings, and this alternative means of expression can make them feel they really have a voice. This aspect of 'giving a voice' is extremely important, especially as children cope and react in different ways to 'hospitalisations' and should never be regarded as a homogeneous group.

Tates *et al.* (2002a, 2002b) describe ways in which adult participants can play a pivotal role in doctor–parent–child interactions at GP surgeries. These researchers looked at the effect on children's opportunities to participate of the parent speaking for the child in a way that is institutionally constructed. They describe a study which aimed at further characterisation of the relationship within this 'Triad' which they describe as a *pas de trois*. They took video footage of 105 interactions between GPs, parents and children, in most of which both the GP and parent displayed non-supportive behaviour to the participation of the child. Some 90% of the consultations followed a pattern which made it difficult or impossible for the children to participate, despite the GPs' initial efforts to involve them. Most disturbingly, during the part of the consultation that involved diagnosis and treatment information, the child's voice was hardly heard. Tates *et al.* conclude that the low degree of child participation should not be seen solely as a consequence of adult behaviour, but rather as a co-construction of all three participants.

McPherson and Thorne (2000) look at the child's voice from a nursing perspective and highlight the importance of this when we consider the role of the nurse as an advocate. They highlight that the issue of voice in the clinical context is notoriously complex, requiring thoughtful reflection and continual critical analysis. They describe how attending to the voice of the child does not necessarily make the decision-making path more self-evident, nor does it ensure that children will always have an equal say in what happens to them. However, by recognising the inherent complexity in the concept of voice and searching for cues to the thoughts and feelings of the child nurses can often begin to develop the conditions under which children can feel more valued, respected and understood.

McPherson and Thorne quote an excerpt from a poem by Sheree Fitch, the 'Eloquent Young Elephant', to illustrate the right of children to formulate and express opinions and to have those opinions taken into account in matters affecting them. This excerpt is very moving and needs to be remembered by everyone caring for children.

> Did you hear the elephants.
> Trumpeting last night?
> They thundered past my bedroom
> The earth rumbled back in fright
>
> They were going to fight a battle
> Thump-galumphing off to war
> Did you hear a wee small voice say
> 'What are we fighting for?'

Tates and colleagues (2000b) argued that one of the ways to encourage children to participate actively in consultations, is for the clinician to provide clarity for the child (as well as for the parent) about the desirable participant roles in triadic encounters, and the importance of active participation on the part of the child.

Accessible and responsive care

C17 The views of patients, their carers and others are sought and taken into account in designing, planning, delivering and improving healthcare services.

When evaluating carers' knowledge and attitude to enuresis services, Cox and Croghan (2001) found that both parents and children placed a high value upon specialist nurse-led services. However, they go on to point out that parents and children tend to be given a lot of conflicting advice, much of it lacking any basis in evidence, about this type of bladder problem before the child is referred to specialist primary care-led enuresis services.

Once again there is a paucity of evidence around the views of parents and children in designing child-focused services.

A positive advance in accessible and responsive care is the ongoing development of Community Children's Services which are designed to meet the needs of all children, including those with long-term conditions. However, the question has to be asked whether these services take into account children's bladder and bowel problems.

It was argued earlier in this chapter that leadership is an important element in service delivery. Leadership in children's services is tending to move from secondary care to primary care as Children's Trusts emerge and develop. However the amount of research evidence behind such initiatives for children tends to be limited. In particular the impact of nursing leadership in the care of the child in a primary care setting is seriously neglected. The problem is compounded by the fact that, at the time of writing, there is only one Nurse Consultant in the UK working within a Community Children's team. Seeing that Nurse Consultants are seen as representing the pinnacle of nursing practice and have a defined role to carry out research this is an area in which it would be hoped that there would be more growth in the next few years.

C18 Healthcare organisations enable all members of the population to access services equally and offer choice in access to services and treatment equitably.

There can be a problem where this standard is concerned, as some particular parts of the community can find it difficult to access specialist services.

There are a number of specialist enuresis and encopresis services around the country; however the level of services for children with other types of bladder or bowel symptoms is poorly documented. Most Primary Care Trusts employ specialist children's services and there is a momentum to develop Children's Trusts. Children's bladder and bowel problems do, however, seem to take a low priority within specialist children's services. This is not surprising given the fact that there are only a couple of specialist courses in the subject around the country. Unfortunately it appears that the subscription rate to these courses is very poor. Children's nurses, and their employers, need to accept that there is a need for them to have some basic education and training to meet the needs of our special group of children, in order to ensure that they have easily accessible services across the board.

There is another obstacle to integrated children's continence services in this dimension. That relates to one of the government's main initiatives, allowing patients to 'choose and book' their care. While this is aimed particularly at secondary care appointment booking, it could have a detrimental effect upon integrated services as primary care physicians may feel that it would be best to direct children to secondary care services rather than to nurse-led primary care services. This is a situation that will need to be monitored and audited in order to see what impact on healthcare delivery 'choose and book' actually has.

D11 Healthcare organisations plan and deliver healthcare which:
    (**a**) reflects the views and health needs of the population served and which is based on nationally agreed evidence or best practice;
    (**b**) maximises patient choice;
    (**c**) ensures access (including equality of access) to services through a range of providers and routes of access; and
    (**d**) uses locally agreed guidance, guidelines and protocols for admission, referral and discharge that accord with the latest national expectations on access to services.

This domain very much links with guidance described in the DH Guidelines for Good Practice in Continence Services, the Children's NSF and Long Term Conditions NSF. It is up to clinicians to ensure that their local health organisations take into account services for children with bladder and bowel problems when developing services, especially those that cross boundaries.

Care environment and amenities

D12 Healthcare is provided in well-designed environments that promote patient and staff well-being, and meet patients' needs and preferences, and staff concerns.

How children feel about their care environment and amenities has been highlighted in a research study conducted by the Child Health Research and Policy Unit at City University (Curtis *et al.* 2003).

One of the most important elements of this study was the need for children's privacy to be respected so that they can maintain their modesty. One area that has been highlighted as being of concern where bladder and bowel problems are involved is the state of toilets in schools.

Another important element, both in hospital situations and outpatient departments, was for age-appropriate conditions. For instance that there should be access to television and magazines and maybe even music.

Conclusion

Governance in all areas of care have become increasingly important in ensuring excellence in healthcare is delivered. This chapter highlights the important elements linked to Department of Health and Heath Care Commission Standards as set out in 2005. These are bound to change, given the ever-changing healthcare environment. All healthcare professionals need to keep up-to-date with the various national drivers that will effect policies, and be able to ensure that they have a postive influence on the delivery of care to children with bladder and bowel problems.

References

Brazzelli M, Griffiths P (2001) Behavioural and cognitive interventions with or without other treatments for defecation disorders in children. *Cochrane Database Systematic Review 4*: CD002240

Butler R, Robinson J, Holland P, Doherty-Williams D (2004) Investigating the three systems approach to complex childhood nocturnal enuresis. *Scandinavian Journal of Urology and Nephrology*, 38(2): 117–21

Cox E, Croghan E (2001) Enuresis services: carers' knowledge and attitudes. *British Journal of Community Nursing*, 6(5): 238–44

Curtis K, Alderson P, Sutcliffe K (2004) Children as partners in their diabetes care. An exploratory research study September – December 2003. Social Science Research Unit (City University)

Daft RL (2002) *The Leadership Experience*. Ohio: South-Western

Erickson D, Ray L (2004) Children with chronic incontinence problems: the challenges for families. *Journal of Wound, Ostomy and Continence Nursing*, 31(4): 215–22

Gaughan AC (2001) Effective leadership behaviour: leading 'the third way' from a primary care group perspective. A study of leadership constructs elicited from members of primary care group management boards. *Journal of Managed Medicine*. 15(1): 67–94

Glazener CMA, Evans JHC, Cheuk DKL (2005) Complementary and miscellaneous interventions for nocturnal enuresis in children. *Cochrane Database Systematic Review 2:* CD005230

Glazener CMA, Evans, JHC, Peto, RE (2005) Alarm interventions for nocturnal enuresis in children. *Cochrane Database Systematic Review 2:* CD002911

Kelleher D, Hillier S (1996) *Researching Cultural Differences in Health*. London: Routledge

Kuther T (2003) Medical decision-making and minors: issues of consent and assent. *Adolescence Summer*; 38(150): 343–58

Laming WH (Chair) (2003) *The Victoria Climbié Inquiry*. Norwich: Crown Copyright. Website: www.victoria-climbie-inquiry.org.uk

Leininger M (1994). Transcultural nursing education: a worldwide imperative. *Nursing Health Care*, 15(5): 254–7

McPherson G, Thorne S (2000) Children's voices: can we hear them? *Journal of Paediatric Nursing*, 15(1): 22–9

National Primary and Care Trust Development Programme (2005) *Competency Framework for Nurses, Midwives and Health Visitors*. London: NHS Modernisation Agency. Website: www.networks.nhs.com

NHS Modernisation Agency (2003) *Essence of Care: Patient Focused Benchmarking for Healthcare Practitioners*. Norwich: The Stationery Office. Website: www.modern.nhs.uk/home/key/docs

Sartain SA, Clarke CL, Heyman R (2000) Hearing the voices of children with chronic illness. *Journal of Advanced Nursing*, 32(4): 913–21

Sureshkumar P, Bower W, Craig JC, Knight JF (2003) Treatment of daytime urinary incontinence in children: A systematic review of randomised controlled trials. *Journal of Urology*, 170: 196–200

Sureshkumar P, Cumming RG, Craig JC (2006) Validity and reliability of parental report of frequency, severity and risk factors of urinary tract infections and urinary incontinence in children. *Journal of Urology*, 175(6): 2254–62

Tates K, Elbers E, Meeuwesen L, Bensing J (2002a) 'I've come for his throat': roles and identities in doctor–parent–child communication. *Child Care Health Development*, 28(1): 109–16

Tates K, Elbers E, Meeuwesen L, Bensing J (2002b) Doctor-parent-child relationships: a 'pas de trois'. *Journal of Patient Education and Counselling*, 48(1): 5–14.

Wells M, Ghosh H, Zannath K, Stannard L (2003), *Bangladeshi Continence Project*: A report on a Scoping Project undertaken by the Continence and Stoma (Bladder and Bowel Care) Services, the Bengali Women's Health Project and the Advocacy Service, August, Islington PCT and Camden PCT

Glossary

adventitia the outer membranous layer of an organ or structure, for example the bladder.

ano-coccygeal sling a supportive sling of muscles forming part of the muscular pelvic floor.

anocutaneous reflex refers to the reflexive contraction of the external anal sphincter when the skin around the anus is stimulated, e.g. by stroking (also referred to as an 'anal wink).

anorectal sampling a phenomenon which occurs as the quantity of faeces builds up in the lower bowel and 'tests' the rectum to see whether it is ready to pass a stool.

anticholinergics a class of drugs which blocks the receptor of the chemical transmitter acetylcholine on the central and peripheral nervous systems making it inactive.

benchmarking an exercise undertaken as part of strategic management, in which organisations evaluate various aspects of their processes in relation to best practice within the sector of operation. Benchmarking enables the status of an organisation's performance to be measured, and realistic objectives for improvement to be set.

clean intermittent catheterisation (CIC) the insertion of a pre-lubricated urinary catheter into the bladder. The catheter is left in position until the bladder has drained, then removed and discarded.

cloacal extrophy a developmental anomaly involving two half-bladders (hemibladders), separated by an area of intestine with a mucosal surface, resembling a large red tumour in the midline of the lower abdomen.

coccygeus a muscle attached to the coccyx and the spine of the ischium, at the back of the pelvic floor.

Common Assessment Framework (CAF) a single assessment for children, which shares information between family members and members of the multidisciplinary team.

Cr-EDTA abbreviation for chromium-ethylenediaminelectraacetic acid, a substance used to evaluate intestinal permeability in bowel disease. Cr-EDTA is therefore the name given to the test that uses this substance.

desmopressin a synthetic analogue of vasopressin with no effect on blood pressure, used as an antidiuretic in primary nocturnal enuresis.

diethylene pantacetic acid (DTPA) a radioactive substance which can be 'traced' as it passed through the body. The name is therefore given to a test which uses this substance to find out what is happening in the renal and urinary systems.

dimercaptosuccinic acid (DMSA) a radioactive substance which can be 'traced' as it passed through the body. The name is therefore given to a test which uses this substance to find out what is happening in the renal and urinary systems.

efferent ducts/ductules part of the testes, connecting the rete testis with the *epididymis.*

Enhanced Disclosure a document resulting from a search of police records which gives details of any legal charges or convictions pertaining to an individual. Anyone working with children or vulnerable adults is now required to have one.

epididymis an elongated cordlike structure along the posterior border of the testis. It is continuous with the ductus deferens and contains space for the storage and maturation of spermatozoa, as well as providing a means for transporting them.

epispadias congenital absence of the upper wall of the urethra, occurring in both sexes. It is more common in males, where it involves a urethral opening somewhere on the side of the penis.

epithelium membranous tissue forming the covering of most internal and external surfaces of the body and its organs. It is made up of one or more closely packed layers of cells.

extrophy of the bladder congenital absence of a portion of the lower anterior abdominal wall and the anterior bladder wall. The posterior bladder wall pushes out through the defect. This is usually accompanied by an open pubic arch, and widely separated ischia connected by a band of fibrous tissue.

glomerular filtration rate (GFR) the number of millilitres of plasma the kidneys are able to filter in one minute, used as a measure of how effectively the kidneys are able to get rid of waste.

gonads a gland that produces gametes, i.e. an ovary or testis.

Hinman syndrome a psychogenic disorder seen in children, imitating a neurogenic bladder. It involves lack of synergy between the detrusor muscle and bladder sphincter but with no accompanying evidence of neural lesion.

Hirschprung's disease a congenital condition, resulting from failure of development of parasympathetic ganglion cells. Megacolon is a possible result.

hydronephrosis distention of the renal pelvis and calices with urine, due to obstruction of the ureter. If untreated, hydronephrosis leads to atrophy of the kidney.

hypospadias a developmental anomaly in which the urethra opens below its normal location. It is more common in males, where it involves a urethral opening on the underside of the penis or on the perineum. In females, it involves the urethra opening into the vagina.

intravenous urography (IVU) X-ray examination of kidneys, ureters, and bladder following the injection of a contrast agent into a vein.

inulin a starch occurring in the rhizome of certain plants, yielding fructose on hydrolysis, and used in tests of renal function.

iohexol a nonionic, water-soluble, low-osmolality radiopaque medium, used in tests of renal function.

Joint Area Review (JAR) a cross-disciplinary inspection carried out in a specified geographical area to examine how well the five outcomes identified by *Every Child Matters* are being met.

leucocyte esterase a urine test for the presence of white blood cells and other abnormalities associated with infection.

levator ani a major striated muscle, part of the pelvic floor. It contains both slow and fast twitch fibres.

magnetic resonance imaging (MRI) a method used for visualising the inside of living organisms, useful for showing pathological or other physiological alterations in body tissues. Former names include magnetic resonance tomography *(MRT)* and nuclear magnetic resonance (NMR).

megaureter ureteral dilatation, which may be either primary (congenital) or secondary to another condition such as *reflux neuropathy*.

mesoderm the middle of the three primary germ layers of the embryo, lying between the ectoderm and endoderm. The mesoderm gives rise to derived the connective tissue, bone, cartilage, muscle, blood and blood vessels, lymphatics, lymphoid organs, notochord, pleura, pericardium, peritoneum, kidneys, and gonads.

mesonephros the excretory organ of the embryo (or 'second kidney', replaced by the fully developed kidney or *metanephros*). Also known as the *Wolffian body*.

metanephros the permanent (post-embryological) kidney in mammals and other higher animals.

micturating cysto-urethrogram (MCUG) a test in which a radioopaque substance (urografin) is instilled into the bladder so that the process of bladder emptying and filling can be observed for abnormalities.

Mitrofanoff stoma a surgically constructed channel into the bladder, through which a catheter can be passed to empty the bladder at regular intervals throughout the day.

Müllerian system a pair of ducts or embryonic tubes which extend along the mesonephros. They become the uterine tubes, uterus, and part of the vagina in the female, and form the prostatic utricle in the male. Also known as the *paramesonephric ducts.*

neuropathic bladder dysfunction failure of the muscles and/or sphincter of the bladder to work properly, usually as a result of a lesion at any level in the nervous system, including the cerebral cortex, spinal cord or the peripheral nervous system.

Ochoa syndrome a rare inherited disorder characterised by inverted facial expressions in association obstructive disease of the urinary tract. Infants with the disorder have an inverted smile, so they appear to be crying when they are actually smiling, in conjunction with uropathy.

PECS abbreviation for Picture Exchange Communication Symbols, a commercially available language package which uses pictures and symbols to augment vocabulary.

pouch of Douglas in men, the region corresponding to the rectouterine pouch, lying between the urinary bladder and rectum. In women it is the deepest point of the peritoneal cavity, behind the uterus and in front of the rectum.

pronephros precursor of the mesonephros and kidney in the embryonic development of the kidney.

rectal compliance the way in which the muscles of the rectal wall change in relation to the amount of faeces being held in the rectum.

reflux nephropathy non-physiological back-flow of urine from the urinary bladder into the ureter or the renal pelvis and the calyces. Also known as *vesico-ureteric reflux (VUR).*

sacral agenesis a rare congenital condition of spinal deformity affecting the caudal partition of the spine, also known as hypoplasia of the sacrum.

trigone a smooth, triangular region of the urinary bladder between the two ureteral orifices and the internal urethral orifice. The area is very sensitive to expansion so, once it has stretched to a certain degree, the brain receives a signal for emptying the bladder. The signals become stronger as the bladder continues to fill.

urachus a fibrous cord stretching from the top of the bladder to the umbilicus. It is the residual form of an embryonic structure the allantoic duct, but in normal development will have ceased to be either patent or tubular.

ureterocele congenital abnormality found in the urinary bladder. In this condition, the distal ureter balloons at its opening into the bladder, forming a sac-like pouch. It is most often associated with a double collector system, where two ureters drain their respective kidneys instead of one.

urodynamics the investigation of functional disorders of the bladder and the urethra often used to refer to a multi-channel cystometrogram. Urodynamics are used for objective confirmation of pathology suggested by symptoms.

uterine didelphys a rare type of deformity of the female reproductive organs, in which some organs are be either split or duplicated. Typically, some of these 'additional' organs are non-functional or semi-functional, though this is not always the case.

Valsalva manoeuvre involves holding the breath then trying to exhale against a closed glottis. This automatically results in bearing down.

vesico-ureteric junction (VUJ) see *reflux nephropathy*.

Vincent's curtsey a manoeuvre adopted by female children in order to avoid leakage of urine by crouching down and pressing the heel of one foot into the perineum.

Widgett a commercially available language package which uses pictures and symbols to augment vocabulary.

Wolffian system see *mesonephros*.

Appendix 1
ERIC and other resources

Penny Dobson

What is ERIC?

ERIC (Education and Resources for Improving Childhood Continence) is a pioneering and an award-winning registered national charity. It was set up in 1988 to provide information, support and resources on childhood continence problems and is the only organisation of its kind in the world.

Formally known as the Enuresis Resource and Information Centre, ERIC has grown from most modest beginnings to being recognised on a global scale and at government level in the UK, and has become the torchbearer for professionals and families in this field. In addition to its core information, educational and unique support services and resources, ERIC aims to 'break the silence' that can prevent families asking for help when a child is bed-wetting, daytime wetting or soiling. ERIC also campaigns to raise public awareness and strives to improve NHS services for children by actively lobbying politicians and key influencers.

Why is ERIC needed?

According to the 2001 Census, out of a population of 8.4 million children:

- Over 500 000 experience bed-wetting;

- Over 125 000 experience daytime wetting;

- Over 100 000 experience regular soiling accidents.

Children with special needs due to physical disability or learning disability can take longer to achieve bowel and bladder control. For some, this may not be possible and they will require help to manage the problem.

There are issues for children and families who are coping with continence difficulties. These include:

- Friendship problems, teasing and the fear of bullying;

- Exclusion from social activities such as school trips and holidays;

- Loss of self-confidence that can continue into adulthood;

- Financial factors;

- Risk of verbal or physical abuse due to the incontinence, and the resulting stress.

Some parents do not know where to turn to for help, or they keep the problem hidden because they fear there is a stigma or shame in having an incontinent child. ERIC can give these parents the confidence to seek advice and encourage them to contact health professionals locally. Young people and families are reassured that they are not alone and that something **can** be done.

What can ERIC offer children, families and health professionals?

- **Confidential Telephone Helpline** for children, parents and professionals, giving information, support and details of local specialist clinics. This is available Monday to Friday between 10 am and 4 pm, and the number is **0845 3708008**. ERIC is a member of the Telephone Helplines Association.

- **Websites** for children, parents and professionals that provide a safe and interactive way of obtaining information, with message board facilities. The main website is www.eric.org.uk, and there is also a specially designed award-winning website for teenagers, www.trusteric.org, that contains frequently asked questions and allows access to a helpline adviser.

- **Telephone support groups** enable parents and young people to share experiences and tips using teleconference facilities from home. These are set up to meet demand. For further information contact the Helpline.

- **Literature.** ERIC has a range of books and leaflets, including guides for parents and guidelines on clinical practice and service delivery for professionals. These can be found on the ERIC Webshop, www.ericshop.org.uk, or in the ERIC catalogue. A copy of the catalogue can be downloaded from the website or obtained by writing to:

ERIC
34 Old School House
Britannia Road
Kingswood
Bristol BS15 8DB
Please enclose a self-addressed A4 envelope with 75p stamp.

- **Products.** The Webshop and Catalogue also contain bedding protection, enuresis alarms, absorbent daytime pants and other helpful products for children and young people. For more information contact the Sales Department on 0117 3012101.

- **Training.** ERIC holds a series of one-day seminars for health professionals around the country covering a variety of topics. All training is CPD approved. Tailor-made days to suit service needs are also available. Contact the Training Department on 0117 3012102 for further information.

- **Subscription service.** ERIC publishes a quarterly subscriber magazine for families, professionals and companies. Professional subscribers also receive a *Research Update* magazine twice a year. This gives details of new research and practice internationally.

- **Research.** ERIC has a database of research references that are available to professionals for a nominal charge. ERIC is involved in research into childhood continence issues through a collaborative study between ERIC and The University of Bristol, based on the experiences of 14,000 families who make up the Avon Longitudinal Study of Parents and Children (ALSPAC). This work will provide valuable data to increase our understanding of wetting and soiling problems in children.

- **Campaigns and materials** The 'Water is Cool in School' Campaign, www.wateriscoolinschool.org.uk, and the 'Bog Standard' Campaign, www.bog-standard.org, were set up to improve provision and access to drinking water and toilet facilities by pupils in UK schools. Health professionals can become involved in promoting these campaigns in their local areas by emailing info@eric.org.uk or by telephoning the ERIC Helpline.

How you can help ERIC to help others

- Tell families about ERIC;

- Display ERIC information locally (leaflets and posters are available on request through the Helpline);

- Become an ERIC subscriber;

- Support ERIC's campaigns and promote them locally;

- Use ERIC's resources and training to share expertise and to maintain standards of practice;

- Give us details of your clinic details and let us know of any changes to your service.

ERIC's plans for the future

Fundraising is a perennial problem but, money permitting, we have many and exciting plans for the future! Some examples are:

- Educational programmes and biennial ERIC Conferences all with a focus upon developing practical skills within the framework of the latest research;

- New publications and resources;

- Updating our informative and interactive websites;

- Putting energy into meeting the goals of our campaigns and political activities.

ERIC looks forward to continuing to support health professionals in the field with their struggles to maintain and improve their continence services. Our goal is to improve the lives of this often neglected group of children and their families.

Other useful organisations

ERIC works closely with other organisations that offer support and information to families and children with continence problems. Organisations are listed in alphabetical order.

British Toilet Association
PO Box 17
Winchester
SO23 9WL
Tel: 01962 850277
Website: www.britloos.co.uk
Campaigns for better public toilets for all.

Contact a Family
209–211 City Road
London EC1V 1JN
Free Helpline 0808 808 3555
(10 am– 4 pm Monday to Friday;
5.30–7.30 pm Mondays only)
Tel: 020 7608 8700
Fax: 020 7608 8701
Email: info@cafamily.org.uk
Website: www.cafamily.org.uk
For families with disabled children.

The Continence Foundation
307 Hatton Square
16 Baldwins Gardens
London EC1N 7RJ
Tel: 0207 404 6875
Helpline: 0845 345 0165
(9.30 am–1 pm)
Website:
www.continence-foundation.org.uk
For adults with bladder and bowel problems.

***In*contact**
SATRA Innovation Park
Rockingham Road
Kettering
Northants NN16 9JH
Tel: 0870 7703246
Website: www.incontact.org
Email: info@incontact.org
Incontact is a leading UK charity committed to helping people with bladder and bowel control problems. Dedicated to raising awareness and improving the understanding of continence issues, it provides user-friendly booklets, offers online support forums and publishes a magazine three times a year.

**PromoCon
(Promoting continence and product awareness)**
Disabled Living
Redbank House
St Chad's Street
Manchester M8 8QA
Tel: 0870 7601580
Helpline: 0161 834 2001
(10 am–3 pm Monday to Friday)
Website: www.promocon.co.uk
Working as part of Disabled Living, Manchester, PromoCon provides a national service by offering product information, advice and practical solutions to both professionals and the general public.

Appendix 2
The part played by incontinence in Victoria Climbié's tragedy

3.2   Victoria was born near Abdijan, Ivory Coast, on 2 November 1991.

3.3   With the agreement of her parents, Victoria was taken by her father's aunt, Marie Thérèse Kouao, to live in France in the Autumn of 1998. She was not quite 7 years old.

3.12   Kouao and Victoria moved to London in April 1999, where they were technically homeless.

3.22   The pair move into a small flat with Kouao's new boyfriend
–32   Manning at the beginning of July. Victoria began to suffer from urinary incontinence very soon after she came to live in Manning's flat. Manning told police that this prompted him to hit Victoria. He recalled that he began by slapping her, but by the end of July he had started to use his fists.

3.38   On 14 July, Victoria was taken to hospital by a concerned childminder. While in hospital, she wet the bed.

3.44   On one occasion she was seen to wet herself while standing to attention in front of Kouoa, who was apparently telling her off.

3.54   Victoria's incontinence had become serious by this stage.

3.57   Kouoa told the pastor of her church about Victoria's incontinence. He formed the view that she was possessed by an evil spirit, and advised that the problem could be resolved by prayer.

3.58   Two weeks after her first visit to his church, Kouoa phoned the pastor and told him that, following a brief improvement, Victoria's incontinence had returned. He claims he reproached her for being insufficiently vigilant and allowing the evil spirit to return. Incontinence continued throughout the rest of September. In October the sofa bed that Victoria had been sleeping on was thrown out and she began to spend her nights in the bathroom.

3.59 The bathroom in Manning's flat was small and the door opened into the living room. There was no window, although there was a heater, it was either broken or unused. When Victoria was inside the door was kept closed and the light switched off. She began to spend her nights alone and in pitch darkness.

3.69 She continued to be forced to sleep in the bath. From November onwards, she was tied up in a black plastic sack in an effort to stop her soiling the bath.

3.70 This meant that Victoria spent extended periods lying in her own urine and faeces. The obvious corrosive effect this was having on her skin may have prompted Manning and Kouoa to abandon this policy in January 2000.

3.71 Despite no longer being kept in a bag, Victoria began to spend more and more of her time in the bathroom. Manning and Kouoa said they left Victoria at home because her incontinence made it difficult to get things done.

3.72 Victoria's meals were served in the bath. Food was placed on a plastic bag, her hands were bound with masking tape she was forced to eat by pushing her face towards the food like a dog.

3.79 Victoria's continence problems were said to be due to possession by an evil spirit. Prayers were said for deliverance from 'withcraft, bad luck and everything bad or evil'.

3.80 Kouao claimed that Victoria's behaviour had 'improved' in that she had ceased to cover the flat in excrement.

Victoria was admitted to hospital, 24 Feb 2000. She died at 3.15 pm on 25 February 2000, aged 8 years 3 months.

Appendix 3
Statement of inter-professional values underpinning work with children and young people

Key attributes

Children and young people value practitioners who enjoy working with them, who treat them with respect and who are good at communicating with them.

Children's practitioners place the interests of children at the heart of their work. They share responsibility for a range of outcomes for children. They are committed to ensuring all children have the chance to: be healthy, stay safe, enjoy and achieve, make a positive contribution, and experience economic well-being. They recognise children's fundamental right to be safe, in order to reach other goals.

Practitioners concern themselves with the whole child, whatever their specialism. Although their own involvement with specific children may be short-term, children's practitioners work to develop the potential and capacities of children for the longer term.

Children's practitioners are committed to equality of opportunity for all children, and actively combat discrimination and its effects through their work. They respond positively and creatively to diversity among children and families, and colleagues.

Practitioners recognise that respect, patience, honesty, reliability, resilience and integrity are valued by children, families and colleagues. By demonstrating these qualities in their work they help to nurture them in others.

Work with children and young people, parents, carers and families

Children's practitioners recognise and uphold children's rights. They involve children in decisions about their lives and take account of their views and preferences. They recognise that childhood and

early adulthood are times of change, and that they need to respond
to changes in children's views, capabilities and circumstances.

Practitioners recognise the fundamental role played by parents in
children's well-being and development, and all this implies for
working in partnership with parents in the interests of children.

Practitioners are committed to engaging children and families
fully in identifying goals, assessing options, and making decisions.
They support children's and families' involvement in issues that
matter to them, including through involvement in the development
and evaluation of children's services.

Children's practitioners respect the right to confidentiality for children,
and for families. They also recognise that their duty to safeguard
children comes first. They acknowledge these commitments sometimes
present dilemmas to be resolved.

Inter-professional work with colleagues

Children's practitioners value the contribution that a range of
colleagues make to children's lives, and form effective relationships
across the children's workforce. Their inter-professional practice is
based on a willingness to bring their own expertise to bear on the
pursuit of shared goals for children, and a respect for the expertise
of others.

Practitioners recognise that children and families, and colleagues,
value transparency and reliability, and strive to make sure that
processes, roles, goals and resources are clear.

Practitioners involved in inter-professional work recognise the need
to be clear about lines of communication, management and accountability as these may be more complex than in their specialist setting.

They uphold the standards, and values of their own professions
in their inter-professional work. They understand that sharing
responsibility for children's outcomes does not mean acting beyond
their competence or responsibilities.

They are committed to taking action if safety or standards are
compromised, whether that means alerting their own manager/
employer or another appropriate authority.

Children's practitioners understand that the knowledge, understanding and skills for inter-professional work may differ from those in their own specialism and they are committed to professional learning in this area as well as in their own field, through training and engagement with research and other evidence.

They are committed to reflecting on and improving their inter-professional practice, and to applying their inter-professional learning to their specialist work with children.

Work with children can be emotionally demanding, and children's practitioners are sensitive to and supportive of each others' well being.

This Statement, currently in the form of a consultation draft, has been jointly prepared by the General Teaching Council for England, the General Social Care Council and the Nursing and Midwifery Council. A chance for professionals to feed back on the content is available through the website, www.nmc-uk.org/aArticle.aspx?ArticleID=2344

Up-to-date information about the progress of this consultation document can be found on any of our websites:
   www.gtce.org.uk
   www.gscc.org.uk
   www.nmc-uk.org

A note on terms: The text uses 'children' for 'children and young people' and 'parents' or 'families' for 'parents, carers and families' for brevity. We have used the terms 'children's practitioner' or 'practitioner' throughout.

Index

Page numbers in *italics* refer to figures or tables. An italic *g* after a number indicates a glossary entry.

Müllerian system 49, 50, *50*, 54,
  347*g*
multi-agency involvement 34,
  35–6
  see also multi-disciplinary
    taskforce
multi-disciplinary taskforce (of
  key stakeholders) 285, 288
  strategy development 289,
    290–92
  Template for Board Report
    288–9, *289*
  Terms of Reference *286–7*, 288
Multi-Professional Assessments
  (MPAs) 242, 243, 246, 247
Muslim families 328, 332

names, using children's 188
nappies
  disposable 108, 123
  removing 265–6
  removing at night 113
  and soiling 138–9
nappy tests 86
National Health Priority Areas
  315, *324*
National Health Service Litigation
  Authority 310
National Occupational Standards
  296
National Qualification
  Frameworks 296
National Service Framework (NSF)
  for Children and Young People
  2, 7, 9–10, 12, 242–3, 280,
  281, 283, 285, 298
  Core Standards 285, *285*
  Markers of Good Practice *283*
National Workforce Development
  Board 297
NE *see* nocturnal enuresis
negative feelings 29–30
neurological examinations 85, 130

neuropathic bladder 161, 347*g*
  assessments 162–3
  bladder training programme
    165–6
  and bowel control 178–9
  bowel training programme
    164–5
  newborns with 166
  physical examination 163–4
  as reason for clean intermittent
    catheterisation 225
  surgical intervention 168–70,
    170, *171*, 172
'New Ofsted' 12
nitrite testing 112
nitrites 145
nitrofurantoin 147, *152*, 166
NMC *see* Nursing and Midwifery
  Council
nocturnal enuresis 103, 104–5
  assessment 110–11
  clinics 110
  and complementary therapies
    119–20
  and constipation 128
  contributory factors 105,
    107–8, *109*
  drug treatment 116–19
  and early life events 106
  and fluid restriction 114
  genetic factors 106
  history taking 111
  initial management 113
  and lifting and/or waking
    schedules 113–14
  prevalence of 105, 108
  Primary Care Trust services 110
  psychosocial factors 106–7
  reward systems 113
  secondary onset 107
  self-help 109–10
  and specialist services 110
  and stress 185

Have you found *Effective Management of Bladder and Bowel Problems in Children* useful and practical? If so, you may be interested in other books from Class Publishing.

Type 1 Diabetes in children, adolescents and young adults
Dr Ragnar Hanas £19.99

Dr Ragnar Hanas shows you step-by-step how to become an expert in your own diabetes. This comprehensive handbook has been written not only for the person with diabetes and their parents but also for members of the diabetes care team.

'It is an incredible book, which deals in depth with every detail of diabetes care in young people and it never ducks any issues.'

Dr Charles Fox
Consultant Physician
at Northampton General Hospital

Type 1 Diabetes:
Answers at your fingertips £14.99

Type 2 Diabetes:
Answers at your fingertips £14.99
Both by Dr Charles Fox and Dr Anne Kilvert

The latest edition of our bestselling reference guide for people with diabetes, has now been split into two books covering the two distinct forms of the disease. These books maintain the popular question-and-answer format, to provide practical advice on every aspect of living with the condition, and giving you the knowledge and reassurance you need to deal confidently with your diabetes.

'I have no hesitation in commending this book'

Sir Steve Redgrave
Vice President
Diabetes UK

Irritable Bowel Syndrome:
Answers at your fingertips £17.99
Dr Udi Shmueli

IBS is a trying problem that can affect confidence and lifestyles. It is also remarkably common.

This practical and reassuring book looks at the science behind the symptoms, examines possible ways of finding relief, and gives advice on taking control of your condition rather than letting it control you.

Eczema:
Answers at your fingertips £14.99
Dr Tim Mitchell and Alison Hepplewhite

With answers to hundreds of questions on every aspect of living with eczema, this book will help you find ways to manage your own eczema – or that of your child.

'What a joy to have a new book which is medically accurate, wide ranging and practical in its approach.'

Margaret Cox, Chief Executive
National Eczema Society

Asthma:
Answers at your fingertips £17.99
Dr Mark Levy, Trisha Weller and Professor Sean Hilton

Contains over 250 real questions from people with asthma and their families – answered by three medical experts. This handbook contains up-to-date, medically accurate and practical advice on living with asthma.

'A helpful and clearly written book'

Dr Martyn Partridge
Chief Medical Adviser
National Asthma Campaign

PRIORITY ORDER FORM

Cut out or photocopy this form and send it (post free in the UK) to:

Class Publishing Priority Service,
FREEPOST 16705   **Tel: 01256 302 699**
Macmillan Distribution   **Fax: 01256 812 558**
Basingstoke, RG 21 6ZZ

Please send me urgently   Post included
(*tick below*)   price per copy (*UK only*)

☐ **Effective Management of Bladder and Bowel Problems in Children**   £32.99
  (ISBN 9781859591659)

☐ **Irritable Bowel Syndrome: Answers at your fingertips**   £20.99
  (ISBN 9781859591567)

☐ **Eczema: Answers at your fingertips**   £17.99
  (ISBN 9781859591253)

☐ **Asthma: Answers at your fingertips**   £20.99
  (ISBN 9781859591116)

☐ **Type 1 Diabetes in children, adolescents and young adults**   £22.99
  (ISBN 9781859591536)

☐ **Type 1 Diabetes: Answers at your fingertips**   £17.99
  (ISBN 9781859591758)

☐ **Type 2 Diabetes: Answers at your fingertips**   £17.99
  (ISBN 9781859591765)

TOTAL _____

Easy ways to pay

Cheque: I enclose a cheque payable to Class Publishing for _____
Credit card: Please debit my   ☐ Mastercard   ☐ Visa   ☐ Amex

Number   Expiry date

Name

My address for delivery is

Town   County   Postcode

Telephone number (*in case of query*)

Credit card billing address if different from above

Town   County   Postcode

Class Publishing's guarantee: remember that if, for any reason, you are not satisfied with these books,
we will refund all your money, without any questions asked. Prices and VAT rates may be altered for reasons
beyond our control.